Palliative and End-of-Life Pearls

Palliative and End-of-Life Pearls

JOHN E. HEFFNER, MD
Professor of Medicine, Executive Medical Director
Medical University of South Carolina
Charleston, South Carolina

IRA R. BYOCK, MD
Research Professor of Philosophy
The Practical Ethics Center
University of Montana
Missoula, Montana

HANLEY & BELFUS, INC. / Philadelphia

Publisher: HANLEY & BELFUS, INC.
Medical Publishers
210 S. 13th Street
Philadelphia, PA 19107
(215) 546-7293, 800-962-1892
FAX (215) 790-9330
Website: http://www.hanleyandbelfus.com

Note to the reader: Although the information in this book has been carefully reviewed for correctness of dosage and indications, neither the authors nor the editors nor the publisher can accept any legal responsibility for any errors or omissions that may be made. Neither the publisher nor the editors make any warranty, expressed or implied, with respect to the material contained herein. Before prescribing any drug, the reader must review the manufacturer's current product information (package inserts) for accepted indications, absolute dosage recommendations, and other information pertinent to the safe and effective use of the product described.

Library of Congress Control Number: 2002103561

PALLIATIVE AND END-OF-LIFE PEARLS   ISBN 1-56053-500-8

Last digit is the print number: 9 8 7 6 5 4 3 2 1

CONTENTS

Patient   **Page**

CONTRIBUTORS

Carla S. Alexander, MD
Clinical Assistant Professor, Department of Medicine, University of Maryland, Baltimore, Maryland

Derek C. Angus, MD, MPH
Associate Professor and Vice Chair for Research, Department of Critical Care Medicine, University of Pittsburgh; Associate Professor, University of Pittsburgh Medical Center, Pittsburgh, Pennsylvania

Robert M. Arnold, MD
Professor of Medicine, Leo H. Criep Chair in Patient Care, Division of General Internal Medicine Section of Palliative Care and Medical Ethics, University of Pittsburgh Medical Center, Pittsburgh, Pennsylvania

Joshua O. Benditt, MD
Associate Professor, Director of Respiratory Care Services, Pulmonary and Critical Care Medicine, University of Washington, Seattle, Washington

Kerry Bowman, MSW, PhD
Assistant Professor, Faculty of Medicine, University of Toronto; Clinical Ethicist, Mount Sinai Hospital, Toronto, Ontario, Canada

Monica A. Branigan, MD, MHSc
Tommy Latner Center for Palliative Care, University of Toronto; Sunnybrook and Women's College Hospital (Sunnybrook Campus), Toronto, Ontario, Canada

Frank Joseph Brescia, MD, MA
Professor of Medicine, Oncology, Medical University of South Carolina; University Hospital, Charleston, South Carolina

Eduardo Bruera, MD
Professor and Chair, Department of Palliative Care and Rehabilitation Medicine, University of Texas; M.D. Anderson Cancer Center, Houston, Texas

Anthony L. Buck, MD
Associate Professor, Department of Medicine, Division of Medical Oncology, University of Washington; VA Puget Sound Health Care System, Seattle, Washington

Ira R. Byock, MD
Research Professor of Philosophy, The Practical Ethics Center, University of Montana; Director, Promoting Excellence in End of Life Care (a national program of the Robert Wood Johnson Foundation), Missoula, Montana

Margaret L. Campbell, RN, MSN, FAAN
Assistant Professor of Medicine, Wayne State University; Nurse Practitioner, Detroit Receiving Hospital, Detroit, Michigan

Alan C. Carver, MD
Assistant Professor, Department of Neurology, Weill Medical College of Cornell University; Clinical Assistant Neurologist, Department of Neurology, Memorial Sloan-Kettering Cancer Center, New York, New York

Elizabeth Chaitin, DHCE
Director of Medical Ethics, Assistant Professor, Palliative Care Services, Department of General Internal Medicine, Section of Palliative Care and Medical Ethics, University of Pittsburgh; Director of Medical Ethics and Palliative Care Services, Greater Pittsburgh Medical Center Shadyside Hospital, Pittsburgh, Pennsylvania

Jason D. Christie, MD
Assistant Professor of Medicine and Epidemiology, Pulmonary, Allergy and Critical Care Medicine, University of Pennsylvania School of Medicine; Attending Physician, University of Pennsylvania Medical Center, Philadelphia, Pennsylvania

Rev. Ralph Ciampa, STM
Director of Pastoral Care, University of Pennsylvania Health System; ACPE Supervisor, Director of University of Philadelphia Health System ACPE Center, Philadelphia, Pennsylvania

Stephen W. Crawford, MD
Commander, Medical Corps, U.S. Navy; Pulmonary Division, Naval Medical Center San Diego, San Diego, California

Ronald J. Crossno, MD
Medical Director, VistaCare Hospice, Temple, Texas

J. Randall Curtis, MD, MPH
Associate Professor, Division of Pulmonary and Critical Care, University of Washington School of Medicine, Seattle, Washington

Marion Danis, MD
Chief, Bioethics Consultation Service, Department of Clinical Bioethics, Warren G. Magnuson Clinical Center, National Institutes of Health, Bethesda, Maryland

Horace M. DeLisser, MD
Assistant Professor of Medicine, University of Pennsylvania, Philadelphia, Pennsylvania

Rosalyn DeWitt-Marshall, MD
Program Coordinator for End-of-Life Project, Medical University of South Carolina—Enterprise End-of-Life Care Program, Charleston, South Carolina

Kenneth J. Doka, PhD
Professor, The Graduate School, The College of New Rochelle; Senior Consultant, The Hospice Foundation of America, New Rochelle, New York

Linda Emanuel, MD, PhD
Professor of Medicine, Northwestern University Medical School; Director, Program in Professionalism, Chicago, Illinois

Jacquelyn R. Evans, MD
Children's Hospital of Philadelphia; Division of Neonatology, University of Pennsylvania, Philadelphia, Pennsylvania

Robin L. Fainsinger, MD
Associate Professor, Division of Palliative Care Medicine, Department of Oncology, University of Alberta; Royal Alexandra Hospital, Edmonton, Alberta, Canada

Bonnie F. Fahy, RN, MN
Pulmonary Clinical Nurse Specialist, Pulmonary Rehabilitation, St. Joseph's Hospital and Medical Center, Phoenix, Arizona

Perry G. Fine, MD
Professor, Department of Anesthesiology, University of Utah; University Hospital, Salt Lake City, Utah

Joseph J. Fins, MD, FACP
Chief, Associate Professor of Medicine and Public Health, Division of Medical Ethics, Weill Medical College of Cornell University; New York Presbyterian Hospital, New York, New York

Michael Frederich, MD
Clinical Instructor (Volunteer), Family and Preventive Medicine, University of California, San Diego; San Diego Hospice Center for Palliative Studies, San Diego, California

Linda Ganzini, MD
Professor of Psychiatry, Department of Psychiatry, Oregon Health and Science University; Portland Veterans Affairs Medical Center and Oregon Health and Science University, Portland, Oregon

David J. Gattas, MB, BS, FRACP
Critical Care Fellow, Department of Critical Care Medicine, Sunnybrook and Women's College Health Sciences Centre, Toronto, Ontario, Canada

Michael J. Germain, MD
Associate Professor of Medicine, Nephrology, Tufts University; Bay State Medical Center, Springfield, Massachusetts

John Hansen-Flaschen, MD
Professor of Medicine, Chief, Pulmonary, Allergy and Critical Care Division, University of Pennsylvania; Hospital of the University of Pennsylvania, Philadelphia, Pennsylvania

Mary Beth Happ, PhD, RN
Assistant Professor, School of Nursing and Center for Bioethics and Health Law, University of Pittsburgh, Pittsburgh, Pennsylvania

John E. Heffner, MD
Professor of Medicine, Executive Medical Director, Medical University of South Carolina; Executive Medical Director, Medical University Hospital, Charleston, South Carolina

Thomas G. Heffron, MD
Associate Professor, Adult and Pediatric Liver Transplantation, Emory University; Emory Hospital and Children's Healthcare of Atlanta, Atlanta, Georgia

Winnie S. Hennessy, RN, MSN
Palliative Care Coordinator, Medical University of South Carolina, Charleston, South Carolina

Sarah Coate Johnston, MD
Associate Professor, Internal Medicine, University of Kansas School of Medicine—Wichita; Via Christi Regional Medical Center and Wesley Medical Center, Wichita, Kansas

Marshall B. Kapp, JD, MPH
Professor, Community Health, Wright State University School of Medicine, Dayton, Ohio

Karin T. Kirchhoff, PhD, RN, FAAN
Rodefer Chair and Professor, School of Nursing, University of Wisconsin, Madison, Wisconsin

Priscilla D. Kissick, RN, MN
Founding Director, Wissahickon Hospice; Adjunct at University of Pennsylvania School of Nursing, Philadelphia, Pennsylvania

Lisa M. Krammer, RN, MSN, ANP, AOCN
Nurse Practitioner, Palliative Care, Northwestern Memorial Hospital, Chicago, Illinois

Jerome E. Kurent, MD, MPH
Associate Professor of Medicine, Neurology and Psychiatry, Department of Medicine, Division of General Internal Medicine/Geriatrics, Medical University of South Carolina; Medical University Hospital, Charleston Memorial Hospital, and Veterans Affairs Medical Center, Charleston, South Carolina

Paul N. Lanken, MD
Professor of Medicine, Pulmonary, Allergy and Critical Care Division, University of Pennsylvania School of Medicine, Hospital of the University of Pennsylvania, Philadelphia, Pennsylvania

Mitchell Levy, MD
Associate Professor of Medicine, Brown University School of Medicine; Medical Director, ICU, Rhoad Island Hospital, Providence, Rhoad Island

Jeanne G. Lewandowski, MD
Medical Director—Pediatrics, Bon Secours Cottage Health Services/Hospices of Henry Ford, Detroit, Michigan

Scott Lorin, MD
Instructor in Medicine, Pulmonary and Critical Care Medicine, Mount Sinai School of Medicine, New York, New York

John M. Luce, MD
Professor, Medicine and Anesthesia, University of California, San Francisco; San Francisco General Hospital, San Francisco, California

Natalie Moryl, MD
Department of Neurology, Memorial Sloan-Kettering Cancer Center, New York, New York

Sheryl B. Movsas, DO
Department of Pain and Palliative Care, Beth Israel Medical Center, New York, New York

J. Cameron Muir, MD
Assistant Professor of Medicine, Northwestern University Medical School; Northwestern Memorial Hospital, Chicago, Illinois

Richard A. Mularski, MD
Fellow in Pulmonary and Critical Care Medicine, Division of Pulmonary and Critical Care Medicine, Oregon Health Sciences University; Consult Chair, Portland Veterans Affairs Medical Center Ethics Commitee, Portland, Oregon

Judith E. Nelson, MD, JD
Assistant Professor in Medicine, Division of Pulmonary and Critical Care Medicine, Department of Medicine, Mount Sinai School of Medicine, New York, New York

Molly Lee Osborne, MD, PhD
Professor, Associate Dean of Student Affairs, Department of Medicine, School of Medicine, Oregon Health and Science University; Oregon Health and Science University and Veterans Affairs Medical Center, Portland, Oregon

Dennis S. Pacl, MD
Clinical Associate Professor, University of Texas Health Sciences Center—San Antonio; Regional Medical Director, VistaCare Hospice, San Antonio, Texas

Steven Z. Pantilat, MD
Assistant Clinical Professor, Department of General Internal Medicine, University of California, San Francisco, San Francisco, California

Barbara Paris, MD
Assistant Professor, Geriatrics, Mount Sinai Hospital, New York, New York

Richard Payne, MD
Professor of Neurology and Pharmacology, Weill Medical College at Cornell University; Memorial Sloan-Kettering Cancer Center, New York, New York

Alexander Peralta, Jr., MD
Vice-President of Medical Sciences, Community Hospice of Texas, Fort Worth, Texas

Todd Pillen, PA-C/SA, MPAS
Manager, Pediatric Liver Transplantation, Solid Organ Transplantation, Children's Healthcare of Atlanta, Atlanta, Georgia

David M. Poppel, MD
Assistant Clinical Professor of Medicine, Tufts University; Bay State Medical Center, Springfield, Massachusetts

Russell K. Portenoy, MD
Chairman, Department of Pain Medicine and Palliative Care, Beth Israel Medical Center; Professor of Neurology, Albert Einstein College of Medicine, New York, New York

Thomas J. Prendergast, MD
Associate Professor of Medicine and Anesthesiology, Section of Pulmonary and Critical Care Medicine, Dartmouth Hitchcock Medical Center, Lebanon, New Hampshire

Bradford Priddy, MD
Clinical Instructor, Department of Internal Medicine, Emory University School of Medicine, Atlanta, Georgia

Christina M. Puchalski, MD
Assistant Professor, Departments of Medicine and Health Care Sciences, George Washington University; Director, The George Washington University Institute for Spirituality and Health (GWish), Washington, DC

Kathleen Puntillo, RN, DNSc, FAAN
Professor and Director, Critical Care/Trauma Graduate Program, Department of Physiological Nursing, University of California, San Francisco; Clinical Nurse Specialist, Critical Care, University of California, San Francisco, Medical Center, San Francisco, California

Timothy E. Quill, MD
Professor of Medicine, Psychiatry and Medical Humanities, Department of Medicine, University of Rochester School of Medicine and Dentistry; Director, Palliative Care Program, Strong Memorial Hospital, Rochester, New York

Michael W. Rabow, MD
Assistant Clinical Professor of Medicine, Division of General Internal Medicine, University of California, San Francisco; Attending Physician, University of California, San Francisco, Moffitt-Long Hospital, San Francisco, California

Jennifer Rhodes-Kropf, MD
Geriatric Fellow, Mount Sinai Hospital, New York, New York

Walter M. Robinson, MD, MPH
Assistant Professor of Pediatrics and Medical Ethics, Division of Medical Ethics, Harvard Medical School; Department of Pediatric Pulmonology, Children's Hospital, Boston, Massachusetts

Graeme Martin Rocker, MA, MHSc, DM, FRCP, FRCPC
Associate Professor, Department of Medicine, Dalhousie University; Queen Elizabeth II Health Sciences Centre, Halifax, Nova Scotia, Canada

Paul Rousseau, MD
Associate Chief of Staff for Geriatrics and Extended Care, Veterans Affairs Medical Center; Adjunct Assistant Professor, Midwestern/Arizona College of Osteopathic Medicine; Medical Director, RTA Hospice and Palliative Care, Phoenix, Arizona

Gordon D. Rubenfeld, MD, MSc
Assistant Professor of Medicine, Division of Pulmonary and Critical Care Medicine, Harborview Medical Center, University of Washington, Seattle, Washington

Cynda Hylton Rushton, DNSc, RN, FAAN
Assistant Professor of Nursing, Faculty Phoebe Berman Bioethics Institute; Program Director, Harriet Lane Compassionate Care Program, The Johns Hopkins University and Children's Center, Baltimore, Maryland

Greg A. Sachs, MD
Associate Professor of Medicine, Chief Section of Geriatrics, Department of Medicine, The University of Chicago, Chicago, Illinois

Rashmin C. Savani, MD
Division of Neonatology, Children's Hospital of Philadelphia, Philadelphia, Pennsylvania

Kava Schafer, MDiv
Hospice and Hospital Chaplain, University of Pennsylvania Medical Center—Hospice Chaplain, Wissahickon Hospice; Staff Chaplain, Hospital of the University of Pennsylvania, Philadelphia, Pennsylvania

Lawrence J. Schneiderman, MD
Professor of Family and Preventive Medicine, University of California, San Diego, School of Medicine; UCSD Medical Center, San Diego, California

Bradley A. Sharpe, MD
Internal Medicine Resident, University of California, San Francisco, San Francisco, California

Joseph W. Shega, MD
Instructor of Clinical Medicine, Department of Medicine, Section of Geriatrics, The University of Chicago, Chicago, Illinois

William J. Sibbald, MD, FRCPC, FCCHSE
Professor of Medicine, Critical Care, Department of Medicine, University of Toronto; Sunnybrook and Women's College Health Sciences Centre, Toronto, Ontario, Canada

Helen M. Sorenson, MA, RRT, FAARC
Assistant Professor, Department of Respiratory Care, University of Texas Health Science Center, San Antonio, Texas

Elizabeth M. Strauch, MD
Medical Director, The Hospice at the Texas Medical Center; Medical Staff, St. Luke's Episcopal Hospital; Consultant, MD Anderson Cancer Center, Houston, Texas

Catherine Sweeney, MB
Research Fellow, Symptom Control and Rehabilitation Medicine, University of Texas M.D. Anderson Cancer Center, Houston, Texas

Peter B. Terry, MD, MA
Professor of Medicine, Division of Pulmonary and Critical Care, Johns Hopkins Hospital, Baltimore, Maryland

Susan W. Tolle, MD
Professor of Medicine and Director, Center for Ethics in Health Care, Oregon Health and Science University, Portland, Oregon

Mark R. Tonelli, MD, MA
Assistant Professor of Medicine, Pulmonary and Critical Care Medicine, University of Washington, Seattle, Washington

Robert D. Truog, MD
Professor, Anesthesia and Medical Ethics, Boston Children's Hospital, Harvard Medical School; Director, MICU, Children's Hospital, Boston, Massachusetts

James A. Tulsky, MD
Associate Professor of Medicine and Director, Program on the Medical Encounter and Palliative Care, Veterans Affairs Medical Center and Duke University, Durham, North Carolina

David B. Waisel, MD
Associate in Anesthesia, Children's Hospital; Assistant Professor of Anaesthesia, Harvard Medical School, Boston, Massachusetts

Kelly A. Wood, MD, MHS
Assistant Professor, Department of Critical Care Medicine, University of Pittsburgh; Assistant Professor, University of Pittsburgh Medical Center, Pittsburgh, Pennsylvania

PREFACE

A commitment to excellence and an unswerving focus on beneficence, acting for the good of those we serve, mark the practice of medicine. Health care clinicians devote not only years of training, but also entire careers to mastering skills necessary to cure disease and assist patients in achieving their highest potential for health. This commitment to excellence and to acting to improve the lives of those who become our patients does not end when disease is advanced and cure is unlikely. Increasingly, patients suffering with pain from terminal disease or searching for ways to prepare for a meaningful death will encounter clinicians whose skills in palliative and end-of-life care extend to alleviating physical distress and providing guidance and support through this inherently difficult time in life. Similarly, even after the death of a patient, health care professionals have roles to play in easing suffering. Support is increasingly available and extended to a wife who is grieving the death of her husband of many years and to young parents and siblings seeking solace in the death of a child. Here too, beneficent intention combined with knowledge, clinical insights, and skills are critically important.

In preparing *Palliative and End-of-Life Pearls,* we have sought the contributions of clinicians who are at the leading edge of these realms of clinical practice. Experts from diverse disciplines were invited to write personal stories of patients and families who are struggling with issues of life-threatening injury, progressive and ultimately terminal illness, and associated grief. *Palliative and End-of-Life Pearls* authors practice in a range of health care settings and health delivery systems. All are active in clinical practice and health care education. Many are advancing the field through research in palliative and end-of-life care. We have selected cases that illustrate and examine key challenges and areas of active discussion, and sometimes controversy, within health care. The patient vignettes presented are compelling and illustrate an array of clinical dilemmas and strategies that provide readers with an opportunity to reflect and enhance their own clinical practices. Readers will not find a cookie-cutter approach to clinical challenges. Rather, the authors' discussions reflect a rich range of perspectives, practice patterns, and clinical strategies. This book follows the format of the earlier books in the *Pearls Series*® by providing a case presentation followed by a succinct, yet inclusive, discussion of the clinical issues at hand. The discussion presents a general overview while including new concepts and recent advances in the field of palliative and end-of-life care. At the conclusion of each discussion, the reader finds a list of the major lessons learned in the form of "clinical pearls." The cases will be familiar to many practitioners; the authors delineate the component issues and principles and offer strategies that have proven effective in their own practices.

We hope these Pearls assist our readers when they find themselves by the bedside of patients who have gone beyond the boundaries of cure. We thank our contributors for sharing their patients' stories—and their Pearls—that will further imbed the commitments to excellence and beneficence within the practice of medicine.

John E. Heffner, MD
Ira R. Byock, MD

Dedication

This book is dedicated to our professors who taught us the science and art of medicine, and to the patients and families who entrust us with their care

FOREWORD

End-of-Life and Palliative Care Pearls is a unique addition to the *Pearls Series*®. Using a case-based method framed around specific questions to be answered, this series presents and discusses the principles and practice of palliative care.

This text of these individual cases mimics the clinical encounter. A brief history, physical examination, and laboratory findings set the stage for a cogent discussion of a clinical problem. This casebook conveys succinct and evidence-based information in a practical and readable format, serving as a pocket palliative-care consultation. It models humane, compassionate care for patients with serious illness and outlines a clinical approach to quality symptom assessment and management, focusing on the patient and family as a unit of care. As appropriate, it recognizes the complex interactions of cultural, religious, and spiritual concerns on end-of-life decision-making.

This book responds to the urgent need identified in the 1997 Institute of Medicine (IOM) report *Approaching Death: Improving Care at the End of Life*. This IOM report strongly emphasized the need to address the existing barriers that cause serious inadequacies in end-of-life care in the United States. These barriers range from inadequate symptom control resulting from clinicians' lack of existing knowledge to significant attitudinal, behavioral, economic, and legal factors that prevent health care professionals from delivering (and patients from receiving) appropriate humane care at the end of life. There are also critical gaps in our scientific understanding of end-of-life care that need further research from medical, social science, and health care investigators, and we lack systems that can demonstrate accountability to ensure patients and their families receive quality palliative care. Other reports, such as surveys of major medical and nursing textbooks, have pointed out that less than 1% of their content focuses on the care of patients with advanced disease.

In its seven recommendations, the IOM strongly urged the translation into clinical practice of evidence-based palliative care, emphasizing the fact that nothing would have a greater impact on the care of dying patients than institutionalizing the knowledge that we have now. This compendium of clinical pearls on end-of-life care begins to fill this educational void. The 71 cases, with their sage advice, serve to emphasize the need to prioritize education about end-of-life care.

Humane, competent, compassionate care of patients with terminal illness is now recognized as an evidence-based discipline. Health care professionals who learn and apply these clinical pearls will surely improve the quality of life for their patients and families. Moreover, they will give voice to the needs of this vulnerable population, enhancing their dignity, autonomy, and personhood.

Kathleen M. Foley, MD
Memorial Sloan-Kettering Cancer Center
New York
foleyk@mskcc.org

Ira Byock, MD

PATIENT 1

A 78-year-old man with a ruptured aortic aneurysm and unfinished business

A 78-year-old man arrives at the emergency department by ambulance with hypotension and severe abdominal and back pain. He describes upper abdominal pain and intense mid-back pain, which he rates at "9 out of 10." He has a history of an abdominal aortic aneurysm that has been shown by ultrasound to be slowly expanding. The patient has a history of non-insulin dependent diabetes, hypertension, coronary artery disease, episodes of transient ischemic attacks, and peripheral vascular disease. His medications include coumadin.

Physical Examination: Blood pressure 90/60, pulse 110, respirations 20, SpO_2 (mask 100% O_2) 93%. General: marked discomfort. Chest: bilateral crackles. Cardiac: S3. Abdomen: diffuse tenderness and rebound, pulsatile epigastric mass with bruit. Neurologic: alert, fully oriented.

Laboratory Findings: Abdominal ultrasound: 8-cm aneurysm with intramural thrombus and retroperitoneal hematoma. EKG: diffuse ischemia.

Course: The emergency physician explains to the patient that he needs emergency surgery for a leaking aneurysm in order to survive. The patient responds that his physician has told him that surgery would be complicated considering his underlying health, and that he would unlikely survive. He has refused surgery in the past and reaffirms his refusal to the emergency physician.

The physician pulls a stool up to the head of the patient's gurney: "I wish I had better news for you. From what you've told me, it sounds like you probably understand the situation. Just like the bleb on a bicycle tire, this aneurysm has been getting bigger over the months. Today, it has begun to leak. As you've said and the doctors have told you, you might well die in surgery. Without surgery, you will almost certainly die within the next few hours. Do you understand?"

The patient listens with his eyes half closed and nods; then, as if by afterthought, he opens his eyes and looks at the physician with an expression of firm resolve, "Yes, I do."

In response, the physician says, "I want to talk with your family and let them know what's happening. Is that OK with you?"

"Yes, please."

Question: How should the physician help prepare the family for the patient's anticipated course?

Diagnosis: Ruptured abdominal aortic aneurysm in a patient who is expected to die who has "unfinished business" with his family.

Discussion: Caring for a patient who is imminently dying can be frustrating for doctors and nurses who are focused on saving lives. In addition to basic ethical and clinical responsibilities, important opportunities can be identified for clinicians to be of service to dying patients and to their loved ones.

Physicians have a primary responsibility for alleviating physical suffering of their patients. In the setting of acute, life-threatening injury or illness, efforts to relieve pain (or dyspnea) must not be ignored, while life-saving measures proceed. By diminishing severe physical distress, a patient's ability to communicate with clinicians and their family and friends often can be enhanced.

Even patients in extremis may retain **decision-making capacity**. It is important that they be informed of their medical condition and be fully involved in guiding therapy. Instructions contained in advance directive documents and existing treatment plans can be reviewed and affirmed or modified with the patient. In situations in which death is anticipated and a life-prolonging intervention is being declined, the patient's family members and any formal proxy decision-makers (whether named in a durable power of attorney for health care or court-appointed) should be apprised of the patient's condition and involved in decisions. Open communication is fundamental for practicing "preventative ethics," helping to avoid later allegations of poor treatment after a patient dies.

Communication is also essential for helping a patient's loved ones through the inherent tragedy of an imminent or sudden death. In clarifying the plan of care and affirming the family's agreement, potential second-guessing and family conflict can be prevented.

In acute care settings, emergency care for patients who are likely to die can extend beyond physiologic treatments. Urgent **psychosocial interventions** are often indicated. Although critical care settings, such as an emergency department, are not conducive to intimate family interaction, careful attention by clinical staff can often create a protected space for families to share poignant, private time.

Even when death is anticipated, meaningful clinical outcomes can be identified. Families need to know that their loved one is receiving the best possible care, consistent with their values and preferences. Every family wants to ensure that their loved one is as comfortable as possible and is treated in a dignified, personable manner. When these basic elements of care are satisfied and the ill or injured person is cognizant, most patients and families value the opportunity to spend time together, in anticipatory grief. This can involve saying the things that matter most, often sharing their sadness and reaffirming their love for one another. Spiritual care may also be valued at such times. Chaplain services or contact with the family's own clergy can be important sources of support.

In caring for the present patient, the emergency physician stepped out of the trauma room and met with the patient's wife, his eldest daughter, and his two sons in a private waiting area. He explained the patient's medical condition and the decision he made to decline surgery. He gently but explicitly informs them that without surgery his death is imminent.

The family is tearful but composed. During the meeting, they frequently comfort one another by holding hands, hugging, or sharing tissues. Each one responds to the doctor, conveying that he or she understands the situation and agrees. The patient's wife asks, "What happens now? Can we see him?"

The physician explains, "Yes, of course. The room is being cleaned, and we'll get you right in. I have a call in to your personal physician, Dr. Jennings. I want him to know what is happening and make sure he agrees. For the moment, your husband is doing okay; we're giving him pain medication, fluids, and treatment to reverse the blood thinner he's on. Hopefully, this will buy a little bit of time. He may have only a matter of minutes to a few hours to live. I realize that this is precious family time, and we'll do all we can to preserve it. I don't know much about your husband and your family, but you seem like a strong and loving family."

One of the patient's sons says, "You got that right."

The physician continues, "I want to suggest something that may seem obvious, but is probably worth saying. Whatever time you have with him today is a chance to say the things that would be left unsaid. In fact, 'stating the obvious' is often important at times like this. Years ago, a colleague taught me that before any important relationship was complete, people had to have said 'the five things': forgive me, I forgive you, thank you, I love you, good-bye. Other things that may be obvious but may have value in being said are 'We'll miss you' and 'We'll never forget you.'"

To this the patient's daughter responds, "You're on the mark again. My father is a man of few words. He loves us and I think he knows how much we love him, but it's not something we've said a lot. Now, there's literally no time like the present."

"We will make sure that he is as comfortable as we can make him. It is important that you let us know if you feel he is hurting too much. As the bleeding continues, his blood pressure will fall and he will become less alert. When his blood pressure falls too low, he will die. It may happen gradually, but it could happen suddenly."

The patient was admitted to a private room. Per his request, a priest was called to administer the Sacrament of the Sick. Three hours after admission, the patient's blood pressure fell to palpable and he became unresponsive. A short while later,

cardiac arrest occurred and he was pronounced dead. His family spent an additional hour with his body and making phone calls to family and friends out of town.

Before leaving the hospital, the patient's daughter stops at the emergency department to express her and her family's appreciation for the care. She says, "This was the best possible way for the worst possible thing to happen. My father was a strong, stoic man. If he had died suddenly, there would have been important things left unsaid. Your advice was right on the mark. He even told each of us kids how proud he was of us. That's something we had never heard him say! Thank you for taking such good care of us all."

Clinical Pearls

1. Even in emergency situations, prospective planning, attention to ethical principles, and clear communication are vitally important.

2. Symptom management is essential to the care of patients with life-threatening injury or illness, preserving the patients' capacity to communicate with clinicians and loved ones.

3. Patients who are imminently dying may still retain decision-making capacity.

4. Clear communication and prospective involvement in decision-making can be thought of as "preventative ethics," helping to avoid potential conflict between families and clinicians and within families.

5. Meaningful clinical outcomes can often be discerned and achieved even when the expected physiologic outcome is death.

6. When death is imminent, urgent psychosocial support may be indicated. Skillful communication and anticipatory guidance can assist patients and families through the difficult process of life completion and life closure.

REFERENCES

1. Wanzer SH, Federman DD, Adelstein SJ, et al: The physician's responsibility toward hopelessly ill patients. N Eng J Med 1984;310:955–999.
2. Byock IR: The nature of suffering and the nature of opportunity at the end of life. Clin Geriatr Med 1996;12:2–10.
3. Brody H, Campbell ML, Faber-Langendoen K, Ogle KS: Withdrawing intensive life-sustaining treatment—recommendations for compassionate clinical management. N Engl J Med 1997;336:652–657.

J. Randall Curtis, MD, MPH

PATIENT 2

A 62-year-old man with lymphoma who develops respiratory failure, renal failure, and hypotension after bone marrow transplantation

A 62-year-old man has with a history of recurrent diffuse large cell lymphoma stage IIIB in his cervical, mediastinal, and retroperitoneal lymph nodes. Following a partial response to salvage combination chemotherapy, he undergoes autologous bone marrow transplantation using his own peripheral blood stem cells. After his preparative regimen for transplantation, he developed pancytopenia, mucositis, and fever, which were treated with transfusions, morphine, and empiric antibiotics. On day 15 after transplantation, his cervical adenopathy has progressed and he develops fever, confusion, increasing dyspnea, and anuria.

Physical Examination: Blood pressure 72/40, pulse 145, respiratory rate 28, temperature 38.9°C. General: confused, lethargic. Cardiac: no murmur. Chest: coarse crackles diffusely.

Laboratory Findings: Hct 22%; WBC 200/μL, platelets 12,000/μL. Electrolytes normal. BUN 62 mg/dL, creatinine 3.9mg/dL; AST 298 IU/L, total bilirubin 1.9 mg/dL. Arterial blood gas (10 L/min oxygen by mask): pH 7.48, $PaCO_2$ 30 mm Hg, PaO_2 52 mm Hg. Chest radiograph: mediastinal widening and diffuse opacities consistent with pulmonary edema.

Course: The patient is admitted to the ICU and placed on high flow, 100% oxygen by facemask. He receives volume resuscitation with intravenous saline, and vancomycin is added empirically to his antibiotic regimen. His blood pressure and urine output remain low despite rapid administration of saline, and he is started on dopamine, which is required at 10 μg/kg/min to maintain a systolic blood pressure over 90 mm Hg. He remains tachypneic with accessory muscle use. A PaO_2 is now 58 mm Hg. In a brief discussion with the ICU team, the patient's wife requests that the team "do everything" to keep him alive.

Question: Is continued life support for this man futile, and if so, should life support be discontinued?

4

Discussion: Clinical situations in which a patient with an underlying terminal or life-limiting illness develops an acute exacerbation or complication commonly arise in the ICU. Families in such situations often express a desire to "do everything," prompting acute care clinicians to feel that they are being asked to provide futile medical care that is, at best, a poor use of medical resources and, at worst, unethical. Frequently, these clinicians use the term **medical futility** to express their dissatisfaction with providing aggressive medical care for patients they believe will not benefit from it.

The concept of medical futility became popular with the growth of high technology in medical science, which created concern that this technology could be misused simply to delay death for short periods rather than restore patients to health. Although some ethicists argue that the principle of "medical futility" has not stood up well under careful scrutiny and should no longer be used in clinical practice, it remains a part of routine clinical discourse in many institutions. Increasing consensus exists, however, that the principle of medical futility should not be used to make unilateral decisions to withhold treatments over the objections of patients or their families. Any clinical utility of the medical futility concept lies in its role in assisting decision-making processes.

If clinicians employ considerations of futility, it is essential they understand its definition and appropriate use. Evidence exists that some clinicians apply the concept of medical futility in circumstances for which it clearly does not apply.

The principle of medical futility defines a therapy as futile if there is no or a very low likelihood that the therapy will achieve the goals of care. The figure below depicts a framework for applying medical futility to think through the indications for initiating or continuing life-sustaining therapy before approaching a patient or family. In this framework, a clinician first elicits from the patient or family **the patient's wishes** for therapy and outcome. These wishes should be formulated into reasonable **therapeutic goals**. Often, goals include discharge from the hospital alive or discharge to home, but for some patients, a goal might include surviving until the arrival of a family member or the birth of a child. Once the goals have been understood, the clinician should use published literature and clinical experience to determine whether the treatment in question can achieve one of the goals. If the treatment can achieve one of the goals, the patient or family should be asked if the patient would want the treatment. If, however, treatment cannot achieve one of the goals, the treatment is determined to be medically futile and, in most instances, should not be offered.

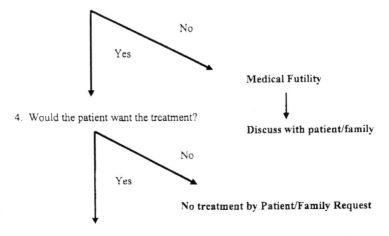

1. Elicit patient's wishes about therapy and outcomes.

2. Formulate these wishes into appropriate therapeutic goals (such as discharge to home with independent living or survive until granddaughter is born).

Treatment Decision:

3. Determine whether treatment can achieve at least one reasonable therapeutic goal

Yes / No

Medical Futility

4. Would the patient want the treatment?

Discuss with patient/family

Yes / No

No treatment by Patient/Family Request

Provide treatment and periodically reassess goals and indications

A clinical and ethical framework for discussing specific interventions and considering the role of medical futility.

When the principle of medical futility is applied and treatments are not offered, the rationale for the decision should be discussed with patients and families. In most instances, patients and families will agree with this determination and will appreciate not being asked to choose to forgo a treatment that is not indicated. In some instances, however, patients and families will not agree with forgoing a futile treatment. In these situations, a process should be initiated **to reconcile these differences**, as described by the Council on Ethical and Judicial Affairs of the American Medical Association. In most instances, the treatment should be provided until differences can be reconciled.

Relatively little is known about patients' attitudes toward the principle of futility. In a recent study of patients with advanced AIDS, over half of the patients believed that it was definitely acceptable for their physician to not offer mechanical ventilation if the physician decided this intervention was futile. Only 10% or less of patients said it was definitely unacceptable for their physician not to offer these therapies under futile circumstances. Although the majority of patients with advanced AIDS accepted the medical futility rationale, a substantial minority did not. These data suggest that clinicians invoking the medical futility rationale need to be aware of this diversity in patient attitudes toward the application of this principle.

Application of medical futility requires skilled caregivers to initiate a dialogue with patients and families as well as relevant members of the clinical staff. Such conferences review prognostic data, establish the goals of care, and compassionately convey information along with recommendations to treat patients with aggressive palliative care rather than life-sustaining treatments. The ability to effectively carry out such conferences is actually as important a skill for clinicians to possess as the ability to review clinical data to determine futility. In most instances, this conference process will be sufficient to achieve consensus. In relatively rare situations when the family does not agree and wishes to continue futile care, life-sustaining treatments are continued and mechanical ventilation initiated while consensus between the medical team and family has time to develop. Often, family members simply need time to come to terms with the prognosis and work through personal "family-centered" issues.

If the family and medical team still cannot achieve consensus, it is helpful to bring additional people into the discussion, such as clergy, a community representative, additional consultants, or hospital ethics committee members. Unresolved disagreements regarding the futility of life-sustaining care are difficult for families and clinicians alike. However, a sensitive and thoughtful approach to families and providing sufficient time to carefully understand the family's perspectives can promote consensus in most instances.

Regarding the present patient, a recent series has demonstrated that no one survived to hospital discharge among 398 patients with lung injury and renal failure requiring vasopressors after bone marrow transplantation. Life-sustaining therapy in this setting, therefore, fulfilled the definition of "futile" care. The ICU team initiated the family dialogue as depicted in the figure. The family called in additional family members and soon accepted comfort care with intravenous morphine. After withdrawal of antibiotics and vasopressors, the patient died peacefully later in the day.

Clinical Pearls

1. The concept of medical futility may be useful in formulating an approach to treatment decisions for an individual patient, but it must only be applied in appropriate circumstances in a manner that assists the decision-making process (see figure) and should not be used to make unilateral decisions to withdraw or withhold treatment.

2. Clinicians should be careful to define medical futility before using it in thinking about an individual patient: e.g., if, based on published data or clinical experience, we can confidently say that a treatment is successful at achieving the desired outcome in less than 1 in 100 cases, then the treatment meets the criteria for medical futility.

3. Clinicians should be aware that many patients support the concept of medical futility, but a substantial minority would not want their clinicians to make unilateral decisions without involving them or their families.

4. In most instances, patients and families will not request a treatment determined to be futile.

5. In the absence of a consensus, treatment should be initiated while a dialogue is maintained. Many families need time to resolve personal and family issues before they can recognize the futility of care.

REFERENCES

1. Lantos JD, Singer PA, Walker RM, et al: The illusion of futility in clinical practice. Am J Med 1989;87:81–84.
2. Schneiderman LJ, Jecker NS, Jonsen AR: Medical futility: its meaning and ethical implications. Ann Intern Med 1990;112:949–954.
3. Schneiderman LJ, Jecker NS. Futility in practice. Arch Intern Med 1993;153:437–441.
4. Curtis JR, Park DR, Krone MR, Pearlman RA: Use of the medical futility rationale in do-not-attempt-resuscitation orders. JAMA 1995;273:124–128.
5. Rubenfeld GR, Crawford SW: Withdrawing life support from mechanically ventilated recipients of bone marrow transplants: a case for evidence-based guidelines. Ann Intern Med 1996;125:625–33.
6. Asch DA, Shea JA, Jedrziewski MK, Bosk CL: The limits of suffering: critical care nurses' views of hospital care at the end of life. Soc Sci Med 1997;45:1661–1668.
7. Council on Ethical and Judicial Affairs, AMA: Medical futility in end-of-life care. JAMA 1999;281:937–941.
8. Helft PR, Siegler M, Lantos J: The rise and fall of the futility movement. N Engl J Med 2000;343:293–296.
9. Curtis JR, Patrick DL, Caldwell E, Collier AC: The attitudes of patients with advanced AIDS towards use of the medical futility rationale in decisions to forego mechanical ventilation. Arch Intern Med 2000;160:1597–1601.
10. Rubenfeld GD, Crawford S: Principles and practice of withdrawing life-sustaining treatments in the ICU. In Curtis JR, Rubenfeld GD (eds): Managing Death in the Intensive Care Unit: The Transition from Cure to Comfort. New York: Oxford University Press; 2001:pp 127–148.
11. Curtis JR, Patrick DL: How to discuss dying and death in the ICU. In Curtis JR, Rubenfeld GD (eds): Managing Death in the Intensive Care Unit: The Transition from Cure to Comfort. New York: Oxford University Press; 2001:pp 85–102.

PATIENT 3

A 14-year-old boy with cystic fibrosis

A 14-year-old boy with cystic fibrosis is admitted to the ICU in impending respiratory failure. He lives at home and attends high school and is managed with pancreatic enzyme replacement therapy, a pulmonary regimen of bronchodilators, and occasional intensive courses of intravenous antibiotic therapy to reduce the bacterial load in his lungs. Over the past 3 years, his pulmonary function has gradually declined. One year ago, his pulmonologist discussed the possibility of lung transplantation with him and his family as the only way to significantly extend his life. He agreed to be placed on the transplant waiting list and had a gastrostomy tube inserted to improve his nutritional status with nighttime feeds. One month ago, a life-long friend of his with cystic fibrosis underwent lung transplantation and died in the immediate postoperative period.

On admission, he is breathing 30 times per minute, with marked retractions and distress. He is placed on noninvasive mechanical ventilation through a facemask, making him comfortable enough to be able to communicate with his clinicians. He is told that he will probably need to be intubated soon. At this point, he tells his clinicians that he has changed his mind about transplantation and that he does not want to be intubated. Although he appears somewhat anxious and frightened, he is lucid and articulate, and he seems to fully appreciate that without intubation he will soon die. His parents are extremely upset, and acknowledge that since the death of his friend, he has told them repeatedly that he has changed his mind about transplantation. Nevertheless, his parents insist that the doctors go ahead and intubate him if necessary, regardless of his refusal. His respiratory status continues to deteriorate.

Question: Should the patient be intubated?

Diagnosis: Respiratory failure due to advanced cystic fibrosis.

Discussion: **Decision-making for minors** is a process that is widely misunderstood. Many clinicians mistakenly believe that until a child reaches the age of majority (18 years in most jurisdictions), the child's parents have full authority regarding medical decision-making. This view fails to account for the ethical and legal implications of the fact that children gradually develop the ability to make decisions for themselves as they mature. Beginning at about age 7, therefore, medical decision-making is a collaborative process between the child, parents, and clinicians.

Guidelines developed by the American Academy of Pediatrics (AAP) state that "the doctrine of 'informed consent' has only limited direct application in pediatrics. Only *patients* who have appropriate decisional capacity and legal empowerment can give their *informed consent* to medical care. In all other situations, parents or other surrogates provide *informed permission* for the diagnosis and treatment of children with the *assent* of the child whenever appropriate" (emphasis in the original).

In other words, traditional understandings of informed consent do not apply in pediatrics. Rather, parents give their informed permission, and children give their assent. The nature of the child's assent depends upon age and maturity, but for adolescents, "assent" should include at least the following elements:

1. Helping the patient achieve a developmentally appropriate awareness of the nature of his or her condition.
2. Telling the patient what he or she can expect with tests and treatment(s).
3. Making a clinical assessment of the patient's understanding of the situation and the factors influencing how he or she is responding (including whether there is inappropriate pressure to accept testing or therapy).
4. Soliciting an expression of the patient's willingness to accept the proposed care. Regarding this final point, the AAP notes that "no one should solicit a patient's views without intending to weigh them seriously. In situations in which the patient will have to receive medical care despite his or her objection, the patient should be told that fact and should not be deceived."

Of necessity, the legal issues surrounding **adolescence** are more clearcut than the ethical considerations. Once a person reaches the age of majority, they have the right to make medical decisions for themselves, unless this is altered through legal process. For adolescents under the age of majority, the law varies by state. Most states recognize "emancipated minors" as having decisional capacity for health care matters. For example, minors who are married or who are serving in the armed forces may be designated as emancipated. In addition, some states have a "mature minor" doctrine that allows a judge to decide that an individual adolescent is mature enough to make a particular decision. This is an area where the law attempts to account for the ethical principles noted above and confers decisional capacity based on developmental maturity and not just chronological age. In actual practice, however, it is rare for clinicians to seek judicial involvement in decision-making for minors.

Some clinicians find the **"rule of sevens"** to be a useful, if only approximate, guide. Based on our understanding of child development, under age 7 most children are not able to participate in a meaningful way in medical decisions. Between 7 and 14 years of age, children should increasingly be involved in decisions about their care, but may often need to have their choices overridden when parents and clinicians perceive that these choices are not in their best interests. By age 14, the assumption should be that the child is fully able to participate in decision-making, and the burden of proof should be on anyone who believes otherwise.

Children with chronic illness require special consideration. Many of them are mature "beyond their years." In particular, by virtue of their need for frequent medical care, they may be very familiar with the pain as well as the benefits of medical tests and treatments. Those with life-threatening illnesses often already have experience with thinking about trade-offs between quality of life and longevity, and they may have developed considered opinions about how they choose to weigh these trade-offs. These generalizations are not always true, however, and some children with chronic illness may be less mature than their healthy peers and more dependent on their parents for emotional support and decision-making.

This case is particularly difficult because of the uncertainties involved and the need to act quickly. Even acknowledging that the choice is not for his parents to make, clinicians must struggle with the question of how best to protect this boy's right to choose for himself. Is he mature enough to make a life or death decision for himself? Even if he is, has his decision-making been clouded by the grief, sadness, and fear that has certainly been triggered by his friend's recent death?

The dilemma presented by the present patient does not have a "right" answer. Thoughtful and compassionate clinicians could choose and defend either path of treatment. The physicians caring for the patient proceeded with intubation for this illness and overrode his refusal. The patient recovered from his acute pulmonary exacerbation, at which time he was engaged in a dialogue regarding his wishes for treatment in the future. He firmly stated his desire to forgo transplantation and future endotracheal intubations. His physicians promised him that with this enhanced understanding of his wishes, they would respect his choices in the future.

Clinical Pearls

1. Decision-making for minors is not the process of seeking the informed consent of the parents. Depending on the developmental maturity of the child, it is a process of seeking the informed permission of the parents and the assent of the child.

2. The process of obtaining assent from a child parallels the process of obtaining informed consent from an adult, with the additional need for tailoring the communication to the developmental level of the child. Assent should not be sought when there is no intention to include the preferences of the child in the decision.

3. Chronically ill children require special consideration, because their illness may significantly alter their emotional and cognitive maturity, and because their life experiences may make them knowledgeable and able to deliberate about their desire for medical interventions.

REFERENCES

1. King NMP, Cross AW: Children as decision-makers: guidelines for pediatricians. J Pediatr 1989;115:10–16.
2. Bartholome WG: A new understanding of consent in pediatric practice: consent, parental permission and child assent. Pediatr Ann 1989;18(4):262–265.
3. Sigman GS, O'Connor C: Exploration for physicians of the mature minor doctrine. J Pediatr 1991;119:520–525.
4. Kohrman A, Wright Clayton E, Frader JE, et al: Informed consent, parental permission, and assent in pediatric practice. Pediatrics 1995;95:314–317.
5. Harrison C, Kenny NP, Sidarous M, Rowell M: Bioethics for clinicians: involving children in medial decisions. CMAJ 1997;156(6):825–828.

Susan W. Tolle, MD

PATIENT 4

A 78-year-old woman with severe pain at the end of life

A 78-year-old woman with advanced squamous cell lung cancer is brought to the emergency department because of increasing dyspnea and fever. She is widowed and lives alone in her own apartment. Her cancer was diagnosed just over 2 years ago, and she completed chemotherapy and full-dose radiation therapy with an initial good response. She has a form signed by her physician and posted in her home with a do-not-resuscitate order. The patient also has an advance directive in which she has appointed her son as her power of attorney.

Physical Examination: Blood pressure 104/72, pulse 128, temperature 39.5°C, respirations 38. General: thin, anxious woman sitting up, leaning forward and gasping for breath. HEENT: nasal oxygen prongs in place. Cardiac: tachycardic without murmur. Chest: dullness and absent breath sounds in the right lung base. Extremities: no edema. Neurologic: oriented.

Laboratory Findings: Chest radiograph: new consolidation in the right middle and lower lobes consistent with post-obstructive pneumonia. CT scan (done 2 weeks earlier): tumor growth compared to previous studies, with near obstruction of the right lower lobe bronchi within the previous radiation port.

Hospital Course: The patient is admitted, and a do-not-resuscitate (DNR) order is written at the patient's request and in line with her wishes and her out-of-hospital DNR order. Her son states the patient's wishes to refuse antibiotics and requests that she be made comfortable. The physician responds, "If she did not want antibiotics, why did she come to the hospital?"

The patient and her son agree on the goal of treatment with a focus on maximizing her comfort. The patient accepts that she will die soon but deeply fears suffocation. Over the next few hours, she becomes more agitated and is even more dyspneic. Her son begs the doctor for more medication, shouting "Who cares if she dies 10 minutes sooner! Give her more medication!" The physician orders 1 mg/hour of IV morphine and refuses to give more when this dose proves ineffective. "I'd like to give her more, but people will think I am killing her."

Question: What makes the physician reluctant to prescribe more pain medication?

Diagnosis: Advanced lung cancer with severe dyspnea and no expectation of survival to hospital discharge.

Discussion: Unfortunately, some physicians mistakenly believe that aggressive use of narcotics and other pain-relieving drugs for palliative care at the end of life may trigger investigations into their professional practices by regulatory agencies. These misunderstandings and fears of investigation contribute to a reluctance to prescribe appropriate palliative measures for their dying patients. One study suggests that these perceived hindrances to palliative care are greatest in acute care hospitals. Families of patients dying in acute care hospitals report having observed their loved ones experiencing more severe pain as compared with observations of patients who die at home or in a nursing home. Although many factors underlie these differences, the greater scrutiny of physician practices in an acute care setting probably contributes to inadequate opioid prescribing. An additional factor may be some physicians' difficulty in accepting death as a natural process.

State regulations for prescribing scheduled drugs also appear to alter physicians' willingness to provide palliative care. Observational studies have demonstrated reduced prescribing of opioids for appropriate use in pain control in states that have the most restrictive prescribing laws. The Institute of Medicine has affirmed that excessive regulations can serve as a barrier to optimal pain management at the end of life. As awareness of the importance of palliative care grows, many states are altering their overly restrictive drug-prescribing regulations to promote the appropriate administration of scheduled drugs for end-of-life care. In the meantime, physicians remain on safe ground in prescribing these medications as long as their palliative intentions are clearly documented. The patients' charts should include a description of the symptoms being treated; the pharmacologic and nonpharmacologic components of care plans, and the reasons for increasing drug doses.

The present patient came to accept that she would not live long and decided not to fight to prolong her life. She was fiercely independent and insisted on staying in her own home as long as possible. Her son lived 50 miles away and visited her often, helping each week with groceries and household tasks. She considered enrolling in hospice but lacked a full-time caregiver, which the home hospice programs she contacted required. She would not consider moving out of her home.

The patient deeply feared being unable to breathe and experiencing a suffocating death. Her request to be taken to the emergency department did not result from a change in mind about accepting life-sustaining treatment, but rather arose from the unbearable severity of her dyspnea. Like his mother, the son had come to accept her inevitable death. He could not bear to see her struggling to breathe and could not understand why her doctor was reluctant to increase her pain medications. The more the son insisted, the more resistant the doctor became.

Misunderstanding the son's intentions had increased the doctor's reluctance to provide pain medications to control the patient's distress. The doctor incorrectly interpreted the son's acceptance of his mother impending death and his desire to aggressively relieve her suffering as a desire to hasten her death.

Acceptance of death is a normal and desirable stage in moving from terminal illness to death. Those who have accepted their impending death often complete advance directives and agree to out-of-hospital DNR orders. They often enroll in home hospice and are less frequently admitted to acute care hospitals in their final weeks of life. As the rates of in-hospital death fall, the experience of hospital-based physicians moves even more toward a patient population in whom the goals of care are focused on prolonging life. A deep acceptance of death may be misperceived as a desire to hurry death. This acceptance and attendant requests for palliative care do not mean that the patient and family are requesting physician-assisted suicide or euthanasia. Desires to hasten death may coexist and deserve specific evaluation.

A social worker was called to meet with the son and spent time both with him and with the patient's physician. The social worker was able to clarify that neither the son nor his mother was asking for a deliberate hastening of her death. With this understanding, the physician then requested consultation from the Comfort Care Team (called the palliative care team in many parts of the country) on managing the patient's pain and dyspnea. The Comfort Care Team provided guidance and reassurance about the goals of care and assisted with medication dosages. They also advised on proper documentation of the physician's intention in using the medications. The physician entered the following note into the hospital record: "terminally ill patient experiencing severe dyspnea, will titrate morphine to comfort." He then wrote an order for morphine at 5 to 10 mg/hr IV to be titrated to comfort. To the son's great relief, the patient relaxed peacefully on her pillow with a respiratory rate of 20. The patient died peacefully in her hospital room the next afternoon, with her son holding her hand.

Clinical Pearls

1. Acceptance of death and a desire for comfort in life's final days should not be interpreted as a request to hasten death.

2. Whether or not a patient and his or her family desire a hastened death, effective palliation of distressing symptoms of terminal illness is imperative.

3. Clear documentation of the physician's purpose in using medications for comfort at life's end reduces the potential for misinterpretation of the palliative intentions.

4. In addition to other comfort measures, doses of opioids and sedatives should be increased until the patient's dyspnea is adequately controlled.

5. In difficult situations, consultation with an individual or team with expertise in symptom management is advisable.

REFERENCES

1. Kübler-Ross E: On Death and Dying. New York: MacMillian; 1969.
2. Tolle SW, Rosenfeld AG, Tilden VP, Park Y: Oregon's low in-hospital death rates: what determines where people die and satisfaction with decisions on place of death? Ann Intern Med 1999;130:681–685.
3. Hickman SE, Tolle SW, Tilden VP: Physicians' and nurses' perspectives on increased family reports of pain in dying hospitalized patients. Palliat Med 2001;3:413–418.
4. Tolle SW, Tilden VP, Hickman SE, Rosenfeld AG: Family reports of pain in dying hospitalized patients: a structured telephone survey. West J Med 2000;172:374–377.
5. Joranson DE, Gilson AM: Regulatory barriers to pain management. Semin Oncol Nurs 1998;14:158–163.
6. Joranson DE: Federal and state regulation of opioids. J Pain Symptom Manage 1990;5(suppl):S12–23.
7. Field MJ, Cassel CK: Approaching Death: Improving Care at the End of Life. Washington, DC: National Academy Press; 1997.

David B. Waisel, MD

PATIENT 5

A 67-year-old man with terminal cancer and a DNR order who needs a surgical procedure

A 67-year-old man with diabetes mellitus and liver cancer with bony metastases requires placement of an indwelling central venous catheter to facilitate pain management at home. He has been unable to tolerate oral or subcutaneous medications. The patient has previously undergone abdominal surgery and chemotherapy for his cancer, but his life expectancy is now estimated to be 3 months. He also suffers from coronary artery disease and underwent coronary artery bypass surgery 5 years ago. The patient has smoked 2 packs of cigarettes a day for 50 years. He currently has a do-not-resuscitate (DNR) order. His durable power of attorney for health care names his son as his health care proxy in the event of his incapacitation. The patient wishes to retain his DNR status during the perioperative period after placement of the central venous catheter.

Question: Should the patient's wishes for no perioperative resuscitation be honored?

Diagnosis: Central venous catheter placement in a patient with terminal liver cancer and a DNR order in place.

Discussion: A DNR order is predicated on the concept that a patient may choose to forgo certain procedures and their possible benefits because he or she rejects the burdens associated with these procedures. This premise is as legitimate in the operating room as it is on the hospital wards or in intensive care. Some patients with terminal conditions may desire the benefits of palliative surgery, such as placement of an indwelling venous catheter or repair of a fractured hip. Many of these patients, however, would not wish to bear the burdens of undergoing a futile cardiopulmonary resuscitation or one that might leave them with diminished functional capacity. Both the American Society of Anesthesiologists and the American College of Surgeons have recently published statements rejecting the automatic perioperative revocation of patients' DNR orders and endorsing the active reevaluation of the DNR order for the perioperative period.

DNR orders should be reevaluated for the perioperative period in light of the patient's goals. In addition to including the patient and family, the reevaluation process should include a dialogue with the healthcare personnel who may contribute to the patient's care. These caregivers include intraoperative personnel, such as anesthesiologists and surgeons, postoperative caregivers, such as intensivists who may be called upon to fulfill agreements with patients to withdraw care, and primary caregivers, such as nurses, internists and oncologists, who may be best prepared to facilitate discussions about end-of-life decisions.

There are three basic options for perioperative management of the DNR order. The first option entails **full resuscitation**. Most of the recent debate on perioperative end-of-life care has focused on the rights of patients to refuse perioperative resuscitation and maintain a preexisting DNR order during treatment in the operating room. This debate has addressed the status quo, or historical "default approach," wherein patients were managed with full resuscitation in the operating room regardless of their preexisting resuscitative status. Readers should not misinterpret the trend toward allowing patients to maintain their DNR status in the operating room to indicate that it is always inappropriate for patients to rescind their DNR status before surgery. Indeed, patients who elect a DNR status on hospital wards may prefer full resuscitation if a life-threatening event occurs during surgery. Such patients may believe that that the benefits of an extended life outweigh the burdens from the resuscitative efforts that are available in the operating room. This viewpoint is supported by the observation that the probability for quality survival after a witnessed arrest in the operating room is greater than after an unwitnessed arrest elsewhere. Withdrawal of a DNR order for a surgical procedure also allows a wider application of anesthetic and surgical interventions to manage complications during surgery.

The second option entails a **procedure-directed perioperative DNR order**. The procedure-directed approach parallels the techniques used for ward DNR orders in some institutions. Patients choose which specific interventions may be used. Physicians advise their patients based on the benefit and burden of the intervention, as well as the likelihood of that intervention allowing the patient to achieve desired goals. Interventions frequently discussed include tracheal intubation or other airway management procedures, postoperative ventilation, chest compressions, defibrillation, vasoactive drugs, and invasive monitoring. When procedures are necessary for the anesthetic and surgery to occur, such as tracheal intubation, patients should be informed whether procedures are "essential" and thus may not be refused. Procedure-directed orders work well for patients who want to unambiguously define which procedures are desired and for those who do not wish to allow perioperative caregivers to customize resuscitative efforts based on clinical circumstances.

The third option entails **goal-directed perioperative DNR orders**. By taking advantage of the operating room environment in which specific physicians take care of a patient for a defined period of time, patients may guide therapy by prioritizing outcomes rather than procedures. After defining desirable outcomes in individual discussions with the physicians who will be in the operating room, patients authorize those physicians to use their clinical judgment to determine how specific interventions will affect the achievement of these goals. Clinical experience indicates that many patients prefer the following as a standard goal-directed order: "The patient desires resuscitative efforts during surgery and in the recovery unit only if the adverse events are believed to be both *temporary* and *reversible*, in the clinical judgment of the attending anesthesiologists and surgeons." A recommendation for this order serves well as the starting point for discussions with the preoperative patient.

The strength of the goal-directed approach is that physicians are better able to honor the patient's desires without having to worry about getting "caught" in a technicality inconsistent with declared desires. Moreover, predictions about the success of interventions that are made at the time of the resuscitation are likely to be more accurate than predictions made preoperatively, when the quality and nature of the problems are not known. Goal-directed orders work well for patients who want their perioperative caregivers to customize the extent of resuscitation based on the caregivers' understanding of the patients' goals for the postoperative period. For this benefit, patients must accept the ambiguity that comes with relying on physicians to apply assessments of the clinical situations to their interpretations of the patients' goals.

A useful concept to assist patients' decision-making about perioperative resuscitation is the ability of physicians to withdraw life-supportive care if it no longer proves beneficial in achieving the patient's goals. The ability to give the patient a trial of therapy, such as mechanical ventilation, is a good way to fulfill patients' end-of-life requests to be the recipient of resuscitative efforts without obligating them to endure undesirable burdens. Following an unsuccessful intervention, decision-makers know with as much certainty as possible that continued therapy would be inconsistent with stated goals, and therapy may then be withdrawn. The opportunity to withdraw care is available for all three options listed above for perioperative resuscitation.

On occasion, patients with acute surgical conditions may present to the operating room unable to communicate their end-of-life wishes, yet have family members who convey a patient preference for forgoing resuscitative care. If a need for immediate surgery does not allow sufficient time to substantiate the patient's end-of-life wishes, then the traditional bias favoring life and providing emergency treatment takes precedence. Following stabilization, the patient's wishes may be clarified and instituted. Although this approach may temporarily circumvent a patient's resuscitative wishes, it provides the best available approach to avoid incorrectly withholding life-saving interventions when a patient's end-of-life wishes are unclear and later prove to favor full resuscitative care.

Patients' resuscitative preferences should be honored even in settings when a life-threatening event is iatrogenic in etiology. Patients make decisions about the desirability of perioperative resuscitation based on the life they want to live and the probability of a worthwhile post-resuscitative functional status. They do not make these decisions on the basis of what caused the life-threatening event to occur. It is irrelevant to patients whether an iatrogenic complication or a natural consequence of their underlying disease causes a cardiopulmonary arrest. What matters is their physical and mental status following recovery from resuscitative care.

The present patient went through a series of four discussions. He first discussed with his son, anesthesiologist, and surgeon the available options and chose a goal-directed DNR order. His physician wrote the following order: "The patient desires resuscitative efforts during surgery and in the post-anesthesia care unit only if the adverse events are believed to be both *temporary* and *reversible*, in the clinical judgment of the attending anesthesiologists and surgeons."

The patient and son then met with a physician in the intensive care unit so that he could clarify his desires for postoperative care. He requested the withdrawal of life-supportive care after several days if the probability of successful extubation appeared unlikely. Recognizing the difficulty in applying such a statement, the patient made clear that he afforded his son decision-making capacity in making this decision. The patient and son then met with his longtime internist and the rest of his family to make clear his wishes regarding both resuscitation and the son's decision-making authority. Finally, the patient met with nurses and technicians who provide operating room care so that they may hear the patient's wishes directly and so may be able to withdraw from providing elective care if they cannot support the patient's desires.

The patient's end-of-life preferences were documented in the medical record and co-signed by the anesthesiologist and surgeon. A copy of the health care proxy was placed in the medical record. He underwent placement of the venous catheter without complication and returned home with improved pain control.

Clinical Pearls

1. DNR orders should be reevaluated for the perioperative period. Resuscitative options include full resuscitation, a procedure-directed order, or a goal-directed order.

2. All relevant caregivers should be involved in discussions about perioperative management, including, when appropriate, primary caregivers, intraoperative personnel, and caregivers who will manage the patient in the postoperative period.

3. Use the option to withdraw care to the patient's advantage. Patients can be managed with full resuscitative and life-supportive care when their end-of-life wishes are unclear. Caregivers can withdraw life support after a period of stabilization allows sufficient time to clarify patients' advance directives.

4. Patients' resuscitative preferences should be honored regardless of the cause of a cardiopulmonary arrest. Patient decisions about the desirability of resuscitation do not differ if a life-threatening event is iatrogenic in nature or a natural consequence of the underlying disease.

REFERENCES

1. Tomlinson T, Brody H. Ethics and communication in do-not-resuscitate orders. N Engl J Med 1988;318:43–46.
2. Cohen CB, Cohen PJ: Do-not-resuscitate orders in the operating room. N Engl J Med 1991;325:1879–1882.
3. Truog RD: "Do-not-resuscitate" orders during anesthesia and surgery. Anesthesiology 1991;74:606–608.
4. Clemency MV, Thompson NJ: Do not resuscitate orders in the perioperative period: patient perspectives. Anesth Analg 1997;84:859–864.
5. Truog RD, Waisel DB, Burns JP: DNR in the OR: a goal-directed approach. Anesthesiology 1999;90:289–295.
6. Casarett DJ, Stocking CB, Siegler M: Would physicians override a do-not-resuscitate order when a cardiac arrest is iatrogenic? J Gen Intern Med 1999;14:35–38.

Paul Rousseau, MD

PATIENT 6

A 55-year-old man with recurrent metastatic esophageal cancer who wants to "just go to sleep" until death occurs

A 55-year-old man with a history of recurrent metastatic esophageal cancer is now unable to swallow medications and is limited to fluids for nutritional sustenance. He is increasingly unable to manage his oral secretions and is dyspneic. He also has begun to experience paroxysms of coughing and choking from presumptive pulmonary aspiration, symptoms which frighten both him and his family. Further chemo- and radiotherapy are considered to offer little benefit, and the patient has declared he wants no further attempts at curative therapies, treatments that reduce his quality of life, or resuscitative measures. He has also refused placement of an esophageal stent or enteral feeding tube and resists placement of analgesics rectally. A continuous subcutaneous infusion of hydromorphone is initiated for pain control, however, the patient and his family request that he be allowed to "just go to sleep" until death occurs.

Physical Examination: Blood pressure 102/60, pulse 100, respirations 28, temperature 37.9°C. General: cachectic and pale with mild-to-moderate respiratory distress. HEENT: normal. Chest: crackles in right lower lobe. Cardiac: regular rhythm with tachycardia, no murmur. Abdomen: nontender without organomegaly. Extremities: 1+ pedal edema bilaterally.

Laboratory Findings: Hct 20%, WBC 15,000/μL, electrolytes normal, BUN 75 mg/dL, creatinine 4.5 mg/dL.

Home Course: A plan of care is devised using pharmacologic interventions in accordance with the patient's goals of care. He refuses antibiotics for a presumed pneumonia, but is aggressively treated with subcutaneous hydromorphone, small volume nebulizer treatments, and oxygen in an effort to alleviate breathlessness. Subcutaneous glycopyrrolate is also administered in an attempt to desiccate oral secretions, while subcutaneous lorazepam is provided to reduce anxiety.

Despite these palliative interventions, his condition continues to deteriorate. The patient and family once again ask for him to be helped to "just go to sleep" until death occurs, instead of suffering with debilitating, dispiriting, and intolerable symptoms. When questioned, the patient denies depression other than sadness at his impending "passing" and reiterates that unrelenting and persistent symptoms are precipitating an undignified and insufferable quality of life.

Question: Should terminal sedation (also referred to as palliative sedation and sedation for intractable distress of a dying patient) be utilized?

Diagnosis: Recurrent metastatic esophageal cancer with persistent physical suffering.

Discussion: The goals of medicine include the improvement of patients' functional status, education regarding their disease and prognosis, and relief of pain, symptoms, and suffering. The latter two pronouncements are cardinal to palliative care, and facilitate comfort and a dignified death for the patient and reassurance for family members. Yet, in many cases, suffering in all its domains cannot be readily palliated, particularly in terminally ill patients. In such circumstances, terminal sedation remains a somewhat controversial, yet valuable therapeutic intervention to manage refractory symptoms and suffering at the end-of-life. Moreover, it was fundamentally sanctioned by the United States Supreme Court decision negating the constitutional right to physician-assisted suicide in 1997. In their judgment summaries, Justices O'Connor and Souter supported the use of medications to alleviate the suffering of terminally ill patients, even if such treatment causes a drug-induced loss of consciousness or hastens death.

Terminal sedation can be defined as the act of intentionally inducing and maintaining a sedated state in dying patients who are experiencing suffering that has been refractory to all standard therapies. The intention of sedation is not to cause death, yet in such situations death is the expected outcome. Ethical and moral justification of terminal sedation derives in part from the doctrine of double effect, a doctrine that is applied in situations in which it is impossible to avoid all harmful actions. The **rule of double effect** stipulates four criteria: 1) the nature of the act must be good; 2) the good effect and not the bad effect must be intended; 3) the bad effect must not be the means to the good effect; and 4) the good effect must outweigh the bad effect.

Controversy arises from assertions by opponents of terminal sedation that the cessation of nutrition and hydration bring about death from malnutrition or dehydration, not the underlying disease. In virtually all instances in which terminal sedation is employed, patients have already limited their oral intake or completely stopped eating and drinking due to the anorexia associated with advanced disease. In such circumstances, beginning artificial nutrition or hydration would seem antithetical to the goals for palliation and allowing natural death. Within contemporary ethical and legal discourse, artificial nutrition and hydration are often considered extraordinary care. In the context of advanced and inevitably fatal illness, there are no ethical or legal requirements for beginning or continuing such interventions. Particularly when artificial hydration and/or enteral nutrition previously have

been initiated, frank discussion must take place regarding the benefits and burdens of nutrition and hydration at the end-of-life, and in particular, the futility of such therapy in terminal sedation.

Minimum clinical guidelines have been proposed to ensure safe and ethical use of terminal sedation as a palliative intervention of last resort. Although use of terminal sedation must be highly individualized to the needs and circumstances of specific patients, categorical guidelines have been developed that mandate basic requirements. Existing guidelines mandate that clinicians must:
- ascertain the presence of a terminal illness;
- screen for depression;
- consider consultation with a mental health professional or ethics consultation committee if psychiatric or ethical issues are of concern;
- exhaust all standard palliative treatments, including treatment for pain, dyspnea, nausea/vomiting, depression, delirium, anxiety, or any other contributing source of distress;
- obtain informed consent from the patient or surrogate decision-maker; and
- establish the presence of a do-not-resuscitate order (DNR).

Medications used for terminal sedation include the benzodiazepines, barbiturates, neuroleptics, and the anesthetic propofol (see table). The benzodiazepines, barbiturates, and neuroleptics can be administered intravenously, subcutaneously, or rectally, whereas propofol must be delivered via an intravenous solution.

In the present patient, all proposed clinical criteria for the use of terminal sedation were met: he suffered from a terminal illness, all standard palliative measures had been exhausted, he gave uncoerced informed consent, and a DNR order was in effect. When asked if he was depressed, he responded that he was sad but not depressed. Such a simple single-item question for depression in terminal illness is more valid than other depression screening inventories, and can be readily used by all clinicians. However, if depression is suspected and potentially contributing to refractory symptoms, treatment is suggested prior to initiating terminal sedation. Any of the antidepressants can be tried, but if waiting 7 to 14 days for the antidepressant effect is not feasible and time is limited, a trial of a rapid-acting psychostimulant such as methylphenidate, 2.5 mg to 5 mg every morning, should be considered.

In extraordinary situations in which physical symptoms are intolerable and inexorable (such as massive hemorrhage, impending tracheal obstruction from a tumor mass), terminal sedation may be

Drugs for Terminal Sedation

	Dose/Bolus	Route
Opioids	Dose varies—increase dose to accomplish sedation; however, myoclonus may develop.	OR, PR, SL, IV, SQ
Lorazepam	0.5–2 mg q 1–2 hr	OR, SL, SQ
Lorazepam	Bolus 1–5 mg, then start CII/CSI at 0.5–1 mg/hr; usual maintenance dose 4–40 mg/day.	IV, SQ
Midazolam	Bolus 0.5–5 mg (higher bolus for SQ), then start CII/CSI at 0.5–1 mg/hr; usual maintenance dose 30–120 mg/day.	IV, SQ
Chlorpromazine	10–25 mg q 2–4 hr	OR, PR, IV
Haloperidol	0.5–5 mg q 2–4 hr	OR, SQ
Haloperidol	Bolus 1–10 mg, then start CII/CSI at 5 mg/day; usual maintenance dose 5–15 mg/day.	IV, SQ
Pentobarbital	60–200 mg q 2–4 hr	PR
Pentobarbital	Bolus 2–3 mg/kg, then start CII at 1 mg/hr, titrate upward to maintain sedation.	IV
Thiopental	Bolus 5–7 mg/kg, then start CII at 20 mg/hr; usual maintenance dose 70–180 mg/hr.	IV
Phenobarbital	Bolus 200 mg, then start CII/CSI at 600 mg/day; usual maintenance dose 600–1600 mg/day.	IV, SQ
Propofol	10 mg/hr CII, may titrate by 10 mg/hr increments every 15–20 minutes; bolus of 20–50 mg may be used for emergent sedation.	IV

OR=oral, SL=sublingual, PR=rectal, IV=intravenous, SQ=subcutaneous, CII=continuous intravenous infusion, CSI=continuous subcutaneous infusion

considered emergent and necessary despite depression. Respite sedation, in which a patient is sedated for a predetermined period of time and then gradually reawakened, can also be considered when existential distress is coupled with progressive physical symptoms. Respite sedation is properly distinguished from terminal sedation, because death is not necessarily the expected, nor the inevitable, outcome. If existential distress is refractory to treatment or contributing to physical suffering, sedation for 24 to 48 hours may allow a deep and restful sleep that allays existential anguish and, in select cases, reduces physical symptoms. In such cases, patients may elect to remain awake, while preserving the option of terminal sedation if it is required later in the disease process.

Because all criteria were met for terminal sedation for the present patient, a continuous subcutaneous infusion of midazolam was begun at 1 mg/hr and titrated accordingly to keep the patient completely sedated. As there is no definitive evidence that unconscious patients do not feel pain, and because the abrupt discontinuation of an opioid can precipitate withdrawal symptoms, the hydromorphone infusion was continued but not titrated upward. The patient's family remained at the bedside in shifts and was present when he died 12 days after starting terminal sedation.

Clinical Pearls

1. Terminal sedation is an ethically and morally acceptable option for refractory suffering at the end of life.

2. Clinical guidelines have been developed for the use of terminal sedation. Such criteria include ascertaining the presence of a terminal illness, screening for depression, considering consultation with a mental health professional or ethics committee if psychiatric or ethical issues are of concern, exhausting all palliative treatments, obtaining uncoerced informed consent, and establishing the presence of a DNR order. If depression is suspected, an attempt at treatment is suggested, unless intolerable and inexorable physical symptoms mandate immediate sedation.

3. Benzodiazepines, barbiturates, neuroleptics, and propofol are the most common medications used for terminal sedation.

4. Opioid analgesics should not be discontinued during terminal sedation. Withdrawal of opioids may cause a patient to experience pain, and sudden opioid withdrawal symptoms can occur.

5. Many patients will die within a few days of instituting terminal sedation. However, patients and their families should be advised that death may take several days up to a few weeks when adequate nutritional and hydration status exist before initiating terminal sedation.

REFERENCES

1. Lynn J: Terminal sedation [letter]. N Engl J Med 1988;338:1230.
2. Cherny NI, Portenoy RK: Sedation in the management of refractory symptoms: guidelines for evaluation and treatment. J Palliat Care 1994;10:31–38.
3. Chochinov HM, Wilson KG, Enns M, Lander S: "Are you depressed?": screening for depression in the terminally ill. Am J Psychiatry 1997;154:674–676.
4. Quill TE, Dresser R, Brock DW: The rule of double-effect—a critique of its role in end-of-life decision making. N Engl J Med 1997;337:1768–1771.
5. Vacco v Quill, No. 117 SCt 2293, 1997.
6. Washington v Glucksberg, No. 117 SCt 2258, 1997.
7. Jonsen AR, Siegler M, Winslade WJ: Clinical Ethics: A Practical Approach to Ethical Decisions in Clinical Medicine, 4th ed. New York, McGraw-Hill, 1998.
8. Quill TE, Byock IA: Responding to intractable terminal suffering: the role of terminal sedation and voluntary refusal of food and fluids. Ann Intern Med 2000;132:408–414.
9. Rousseau PC: The ethical validity and clinical experience of palliative sedation. Mayo Clin Proc 2000;75:1064–1069.
10. Rousseau PC: Existential suffering and palliative sedation: a brief commentary with a proposal for clinical guidelines. Am J Hosp Palliat Care 2001;18:151–153.

Walter M. Robinson, MD, MPH

PATIENT 7

A 10-year-old child on mechanical ventilation and pharmacologic paralysis whose parents request discontinuation of ventilator support

A 10-year-old boy has been treated with mechanical ventilation in the intensive care unit for a respiratory infection with respiratory syncitial virus (RSV). Despite multiple efforts, the patient has not improved sufficiently to allow weaning from the ventilator. He now requires complete neuromuscular blockade with vecuronium to assist ventilatory support. Recently, moderate renal insufficiency as well as moderate liver dysfunction has developed.

He had been healthy until a near-fatal motor vehicle accident at age 6 years. His injuries were severe, with a lacerated liver, crush fractures of the pelvis, cardiac contusions with rib fractures, and severe head trauma. After a lengthy hospital course, he was discharged to a rehabilitation facility, where he regained only minimal communication skills. He can recognize his parents and smile when they enter the room but cannot speak, walk, or feed himself. He had been living at home with his parents and older brother. The patient has moderate to severe pulmonary parenchymal scarring secondary to acute respiratory distress syndrome that occurred at the time of the motor vehicle accident. He has had two previous episodes of RSV infection, each requiring intubation and mechanical ventilation for 1 week.

In consultation with the medical team, the parents decide that the likelihood of their son's survival without mechanical ventilation is slim, and they see continuation of the ventilator as not in his best interests considering his already restricted quality of life. The parents request removal of mechanical ventilation to allow their child to die. The physicians agree with the parents' decision and make plans to remove the ventilator.

Question: Should the paralytic agent be continued or stopped, and if stopped, is it necessary to wait until neuromuscular function returns before removing the ventilator?

Diagnosis: Respiratory failure and pharmacologic paralysis in the setting of ventilator withdrawal[0].

Discussion: The right of a patient or surrogate to refuse treatment, including life-sustaining mechanical ventilation, is firmly established in American medical ethics and law. At issue in the present case is not the right to refuse medical interventions, but the appropriate use of neuromuscular blocking agents by the physician in honoring the legitimate request of the patient or surrogate.

The use of neuromuscular blocking agents at the end of life is controversial but by no means exceptional. In one study[1], 9% of patients continued to receive neuromuscular blocking agents during withdrawal of life support. In another study[2], 26% of children received neuromuscular blocking agents at some time during the 4 hours preceding withdrawal of the ventilator. A survey of critical care physicians[3] has found that 6% report using neuromuscular blocking agents at least occasionally in patients at the end of life, and a survey of pediatric ICU specialists in Britain[4] found that 12% would continue the administration of these agents during removal of the ventilator. A Dutch study[5] reported the use of neuromuscular blocking agents in 7% of dying infants "because of a very prolonged dying process."

Neuromuscular blocking agents are commonly used in intensive care. They are most often given over a limited time to facilitate endotracheal intubation, yet they are also administered continuously to those patients who require high ventilator settings. Neuromuscular blocking agents have **no sedative or analgesic effects** and therefore should never be used in the absence of adequate sedation or analgesia. Although the usual half-life of the common neuromuscular blocking agents ranges from minutes to hours, the half-life can be extended in patients with hepatic or renal dysfunction, leading to prolonged neuromuscular blockade after infusion of the agents is ceased[6]. Because it does not provide any relief of pain or discomfort, neuromuscular blockade **should never be added** at the time of ventilator withdrawal in order to provide the appearance of comfort.

At issue here are the conditions in which withdrawal of a ventilator might be ethically permissible if neuromuscular blockade is already present and cannot be completely reversed. There are three concerns about the use of pharmacologic paralysis during withdrawal of the ventilator:

1. that the patient might have otherwise survived withdrawal of the ventilator if pharmacologic paralysis had not been present;
2. that pharmacologic paralysis may prevent assessment of the patient's comfort during ventilator withdrawal; and

3. that pharmacologic paralysis will reduce the possibility of interaction between the patient and his or her family when the patient is dying.

The first concern, that pharmacologic paralysis will prevent spontaneous breathing by the patient when the ventilator is removed, is most certainly valid but only rarely applies to these types of cases. Occasionally, physicians and families may view ventilator withdrawal as one last chance for the patient to demonstrate the potential to survive[7]; at the extreme end of the spectrum, families (and physicians) may view the withdrawal of the ventilator as the last chance for a miracle to occur. If this is the case, then paralysis must *always* be reversed prior to removal of mechanical ventilation. As well, care must be taken so that respiratory suppressants, such as opioids, are stopped (or dose adjusted if needed for pain management) to allow adequate ventilation. Other necessary steps are taken to ensure the best possible chance that spontaneous breathing will be successful.

Yet in most cases, it is clear to all involved that the patient cannot survive without the ventilator, and there is no realistic expectation of spontaneous breathing. In many cases, there is virtual certainty that a patient cannot survive even for a brief period of time without the ventilator. This has been demonstrated in several trials of ventilator weaning or in patients currently surviving only due to nonphysiologic ventilation modes. If this is the case, the additional presence of pharmacologic paralysis is unlikely to reduce the chances of survival off the ventilator.

The second concern, that neuromuscular blockade makes assessment and treatment of symptoms of dying more difficult, is also valid and is the best reason that blockade should be reversed, if possible, before the ventilator is removed. Although direct assessment of a patient's comfort is preferable, direct assessment is not always necessary to guarantee the patient's comfort. Skilled anesthesiologists use neuromuscular blockers during routine surgeries and are highly confident that the patient's comfort can be ensured, even in the setting of rapidly fluctuating noxious stimuli such as might be expected during ventilator withdrawal. However, the ability of a skilled anesthesiologist to ensure comfort without direct assessment does not mean that all other clinicians are able to do so.

There is clear evidence that many physicians currently under-treat pain[8], even when the patient can directly express his or her discomfort. In many ICUs, the withdrawal of ventilators is a job delegated to respiratory therapists and nurses. If physicians do not always have the skills to treat pain adequately when there is no paralysis, then it would be unreasonable to expect nonphysician caregivers to be able to do so when paralysis is present. Thus, if withdrawal will be performed in the setting of neuromuscular blockade, consultation with clinicians with expertise in the assessment and management of symptoms in paralyzed patients is ethically mandatory. In training institutions, the withdrawal of life-supportive care requires the presence of an experienced attending physician.

The third concern is that neuromuscular blockade may eliminate the possibility for interaction between a dying patient and his or her family. This concern is also valid but again may not apply to situations of the sort illustrated by the present case. Most patients in whom neuromuscular blockade cannot be reversed are desperately ill, and the possibilities for meaningful verbal communication with family members are very limited. This does not mean that the patient cannot be held or talked to as the end of life nears, or that other steps cannot be taken to facilitate the human connection of families and their dying loved ones[9]. The decreased possibility of the patient communicating with the family should be weighed against the discomfort that the family may experience while waiting for the possible return of muscle function. Open discussion with the family of the presence of neuromuscular blockade is important in these settings.

In the present patient, the infusion of vecuronium was stopped, and recovery of neuromuscular function was evident 30 minutes later. After appropriate sedation and analgesia were administered, the ventilator was withdrawn, and he died resting in his mother's arms.

Clinical Pearls

1. Neuromuscular blocking agents should never be added to a patient's therapeutic regimen at the end of life in order to produce the appearance of comfort. Because neuromuscular blockers do not have sedative or analgesic properties, their addition during withdrawal of a ventilator may result in the silent suffering of a patient unable to demonstrate his discomfort.

2. When possible, neuromuscular blockade should be reversed when withdrawing a ventilator so that the best possible assessment and treatment of the patient's symptoms can be performed.

3. It is ethically permissible to withdraw a ventilator while the effects of pharmacologic paralysis are still evident, but only when the following four provisions have been met: (a) reversal of paralysis is not possible in a reasonable period of time; (b) there is a very high degree of certainty that the patient cannot survive without mechanical ventilation; (c) continuing to wait for reversal of pharmacologic paralysis causes the patient's family significant distress; and (d) assurance of adequate analgesia and/or sedation can be provided by those with expertise in managing symptoms in paralyzed patients.

REFERENCES

0. Truog RD, Burns, JP, Mitchell C, et al: Pharmacologic paralysis and withdrawal of mechanical ventilation at the end of life. N Engl J Med 2000;342:508–511.
1. Wilson WC, Smedira NG, Fink C, et al: Ordering and administration of sedatives and analgesics during the withholding and withdrawing of life support form critically ill patients. JAMA 1992;267:949–53.
2. Burns JP, Mitchell C, Outwater KM, et al: End of life care in the pediatric intensive care unit following the forgoing of life sustaining treatment. Crit Care Med 2000;28:3060–3066.
3. Faber-Langendoen K: The clinical management of dying patients receiving mechanical ventilation: a survey of physician practices. Chest 1994;106:880–888.
4. Hatherill M, Tibby SM, Sykes K, Murdoch IA: Dilemmas exist in withdrawing ventilation from dying children. BMJ 1998;317:80.
5. DeLeeuwR, deBeaufort AJ, de Kleine MJ, et al: Forgoing intensive care treatment in newborn infants with extremely poor prognosis: a study in four neonatal intensive care units in the Netherlands. J Pediatr 1996;129:661–666.
6. Segredo V, Caldwell JE, Mathay MA, et al: Persistent paralysis in critically ill patients after long term administration of vecuronium. N Engl J Med 1992;327:524–528.
7. Hatherill M, Tibby SM, Sykes K, Murdoch IA: Dilemmas exist in withdrawing ventilation from dying children. BMJ 1998;317:80.
8. The SUPPORT Principal Investigators: A controlled trial to improve care for seriously ill hospitalized patients: the Study to Understand Prognoses and Preferences for Outcomes and Risks of Treatment. JAMA 1995;274:1591–8. [Erratum appears in JAMA 1996;275:1232.]
9. Curtis JR , Rubenfeld GD (eds): Managing Death in the Intensive Care Unit: The Transition from Cure to Comfort. Oxford, Oxford University Press, 2001.

John Hansen-Flaschen, MD

PATIENT 8

A 56-year-old ventilator-dependent man with a previously expressed wish to avoid prolonged mechanical ventilation

A 56-year-old man with a history of dementia and progressive dyspnea attributed to chronic obstructive pulmonary disease (COPD) is transferred to a teaching hospital after 13 days of care in a community hospital. There, he had been treated for pneumonia and hypercapneic respiratory failure.

On admission to the community hospital, he required intubation and mechanical ventilation. Three days after admission, his wife produced a medical advance directive legally executed by her husband months earlier when the diagnosis of dementia had been confirmed by a consultant. The document directed that he not undergo cardiopulmonary resuscitation and that invasive life-supportive care should not be continued beyond 3 days. The patient's physician at the community hospital, however, refused to withdraw mechanical ventilation because the man "still had a chance" to recover from pneumonia. His course was complicated by intermittent agitation that prompted the use of intravenous benzodiazepine sedation. Thirteen days later, after two unsuccessful attempts at extubation, the patient was transferred to a nearby teaching hospital at the request of his wife.

The patient had been active until 14 months earlier, when he stopped working because of exertional dyspnea. Five months ago, impairment of memory and concentration lead to a diagnosis of dementia. During the last several months, the patient had become socially withdrawn and increasingly inactive, rarely venturing from his bedroom. Supplemental oxygen and furosemide were prescribed for arterial oxygen desaturation and peripheral edema. A third episode of bronchitis in 3 months progressed to pneumonia. His earlier medical history was unremarkable, except for an episode of polio at age 15 from which he recovered completely.

On arrival to the teaching hospital, the patient is mechanically ventilated and unresponsive while receiving large doses of sedating drugs. A chest radiograph shows near complete resolution of his pneumonia. On the day of admission, the patient's wife meets with the attending physician, and she asks that her husband's written directive be honored before morning. The physician responds that it is his custom to evaluate new patients thoroughly before acquiescing to requests for terminal withdrawal of life support. This evaluation might take 2 or 3 days in this instance. The woman becomes distraught: "The other doctors did the same thing. They delayed and delayed. His wishes are clear. He did not want mechanical ventilation beyond 3 days."

Question: Should the doctor comply with the request for immediate withdrawal of life support?

Diagnosis: Progressive dyspnea secondary to bilateral vocal cord paralysis and resolving pneumonia, which mimicked severe COPD and dementia, in a patient with a potential for functional recovery.

Discussion: Respect for patient autonomy is a pillar of modern medical ethics. Patients may refuse any or all medical interventions including life support, even if they are expected to die as a result. Physicians should not impose diagnostic studies or treatment over the objections of a patient who possesses decision-making capacity or an appropriate surrogate decision-maker who acts in apparent good faith on behalf of the patient.

Are there any reasonable limits or exceptions to this precept? George Annas, a noted Boston law professor, has argued no, as have others. Justifications for exceptions to patient autonomy start us on a slippery slope and lead quickly to an avalanche of abuse, they argue. History and current practice are replete with instances in which physicians have "protected" competent, aware patients from their own personal preferences regarding health care. How many lives have been prolonged in critical care units, against the will of patients, by physicians or surgeons who argue that they "still have a chance" to recover?

Some physicians hold a contrary view. They argue that human life is too precious for unquestioned adherence to general rules. The determination of a patient's decision-making capacity sometimes requires repeated observations over time. Also, many personal decisions regarding health care are conditional or are based on certain assumptions, whether stated or implied. When there is reason to doubt a patient's decision-making capacity, the motives of a surrogate decision-maker, or the factual basis of life-or-death decisions, these commentators recommend that physicians "err on the side of life," while gathering additional information and continuing discussions with the patient or surrogate.

In the present case, one may recognize a reason to doubt the applicability of the patient's advance directive. On the evening of hospital transfer, the receiving physician did not withdraw mechanical ventilation as requested by the wife; but instead, without further explanation, he continued his diagnostic evaluation. Laryngoscopy performed the next day revealed paralysis of both vocal cords with near-complete obstruction of the airway. On the third hospital day, the patient was able to sustain adequate ventilation through an endotracheal tube without the benefit of mechanical assistance. An electromyogram, performed by a consulting neurologist, showed abnormal function of the phrenic nerves.

The physician met again with the wife and her three sons. He advised that the patient's recent medical problems, including his shortness of breath on exertion, progressive cognitive impairment, and recurrent respiratory infections might have been caused by postpolio syndrome involving primarily nerves of the pharynx, larynx, and diaphragm. The doctor predicted that the man might do well with a tracheostomy and long-term, nocturnal mechanical ventilation. After lengthy discussion, the wife consented to a trial of the proposed treatment plan.

About half of patients who survive poliomyelitis develop the postpolio syndrome 30 to 40 years after initial recovery. This condition presents with insidious onset of focal muscle weakness, apparently caused by accelerated loss of remaining functional motor neurons in previously affected nerves. The present patient developed progressive respiratory insufficiency because of bilateral vocal cord paralysis and weakness of the diaphragm. Chronic respiratory insufficiency caused shortness of breath, fluid retention, and ultimately, a dementia-like condition. Pharyngeal dysfunction caused occult aspiration and recurrent respiratory infections. All of these manifestations reversed after initiation of appropriate therapy.

Those who teach unqualified conformance to medical advance directives might fault the physicians at both hospitals equally in this case, regardless of the outcome. Both doctors superseded the clearly expressed wishes of the patient with an alternative plan of their own. Some would argue that occasional reports of unexpected recoveries do not excuse physicians who impose life support that is not wanted. Otherwise, there is little hope for medical advance decision-making.

This argument, although straightforward, misses or ignores important differences in the reasons for the actions of the two physicians. The doctor at the first hospital was unaware of the previous diagnostic error. He continued life support because he believed that 3 days were just a few days short of the time that the patient might require to recover from pneumonia. Never mind that the man might have welcomed death as an escape from progressive dementia. The physician at the second hospital considered postpolio syndrome on the day of the transfer. Like the first physician, but for different reasons, he also thought that the patient might be able to recover from dependence on intensive care. If the patient suffered not from COPD and dementia, but from postpolio syndrome, then his medical advance directive was based on **false diagnoses** and an **incorrect prognosis**. Thus, the second doctor did not act immediately on the advance directive because he suspected that it was invalid.

Why did the second physician not discuss his diagnostic theory with the patient's wife on the evening of the hospital transfer? Afterwards, he explained that the woman was adamantly determined to withdraw life support that night. He feared that she would be distrustful of an unfamiliar physician proposing a new, admittedly improbable, diagnostic possibility. The hospital ethics committee criticized the second physician for not disclosing his diagnostic reasoning promptly to the wife. People expect doctors to be forthright as well as honest. However, the committee supported the doctor's decision to continue life support pending the results of a focused diagnostic evaluation. What if the wife had declined further testing even after hearing about the possibility of postpolio syndrome? Some thought that the wife's request should be respected. The majority disagreed. On the argument that surrogate decision-makers do not have quite the same authority as patients themselves, most members of the committee indicated that they would have supported an expedited work-up to test the diagnostic basis of the man's advanced directive, even if the wife did not concur.

Ultimately, this case is about **medical competence**. Neither the most ethical conduct, nor the most compassionate bedside manner can compensate for major errors in medical diagnosis or therapy. The Hippocratic Precepts contain a passage that rings true today: "Conclusions that are mere words cannot bear fruit, but only those based on demonstrated fact. One must hold fast to generalizable fact and occupy oneself with facts persistently if one is to acquire that ready and sure habit we call the art of medicine." Until an accurate diagnosis is offered and all reasonable therapeutic options are presented, patient autonomy is largely illusionary. In this unusual case, a doctor temporarily defied a request for withdrawal of life support to confirm a previously unsuspected diagnosis, which effectively invalidated the patient's advanced directive and pointed the way to medical interventions that were greatly appreciated by the patient.

In this case, with the consent of the man's wife, a tracheostomy was performed and the patient was awakened from sedation. He was weaned uneventfully off mechanical ventilation, which was continued at night only. Over the next 3 months, the patient recovered cognitive function with complete resolution of his dementia. He also demonstrated improved muscle strength. On return to the physician's office, a capped tracheostomy was hidden under a turtleneck. In a clear, soft voice while his wife sat smiling beside him, he thanked God and the doctor for every day of his extended life.

Clinical Pearls

1. Patients may refuse any or all medical interventions including life support. Physicians should not impose diagnostic studies or treatment over the objections of a patient who possesses decision-making capacity or an appropriate surrogate decision-maker who acts in apparent good faith on behalf of a patient.

2. There are occasional exceptions to nearly all rules of medicine, including the principle of patient autonomy.

3. One such exception occurs if the preferences expressed by a patient or surrogate are based on misinformation. In such situations, irreversible measures should be deferred until the material facts are clarified and discussed anew with the decision-maker.

4. Clinical competence is the first and arguably the most important precept of medical ethics: without competence, there is little expectation of medical beneficence, nonmalfeasance, or respect for patient autonomy.

REFERENCES

1. Hansen-Flaschen J: Advanced lung disease: palliation and terminal care. Clin Chest Med 1977;18:645–655.
2. Chadwick J, Mann WN (trans): Hippocratic Writings. London, Penguin Books, 1983.
3. President's Commission for the Study of Ethical Problems in Medicine and in Biomedical and Behavioral Research: Deciding to Forgo Life-Sustaining Treatment. Washington, DC, U.S. Government Printing Office, 1983.
4. Annas GJ: The Rights of Patients. Southern Illinois University Press, 1989.
5. Jonsen AR: The New Medicine and the Old Ethics. Cambridge, MA, Harvard University Press, 1990.
6. American Thoracic Society Bioethics Task Force: Position statement: withholding and withdrawing life-sustaining therapy. Am Rev Respir Dis 1991;144:726–732.

Marion Danis, MD

PATIENT 9

A 77-year-old woman who expresses a need to discuss her end-of-life care during a routine office visit

A 77-year-old woman asks her physician to discuss her end-of-life care during a routine office visit. During the last few years, she has gradually been more restricted in her activity because of shortness of breath. She is a retired schoolteacher with a long history of smoking that began when her husband was in the service in World War II. She has been widowed for the last 4 years. Her husband died of colon cancer after a protracted and painful illness. The patient lives near one of her two daughters, but her other daughter and her son live across the country.

Question: How would you proceed in discussing end-of-life care and making treatment decisions with this patient?

Diagnosis: Chronic obstructive pulmonary disease.

Discussion: The aim of advance care discussions is to plan for care at the end of life that will be most consistent with an individual's values and goals. There are several obstacles and limitations to achieving this aim. Clinicians should be aware of this reality in order to minimize the obstacles when possible and to provide realistic expectations for patients and families.

Few patients are able to participate fully in medical decisions when they experience life-threatening events, so it is advisable for clinicians to encourage patients to discuss and document their wishes beforehand. The difficulty lies both in encouraging patients, families, and physicians to engage in such a planning process and in translating plans into the desired care.

Most clinical trials have shown that educational interventions can help increase the number of patients who prepare advance directives. The most successful interventions involve the use of teaching materials along with repeated discussions with a physician, patient advocate, or social worker. The Patient Self-Determination Act requires that healthcare organizations notify patients, as they are being hospitalized, about their right to have an advance directive. Many experts, however, believe that it is preferable to ask patients about their wishes for end-of-life care at a less stressful time, such as a routine clinic visit.

Talking with the patient should not be an abrupt process. Talking about dying is a scary topic for most people. An experienced clinician is likely to begin by explaining the process in a nonthreatening way. The patient is likely to be appreciative and willing to talk if the clinician explains that the purpose of the discussion is to find out, in advance, how that patient would want to be treated if he or she becomes critically ill and is unable to communicate his or her wishes.

The discussion might begin by asking the patient about prior encounters with terminal illness among family members and about her assessment of how those illnesses were handled. The discussion may include a review of the things that have mattered to her in her life history and how these things might shape the end of her life. How much does it matter to her whether the end of her life occurs at home or in the hospital? Does it matter most that she live as long as possible or that she live only so long as she maintains a certain quality of life? Is she inclined to try aggressive life-saving treatments or is she more inclined to let go at the end of life and avoid such treatments? This approach to end-of-life discussions permits the patient to do much of the talking. The interaction provides a chance to focus on psychosocial and lifestyle issues and allows the patient and clinician to develop a context within which to build a partnership in planning for end-of-life care. Despite the serious nature of the discussion and the focus on the patient's underlying values, a clinical interaction of this nature can usually be accomplished within approximately 15 minutes.

At the end of this discussion, the patient and physician are likely to have a shared understanding of the kind of care that would be in keeping with the patient's treatment preferences at the end of life. A useful written document will convey the patient's attitudes about the importance of quality of life and her inclinations about prolonging life through the use of life-sustaining treatments. Whether or not the patient is willing to sign a living will, it is easy to obtain the appropriate documents for every state in the United States by searching the website www.partnershipforcaring.org. If the patient does not want to sign an advance directive giving directions for care, she should be encouraged to prepare an advance directive assigning durable power of attorney for health care to the person of her choice. If the patient does not want to prepare a document, it is useful for the clinician to write a note in the medical record conveying the essence of the discussion. Such a note would suffice as convincing evidence of the patient's preferences at some future time if or when such evidence is needed.

It can be useful to tailor advance care discussions to the various stages in a patient's life. For instance, the healthy patient should be advised to assign durable power of attorney, discuss possible emergencies, and discuss preferences with a chosen surrogate and to document these preferences. In contrast, a person who is much older would be encouraged to locate advance directive documents if they have already been prepared, discuss and record preferences for care if not already documented, discuss hopes for the last stage of life, and make specific plans for complications or urgent situations.

The type of discussion described here is intended to overcome many of the barriers to considering end-of-life preferences and preparing advance directives. Other obstacles in advance care planning relate to the translation of a patient's expressed wishes into practice. If the patient prepares a written advance directive, it may be unavailable when it is needed. To address this problem, it is important to encourage the patient to prepare several copies of the advance directive and to give copies to her clinician and family members as well as keeping a copy in her own personal records. If the patient assigns durable power of attorney to someone, it is important to encourage her to discuss her treatment preferences with that individual and to seek agreement among her family members and significant others about the types of care she would want. We know that too often conversations of this nature do not occur, resulting in lack of knowledge and potential for conflict among patients' families and friends. It is also useful to ask patients how strictly they want their directive to be followed, because it is known that patients vary in this regard. Many patients want their chosen surrogates or family members to use their best judgment, informed by previously stated preferences.

While advance directives can be very helpful in providing clues about the patient's preferences and guiding the direction of care, each document needs to be interpreted in light of the actual circumstances of the patient's illness, which cannot be entirely anticipated beforehand. The clinician and family will need to negotiate the plan of care in ways that cannot be fully anticipated by any advance directive. Patients should be made aware that their wishes are less likely to be followed if their wishes are too restrictive to allow care that the family or care provider believe is warranted. At the opposite extreme, wishes are less likely to be followed when the care requested in a directive does not seem to the family or provider to have any chance of being beneficial.

Physicians can do several things to improve the likelihood that advance directives will effectively guide care at the end of life. These include encouraging patients to be sure that there are multiple copies of advance directives and that all relevant parties have copies; encouraging patients to carry on a conversation with their families about their preferences along with preparing a written document; and reviewing patients' preferences with them on occasions of significant changes in health status. Clinicians should ensure that a patient's advance directives and preferences for care are retained in a prominent part of the medical record and that copies are distributed to relevant specialists involved in the patient's care. Clinicians can also help by fostering a commitment in the hospitals and health systems in which they practice to maintain, retrieve, and honor advance directives.

The present patient is unusual in taking the initiative to discuss end-of-life care with her physician. In this talk, it proved useful to begin by letting her talk about her husband's death and then help her formulate her wishes for care at the time of her own eventual advanced illness and impending death. The physician pointed out that events in her life will not necessarily be like those in her husband's or other relatives' lives. Because the present patient has chronic obstructive pulmonary disease, some of the discussion focused on likely scenarios for her, particularly respiratory insufficiency. The physician asked whether she would want to be put on a ventilator either for a brief, potentially reversible episode of acute illness, such as pneumonia, or more permanently for end-stage lung disease. While talking about such specific treatments, the physician emphasized the patient's overall goals, explaining that these would guide her care if situations occurred that could not be anticipated precisely.

Aside from thinking about specific instructions for her future care, this patient should also consider a person to whom she would assign durable power of attorney for healthcare. She expressed concern that her daughter who lives close by may not be the most capable of making decisions or may not make decisions that are the most consonant with the patient's wishes. She nevertheless decided to ask this daughter to become her power of attorney. However, in order to avoid any discord among her children, she specified in writing and in subsequent conversation with her family that she wished for all her children to consult each other before making any decisions about care and to support one another in whatever decisions they ultimately made.

Clinical Pearls

1. Advance care planning should be considered an ongoing process and should not focus exclusively on preparation of a written document, because the paper itself is not likely to increase the likelihood that care will be consistent with the patients wishes.

2. Advance care planning is an effort to respect patient wishes, and to the extent possible, the planning process itself should be respectful of the patient. Patients can be approached in a manner that suits them and is respectful of their own personal style. Patients who prefer not to explicitly discuss their end-of-life care should have their wishes respected. Patients unwilling to talk about their death may be willing to designate someone who can make decisions on their behalf and to whom clinicians can direct questions.

3. Advance care planning can serve as a guide for care at the end of life, but because factors other than patient autonomy also comprise optimal patient care, treatment in life-threatening situations cannot be expected to always conform precisely with previously expressed wishes.

REFERENCES

1. Uhlmann R, Pearlman R, Cain K: Physicians' and spouses predictions of elderly patients' resuscitation preferences. J Am Geriatric Soc 1988;43:M115-M121.
2. Danis M, Southerland L, Garrett J, et al: A prospective study of advance directives for life-sustaining care. N Engl J Med 1991;324:882–888.
3. Sehgal A, Galbraith A, Chesney M, et al: How strictly do dialysis patients want their advance directives followed? JAMA 1992;267:59–63.
4. Danis M: Following advance directives. Hastings Cent Rep 1994;24:S21-S23.
5. Emanuel L, Danis M, Pearlman R, Singer P. Advance care planning as a process: structuring the discussion in practice. J Am Geriatric Soc 1995;43:440–446.4.
6. Field, MJ, Cassel CK (eds): Approaching Death: Improving Care at the End of Life. Washington, DC, Institute of Medicine, National Academy Press, 1997.
7. Hanson L, Tulsky J, Danis M: Can clinical interventions change care at the end of life? Ann Intern Med 1997;126:381–388.
8. Danis M, Federman D, Fins J, et al: Incorporating palliative care into critical care education: principles, challenges, and opportunities. Crit Care Med 1999;27:2005–2013.
9. Roter D, Larson S, Fischer G, et al: Experts practice what they preach: a descriptive study of best and normative practices on end-of-life discussions. Arch Intern Med 2000;160:3477–3485.

Molly Osborne, MD, PhD
Linda Ganzini, MD

PATIENT 10

A 74-year-old man with non-small cell carcinoma who requests physician-assisted suicide

A 74-year-old man from Oregon with non-small cell carcinoma of the lung returns to clinic with ongoing pain. His carcinoma was diagnosed several months ago and is stage IIIb (T4 N2 M0 with vertebral invasion). He has received both chemotherapy and radiotherapy. He has moderate pain but continues to decline higher morphine dosages because he does not like the sedation and effect on his thinking. The physician explains that considering the poor response, the patient probably will not benefit from further chemotherapy. The physician wants to focus in improving his patient's symptoms and comfort. The patient had actively worked his ranch until the recent diagnosis of his lung cancer.

The patient responds somewhat irritably, "Doc, stop beating around the bush. You're telling me I am going to die. If you cannot help me any more, then let's talk about this physician-assisted suicide pill. My wife died from cancer, and I would not let a dog suffer as much as they let her suffer. I have been talking to my sons about this and they agree."

Question: How does the physician assess this patient?

Diagnosis: Nonresectable non-small cell carcinoma of the lung with likely survival less than 6 months.

Discussion: In 1997, a physician-assisted suicide law, the Death with Dignity Act, was enacted in Oregon. The law allows a physician to prescribe a lethal medication for a terminally ill patient. Several requirements meant to constitute procedural "safeguards" restrict this option to those who meet the following criteria: The patient must have an illness that is expected to lead to death within 6 months, as confirmed by both the patient's physician and a second physician consultant. The patient must make two oral and one written request over 15 days, and must be informed of alternatives including hospice care.

All lethal medications prescribed under the Death with Dignity Act are reported to the Oregon Health Division, which has published interviews with prescribing physicians between 1998 and 2000. Assisted suicide accounted for 9 in 10,000 deaths in Oregon in 1999 and 2000, which represents approximately 40 in 10,000 cancer deaths in the state. Although no state other than Oregon has legalized physician-assisted suicide, studies suggest this practice exists elsewhere but is rarely invoked.

Patients who request assisted suicide under legalized conditions often have negative expectations and even dread about the dying process, difficulty tolerating the thought of others taking care of them, difficulty finding meaning and opportunity in the remaining weeks of life, and a strong desire to remain in control. Physicians faced with a request for assisted suicide should clarify whether the request fits with the patient's values, assess the patient for depressive or other psychiatric disorders, explore and correct misperceptions about the dying process, improve symptom management, and refer the patient to hospice. It is fundamentally important that patients who are considering assisted suicide understand all of their options. Some Oregon physicians recommend voluntary refusal of food and fluids as an alternative to assisted suicide.

The Oregon Death with Dignity Act is explicit in regard to the process of physician-assisted suicide. Euthanasia administered by others and lethal injections are not allowed under the Oregon law. Patients who cannot swallow or otherwise self-administer a medication may not be eligible under the law. Whether in Oregon or elsewhere, patients must be assured that they can receive medications to treat pain, even if the necessary dosages of medications for pain relief have an unintended consequence of hastening death (the principle of double effect).

Pain and other distressing symptoms related to the terminal stages of disease are rarely the only reasons patients request assisted suicide. Pain and suffering, however, present potentially treatable conditions that often promote a patient's desire to hasten death. Patients who request assisted suicide usually value control and independence and do not easily accept treatments that impair cognition. Many sources of pain at the end of life, such as bone metastases and neuropathic pain, have specific medical therapies and may only partially respond to opioids. Physicians need to have a clear understanding of palliative care to assist patients who are making decisions about physician-assisted suicide.

It is important to determine whether or not a patient is depressed before decisions about physician-assisted suicide are made. Studies in cancer and palliative care populations demonstrate that the prevalence of depressive disorders is increased in surveyed patients who endorse an interest in hastened death, assisted suicide, or euthanasia. In one study of patients with advanced cancer, a single question—"Are you depressed"—has been shown to identify most patients with major depressive disorders. Hopelessness, a pervasive negative expectation of the future, may have a stronger relationship to desire for death in dying patients than other components of depression. Hopelessness may exist to a profound degree even in the absence of depression.

Previous observations of "bad" deaths frequently influence a patient's views of his or her own terminal illness and dying. Patients requesting assisted suicide tend to focus intensely on and to carefully plan for the future. Unlike most ill people, they tend to carefully plan for the future. Structured advance care planning can help such patients share the burdens of planning for their deaths. For example, a patient can be approached by saying, "Today, we are going to talk about your options and concerns, including those related to assisted suicide. I know that you think about this a lot. I hope that if we review this today, you will feel settled and freer to attend to other things in your planning and in your life."

Patients requesting assisted suicide often perceive their care as a burden to others' even though their family members may wish to participate in their care and find personal meaning in assisting their loved ones face the final stages of life. Patients requesting assisted suicide, however, often see nothing meaningful in the dying process and tend to hold their views strongly. Consequently, they may have difficulty appreciating the different perspectives and needs of their family. Family meetings and the assistance of a social worker may help patients better understand and appreciate their family's desires to provide care. Through this understanding, dying patients may offer important opportunities for family members to participate in care in ways that will comfort them after the patient's death.

Hospice referral is an effective intervention for patients requesting assisted suicide. In a study of requesting patients in Oregon, 46% of patients who received palliative interventions changed their mind about assisted suicide, as compared with 15% of those for whom no palliative interventions were provided. Among different types of palliative care, hospice referral and social work referral were the most effective interventions. Patients requesting assisted suicide may decline hospice if they perceive it as diminishing their autonomy. It is often helpful to point out that patients often feel more in control after they are enrolled in hospice.

The present patient was referred to hospice and accepted. Nonsteroidal anti-inflammatory agents and bisphosphonates were begun and proved to be effective adjuncts to opioids in managing his bone pain. The hospice social worker met with the patient and his sons. He expressed his greatest fears were being a burden and the embarrassment at the intimate physical care he required. His family responded poignantly that they supported his decision to end his life, but said forcefully that they would prefer to care for him at home until he died naturally. His physician agreed to remain open to considering the patient's request for assistance in suicide, either directly or through a referral to another physician.

After several meetings, the patient was able to hear that his family wanted to care for him. With improved pain control, he was able to outline and pursue a set of goals for his remaining weeks. The physician discussed with the patient his fears of a bad death based on his experiences with his wife's terminal illness. The physician outlined a variety of interventions that addressed these fears. The patient withdrew his request for assisted suicide and died at home several weeks later.

Clinical Pearls

1. Physician-assisted suicide is legal in Oregon, but not in any other state.

2. When a patient requests physician-assisted suicide, it is essential to identify any negative expectations about the future, especially a concern about a loss of control, that the patient may harbor.

3. Hopelessness is an important component of depression that causes people to seek an early death.

4. Hospice referral is an effective intervention for patients requesting physician-assisted suicide.

5. A single question, "Are you depressed," is a sensitive screen for depression in terminally ill patients.

6. Patients and their physicians may have a poor understanding of the options available for assisting patients with end-of-life care. These options include treatment for pain, hospice referral, advance care planning, and spiritual support.

REFERENCES

1. Back AL, Wallace JI, Starks HE, Pearlman RA. Physician-assisted suicide and euthanasia in Washington State: patient requests and physician responses. JAMA 1996; 275:919–25.
2. Chochinov HM, Wilson KG, Enns M, Lander S. 'Are you depressed?': screening for depression in the terminally ill. Am J Psychiatry 1997; 154:674–6.
3. Chochinov HMM, Wilson KG, Enns M, Lander S. Depression, hopelessness, and suicidal ideation in the terminally ill. Psychosomatics 1998; 39:366–70.
4. Meier DE, Emmons C-A, Wallenstein S, et al. A national survey of physician-assisted suicide and euthanasia in the United States. N Engl J Med 1998; 338:1193–201.
5. Ganzini L, Nelson HHD, Schmidt T, et al. Physicians' experiences with the Oregon Death with Dignity Act. N Engl J Med 2000; 342:557–63.
6. Silviera MJ, DiPiero A, Gerrity MS, Feudtner C. Patients' knowledge of options at the end of life: ignorance in the face of death. JAMA 2000; 284:2483–8.
7. Sullivan AD, Hedberg K, Fleming DW. Legalized physician-suicide in Oregon—the second year. N Engl J Med 2000; 342:598–604.
8. Sullivan AD, Hedberg K, Hopkins D. Legalized physician-assisted suicide in Oregon, 1998–2000. N Engl J Med 2001; 344:605–7.

Perry G. Fine, MD

PATIENT 11

A 34-year-old woman with end-stage adenocarcinoma of the cervix with intractable neuropathic pain

A 34-year-old woman with Stage IVB adenocarcinoma of the cervix is experiencing excruciating pain in her low back, pelvis, and lower extremities. Recent attempts at palliation with combined chemoradiotherapy have not diminished her pain symptoms. She is bed-ridden, cachectic, and completely dependent on professional and family caregivers. She is receiving hospice care at home. She is still able to enjoy small soft-substance meals such as milkshakes. Spending time with her two children, ages 13 and 15, is what she values above all. The patient does not want to have her husband or children see her suffer, and she prefers, if at all possible, to stay at home through the time of her death. She has ureteral stents for urinary drainage, a diversion colostomy, and a right subclavian Hickman catheter that has been left in place, post-chemotherapy, for administration of intravenous medications.

Her pain is described as both deep and aching in the pelvis and low back areas (rated as 5–6/10) and burning in the perineum, radiating posteriorly down her legs to the soles of her feet (rated as 8/10). She has allodynia (pain to light touch), making bedclothes very uncomfortable. Pain is continuous, with breakthrough episodes of incident pain related to movement associated with basic care. She occasionally experiences spontaneous, brief episodes of jolting, electric-like sensations through both legs (rated as "12" on a 10-point scale).

Pain management has consisted of multiple opioid trials (opioid rotation with morphine, fentanyl, oxycodone, and methadone) with nonopioid analgesics and adjunctive medications, including nonsteroidal anti-inflammatory drugs, tricyclic antidepressants, benzodiazepines, corticosteroids, and antiepileptics. Her current opioid regimen includes hydromorphone via a patient-controlled analgesia pump that delivers a continuous infusion (10 mg/hr) and allows bolus dosing for breakthrough pain. Additionally, she is taking gabapentin, 900 mg three times a day, and low-dose desipramine at night for pain and to help with sleep. Attempts at increasing her opioid and non-opioid pain-modulating drugs have led to significant mental clouding, dysphoria, and myoclonus which have been intolerable.

Question: What other forms of pain therapy are possible?

Diagnosis: Severe nociceptive and neuropathic pain due to lumbosacral tumor infiltration, typical of metastatic adenocarcinoma of the cervix.

Discussion: Severe neuropathic pain is common with far-advanced cervical cancer due to soft tissue and neural infiltration, especially of the lumbosacral nerves. Palliative radiotherapy can be helpful in combination with corticosteroids, opioids, and other pain modulating (adjunctive) drugs such as tricyclic antidepressants and antiepileptic drugs. However, there remain patients, especially those with severe neuropathic pain, for whom dose-limiting side effects preclude adequate symptom relief with the standard "stepladder" approach to treatment. Either pain relief proves to be insufficient with conventional drug therapies, or sedation (or other undesirable psychological effects) interferes with the patients' expressed goals of comfort with cognizance.

With this in mind, a thorough assessment of pain etiologies and psychosocial issues is critical in order to direct therapies appropriately. It is not uncommon that emotional stressors contribute significantly to the pain experience. Supportive therapies for both the patient and family should be applied to minimize these factors.

Neuropathic pain symptoms as demonstrated by the present patient are pathognomonic of lumbosacral plexus infiltration by tumor, characterized by burning pain, allodynia, and paroxysms of excruciating "shock-like" sensations in the distribution of these nerves. Additional examination findings might include dermatomal sensory loss, decreased motor strength with atrophy, hypoactive reflexes, and a cold, clammy, discolored lower extremity due to sympathetic overactivity. Conversely, a hot lower extremity might signal sympathetic deafferentation.

When trials of titrated opioid rotation and supplementation with pain-modulating drugs fail to provide adequate symptom relief, other approaches are indicated. Potent analgesic-anesthetic drugs, such as ketamine and propofol, can reliably relieve otherwise intractable pain. Ketamine has potent analgesic qualities at subanesthetic doses, coupled with a potential to greatly enhance opioid efficacy, secondary to N-methyl-D-aspartate receptor-binding properties. Subanesthetic doses of ketamine have been shown to obviate severe neuropathic pain, while maintaining patient awareness and communicative capacity, especially in the face of exigent opioid analgesia. Ketamine is relatively easy to titrate in the home environment, especially when there is intravenous access. There is very little risk of respiratory compromise or hemodynamic instability. Patients must be told that they might experience a sense of "dreaminess." When using anything more than ultra-low-dose ketamine (5–10 mg/hr), concomitant administration of a benzodiazepine (e.g., diazepam 5 mg q 6h) as a maintenance dose may be necessary to mitigate potentially distressing psychomimetic effects of ketamine, including hallucinations and nightmares. Similarly, an anticholinergic drug, such as scopolamine or glycopyrrolate, may be necessary to prevent excessive salivation.

Before using a drug that might cloud the sensorium (unless sedation is explicitly desired by the patient), regional analgesia-anesthesia approaches that do not have supraspinal CNS effects should be considered and discussed with patients. Continuous epidural or intrathecal delivery of pain-relieving drugs (opioids, clonidine, local anesthetics) via a tunneled catheter can be a useful approach to mitigate symptoms of lumbosacral plexopathy. For patients with bladder catheters and colostomies, regional analgesia is unlikely to induce fecal or urinary retention. When patients are likely to have several weeks of remaining life, epidural and intrathecal catheters to enhance symptom relief may promote the patients' functional status and improve quality of life. Such care supports the wishes of patients who choose to extend life maximally while maintaining intact cognition.

When patients appear likely to survive beyond a few days or weeks, intrathecal catheters are preferred because they remain in place and retain function longer than epidural catheters. Mechanical complications (e.g., displacement, leaking) and infection are the greatest risks of this intervention, but the therapeutic benefits generally outweigh these potential pitfalls. Optimally, placement of a spinal catheter system is performed in an operating room setting, allowing for the provision of maximal patient comfort, radiographic confirmation, and aseptic technique to minimize the risk of infection. In certain cases, where the patient has a very short prognosis and transport to such a facility is excessively burdensome, a neuraxial catheter can be implanted by a skilled anesthesiologist, with the patient at home. When implanted at home, prophylactic antibiotics should be given at the time of catheter placement and for several days thereafter, because cellulitis or a deep-space infection (epidural abscess, meningitis) may prevent effective analgesia and, in and of itself, can greatly add to the patient's overall symptom burden.

In the present case, the patient and her husband considered the pros and cons of an intrathecal catheter for pain relief. Despite the potential benefits of regional, spinal anesthesia, they decided to avoid even this relatively minor surgical procedure. They both agreed that they preferred interventions for pain relief that did not require placement of catheters, even if these interventions diminished her cognitive acuity.

After a discussion with their physician, ketamine was chosen for pain relief. A test dose of ketamine, 5 mg (0.1 mg/kg), was given intravenously. After about 5 minutes, the patient appeared to relax her tensed, guarding posture and stated that she felt very calm, with minimal pain. She preferred to rest with her eyes closed, but she was able to interact in a cogent manner with her family members. Most important to her and them, they were able to sit closely by her without fear of increasing her pain.

The nurse in attendance was able to provide a soothing sponge bath without causing additional pain.

This dose lasted approximately 30 minutes. Therefore, an intravenous infusion of ketamine, 10 mg/hr, was begun after a re-bolus of 5 mg. No change was made in the opioid infusion dose because the patient's level of comfort and wakefulness were deemed by her to be adequate. Several days later, she lost interest in eating and began sleeping most of the time. When it became difficult to arouse her, at the suggestion of the hospice nurse, the family gathered to say goodbye. Ten days after initiation of ketamine therapy, the patient died. Bereavement counseling was continued over the following several months.

Clinical Pearls

1. Comprehensive pain assessment and management are medical and ethical imperatives in the overall care of patients, especially those with far-advanced disease and debilitating pain.

2. A certain percentage of patients develop pain that is intractable to basic approaches, such as those recommended by the World Health Organization.

3. The role of interventional pain management techniques, including regional and neuroaxial anesthesia and the use of drugs such as ketamine or propofol, must be well understood and considered in the care of patients with pain otherwise intractable to conventional approaches.

4. Hospice and palliative care programs must educate their staff members in the indications and management of these advanced techniques. Relationships with interested, capable consultants should be established and maintained for times when these techniques are indicated.

REFERENCES

1. Fine PG: Advances in cancer pain management. In Lake C, Rice LJ, Sperry R (eds): Advances in Anesthesia. St. Louis, Mosby-Year Book, 1995.
2. Fine PG: Low-dose ketamine in the management of opioid resistant terminal cancer pain. J Pain Symptom Manage 1999;17:296–300.
3. Berger JM, Ryan A, Vadivelu N, et al: Ketamine-fentanyl-midazolam infusion for the control of symptoms in terminal life care. Am J Hosp Palliat Care 2000;17:127–132.
4. Ready BL: Regional analgesia with intraspinal opioids. In Loeser JD (ed): Bonica's Management of Pain, 2nd ed. Philadelphia, Lippincott/Williams & Wilkins, 2001, pp 1953–1966.

Chaplain Ralph Ciampa
Chaplain Kava Schafer

PATIENT 12

A 62-year-old woman with a second cancer who has abandoned a belief in God

A 62-year-old woman is admitted for a clinical evaluation of abdominal pain, which confirms the presence of widely metastatic ovarian cancer. She had been treated for breast cancer 3 years ago with a mastectomy and chemotherapy. The patient had returned to work as a schoolteacher until 2 months ago, when diffuse symptoms forced her to take sick time. Although she had been relatively attentive to monitoring her medical condition during her remission from breast cancer, she delayed seeking medical care at the appearance of her abdominal pain.

The patient is estranged from her two adult children, who live out of state. She had raised them as a single mother since her divorce when they were in elementary school. Her mother had died of breast cancer when the patient was 8 years old. Although several of her ancestors and extended family were ministers, the patient had rejected religious belief in reaction to her mother's untimely death. She informs a chaplain during her present admission that she does not "believe in any God who takes away the mothers of young children." She states that she has been battling cancer for 4 years but says, "I don't expect to make it this time."

The patient is well kempt but appears to the medical staff to be depressed and to have lost all hope. Several friends who visit seem surprised and troubled by her lack of verbal responsiveness and emotional withdrawal.

Question: How might the attitudes, moods, and behaviors of this patient be explored to reach the root cause of her discomfort?

Diagnosis: Unmet spiritual needs in a patient with metastatic cancer who is experiencing "psychic pain."

Discussion: At the end of life, many of the questions with which patients want and need to be engaged are spiritual in nature. If the patient has no forum or permission to engage these questions, they often manifest emotional or spiritual distress. If left unaddressed, spiritual suffering may complicate the dying process. Whether or not a person has a religion or believes in a god, every human being possesses a spiritual dimension. One is in the realm of the spiritual when questions of meaning and purpose arise, especially in the context of a relationship with "something greater than" the individually lived life. Human beings express that dimension in a variety of ways. Some people express this dimension in overt religious practices emerging from religious beliefs and value systems rooted in a faith community. Other people relate to the transcendent through a relationship with nature or art, for example.

In the course of his or her life, often a patient has collected valuable spiritual resources on which to draw for comfort and guidance. An attentive caregiver might seek means to enable the patient to "engage and enhance" the wisdom to be found in those personal and collective spiritual resources. Spiritual interventions may take a variety of forms, but each rests on the intention of empowering the patient to connect with the healing sources that are significant for that individual. In providing a nonjudgmental, compassionate presence, caregivers can create a safe space for the patient to explore the strength and flexibility of his or her spiritual (including religious) beliefs and value system and, in this manner, support spiritual healing at the end of life.

Not infrequently, a chasm may open up between a patient's experience of intense emotions during the dying process and a set of personal cherished beliefs and values. Spiritual distress may occur when one's belief and value system do not possess the flexibility to encompass and engage questions of meaning and purpose or when a patient has unresolved past or present conflicts. Untreated psychic pain, or soul suffering, may be comparable in intensity with poorly managed physiological pain and may complicate the beneficial effects of pain medication. The medical team may do their utmost to preserve the bodily comfort of a patient, but a patient may still suffer if there is unfinished life-business awaiting resolution. A patient may seek reconciliation from estranged family or friends, or a patient may experience intense guilt over a past action for which absolution in the religious sense or forgiveness in

a secular sense was never obtained. Unresolved guilt is corrosive and at the end of life can exert a poisonous power to rob people of a sense of peace. A further complicating factor may arise if the patient has become alienated from a faith tradition and feels thwarted in any effort to pursue forgiveness from God because of the estrangement. A nonjudgmental, accepting pastoral care presence may encourage the patient to move through the religious gridlock and approach his or her God directly. An inability to forgive one's self might also be at the heart of the distress.

A pastoral caregiver gives spiritual permission to the patient to engage these discrepancies and provides comfort by normalizing the extreme feelings that death and dying evoke. Anger towards God is a frequent response to the powerful emotions triggered by news of a terminal diagnosis. A helpful spiritual intervention might involve an implicit reframing of values and concepts that had different meanings when cure was possible. For instance, "hope" for a cure may need to be replaced with "hope" for a broader understanding of healing, which may include comfort, peace, reconciliation with family and friends, hope to be remembered in a loving way, or hope for a peaceful death. Or, if suffering and hopelessness obscure the meaning of a patient's existence, a caregiver may intervene spiritually by expressing the willingness to accompany a patient during a life-review process. Through attentive listening, the scope and depth of the patient's life may gain new perspective when viewed against the ground of impending death.

Further exploration of a patient's unmet spiritual needs may uncover the need for explicit sacramental or religious rituals. Even for people who have rejected religion, the faith tradition in which they were raised may acquire new relevance and vital importance as they approach life's end. Often, a patient's faith tradition may yield the nourishment required for the journey into the unknown; it is the task of a pastoral care provider to facilitate connection with the community. If there is no communal framework, then the creation of new rituals or new practices may foster felt connection to a sense of wholeness.

The present patient's situation was analyzed with these concepts and assumptions about spiritual needs. Severe early loss seems to have caused alienation of this patient from the religious community and their beliefs and practices that failed to help her cope with such loss. Although she may have found some implicit spiritual grounding in life, contributing to a meaningful adult life, she remained alienated from an explicit coherent sense of relationship to transcendent realities. A persistent spiritual tension may have contributed to the alienation in important relationships with her adult children and to the current withdrawal from her friends.

Although health care providers of many disciplines can effectively respond to spiritual needs, in this patient a nonjudgmental chaplain provided her the opportunity to revisit the experience of loss and related alienation, which brought her significant resolution and comfort. The patient reviewed her early loss in light of a lifetime of experience and discovered a less rigid religious perspective than was originally available to her. She was assisted in her desire to reconcile with her children and to resolve long-standing guilt and hurt arising out of the past alienation from her children. The patient showed interest in the spiritual world-view of the chaplain and became progressively appreciative of prayer offered by the chaplain.

When the patient was discharged to home hospice care, she expressed interest in the congregation to which the chaplain belonged and asked if the chaplain could participate in her funeral. A sense of peace had begun to replace psychic and spiritual pain.

Clinical Pearls

1. Spiritual needs may or may not be reflected in traditional religious language.

2. Central to spiritual needs are questions of relationships, often touching on both human and transcendent dimensions, and often involving unresolved loss and grief of a lifetime.

3. Interventions that invite full sharing of a wide range of strong feelings in a nonjudgmental atmosphere often contribute to a sense of relatedness and peace in the process of dying.

4. Specific religious rituals or practices may be a powerful means for patients to engage and enhance their spiritual resources.

5. Attention to families, in both traditional and nontraditional configurations, may be an important context and component of good spiritual care at end of life.

REFERENCES

1, Pruyser PW. The Minister as Diagnostician. Philadelphia: Westminster Press; 1976.
2. Oates WE. Pastoral Care and Counseling in Grief and Separation. Philadelphia: Fortress Press; 1980.
3. Holst LE. Hospital Ministry: The Role of the Chaplain Today. New York: Crossroad; 1987.
4. Doka KJ, Morgan JD. Death and Spirituality. Amityville, NY: Baywood Publishing Co.; 1993.
5. Rantz MJ, LeMone P (eds). Classification of Nursing Diagnoses: Proceedings of the Eleventh Conference. Glendale, CA: CINAHL Information Systems; 1995: pp 112, 115–24, 136–149.
6. Meyer C. Surviving Death: A Practical Guide to Caring for the Dying and Bereaved, 2nd ed. Mystic, CT: Twenty-Third Publications; 1997.
7. Ehman JW, Ott BB, Short TH, et al. Do patients want physicians to inquire about their spiritual or religious beliefs if they become gravely ill? Arch Intern Med 1999;159:1803–6.
8. Ahlskog G, Sands H (eds). The Guide to Pastoral Care and Counseling. Madison, CT: Psychosocial Press; 2000.
9. Friedman DA (ed). Jewish Pastoral Care [Hatlavut Ruhanit]: A Practical Handbook from Traditional and Contemporary Sources. Woodstock, VT: Jewish Lights Publishing; 2001.

Margaret L. Campbell, RN, MSN, FAAN

PATIENT 13

An 82-year-old woman is dying in the ICU and the team does not know how to withdraw curative care for her

An 82-year-old woman is admitted to the medical ICU with an acute exacerbation of COPD requiring intubation and mechanical ventilation. In the past year, she has been hospitalized three times, and on the most recent two admissions, she required mechanical ventilation. At baseline, she is alert and able to take care of herself at home. She uses nasal oxygen continuously but becomes dyspneic with minimal physical exertion. Her adult children do her shopping, laundry, and housekeeping.

The patient is stabilized with conventional treatment, and a protocol for weaning from mechanical ventilation is initiated on the second hospital day. On the third day, she becomes less responsive, with left-sided hemiplegia and facial asymmetry. The CT scan reveals a right middle cerebral artery infarction. Over the next 2 days she becomes comatose, and a second CT scan shows cerebral edema and midline shift. Her children, when apprised of the complications, disclose the patient's previously stated preferences for no aggressive life-prolonging treatment if she were unconscious or terminally ill. The children expect the ICU team to stop the aggressive treatment and keep their mother comfortable. None of the ICU staff had ever participated in withdrawal of treatment and were uncomfortable about changing the treatment goals to "comfort measures only." Some members of the team were frustrated by their limitations in this area.

Question: Would a palliative care consultant be useful to the ICU team?

Diagnosis: A terminal, elderly patient who would benefit from a palliative care consultation.

Discussion: Gaps between what patients and their families expect at the end of life and what clinicians are prepared to provide persist in many hospitals despite growing knowledge in this area of care. Clinicians who have never been taught about end-of-life care will provide the treatment that they are more familiar with, i.e., curative and life-prolonging measures. Discomfort with treatment withdrawal and fears about patient discomfort if palliation is not optimized may contribute to avoidance of these patient circumstances. Additionally, clinicians may have misconceptions about the legal and ethical standards that ground end-of-life care. All of these factors contribute to overtreatment of dying patients, especially in the ICU. These factors result in prolonged hospital and ICU lengths of stay, wasteful consumption of nonbeneficial, expensive, or scarce resources, and unnecessary patient and family suffering. Until all clinicians have sufficient educational preparation, knowledge, and comfort with delivering optimal end-of-life care, a palliative care consultant will bridge the gap.

An ideal inpatient palliative care consultant provides many services. Components of care include identification or validation of the patient's poor prognosis, facilitation of communication of the prognosis and treatment options to the patient or surrogate, advice about palliative care treatment options, assistance with implementation of the palliative care treatment plan, advice about hospice options in the community if discharge is possible, and education of hospital staff, residents, and students.

Clinicians must stay abreast of rapidly changing information that comprises the knowledge base for their area of practice. A palliative care consultant will provide the primary physician or physician-resident team with prognosis information and predictors of mortality about which the clinician may not otherwise be aware. Concerns about the reliability of the patient's prognosis can be reduced or validated by the consultant.

Communicating a terminal prognosis to the patient or family is one of the most difficult tasks for any clinician. Inadequate communication contributes to delays in making relevant care decisions, protracted aggressive treatment, and patient and family dissatisfaction. Patients or their surrogates are able to make good decisions about treatment when they are given comprehensive, comprehensible, honest information in a compassionate manner. The palliative care consultant is able to conduct this type of discussion and model the desirable communication behaviors for the inexperienced residents.

The palliative care consultant is an expert in the treatment of symptoms and the development of a treatment plan that reduces superfluous, nonbeneficial interventions. A number of standing interventions are common in hospital and ICU care, which may not be indicated in the care of a patient who is expected to die. The palliative care consultant is able to assist the primary team with their identification and elimination from the treatment plan. When treatment goals change from an aggressive, life-prolonging focus to a focus on palliation, a reduction of more than 50% should be evident in the use of hospital resources, such as diagnostic tests and procedures, prophylactic medications, invasive lines and catheters, and other nonbeneficial interventions. Advice about symptom management and processes for the withdrawal of life-sustaining therapies can also be expected from the palliative care consultant.

The residents caring for the present patient needed assistance with the withdrawal of life support and management of the patient's comfort. The consultant may offer advice or provide bedside support in the implementation of the treatment plan by demonstrating withdrawal procedures. This allows the consultant to teach the residents about the process, while providing the service to the patient and attendant family.

After the withdrawal of life supports, a few patients can be discharged from the ICU and, if death is not imminent, even sent home. The palliative care consultant provides advice about the likely interval before death and options for patient discharge.

The palliative care consultant can provide continuing education offerings or standing lectures in the residency curriculum. Maintaining a relationship with the hospital ethics committee ensures knowledgeable consultation that is consistent with institutional policy, ethical and legal standards, and state and federal statutes. Additionally, the palliative care consultant can participate in or conduct clinical research, facilitate institutional process improvement, and measure and report outcomes.

The palliative care consultant in this case reviewed the patient's record with the residents and conducted a directed exam of the patient. Together, the consultant and resident met with the patient's family. The consultant told the family that the magnitude of the stroke and brain swelling, combined with the patient's underlying end-stage lung disease, meant that the patient was terminally ill with almost no chance of regaining functional consciousness. The plan of care and orders were discussed again and found to be consistent with the patient's preferences and prognosis. Withdrawal of life-sustaining therapy was discussed, and a decision was made to postpone withdrawal until later in the day when the patient's extended family members could be present. Preferences about being at the bedside, spiritual support, or other family-specific rituals were determined.

After prayers at the bedside presided over by the hospital chaplain, some of the family retired to a private waiting area near the ICU. The consultant explained the process about withdrawal of ventilation and other nonbeneficial life supports to the family and the residents who were observing. This patient had no signs of distress before, during, or after the removal of life supports. She remained unconscious and died 2 hours after the withdrawal, with her children at her bedside. Signs of imminent death precluded discharge from the ICU, and all attempts were made by the ICU staff to provide a quiet, private, unrestricted environment for the family. The family expressed their satisfaction and gratitude to the ICU staff before departing from the hospital after the patient's death.

The residents and nursing staff caring for the present patient had a debriefing session with the consultant the next day to discuss the case and its outcome. Plans were made for continuing education topics and readings for the team. All parties involved were satisfied, and the residents expected to be more comfortable the next time a terminal care case occurred.

Clinical Pearls

1. An inpatient palliative care consultant can facilitate optimal end-of-life care in the hospital when hospital staff are not knowledgeable or comfortable with this type of care.

2. An ideal consultant provides advice and mentoring about prognosis determination, communication, symptom management, use of resources, and discharge options.

3. Reductions in hospital and ICU lengths of stay and the use of nonbeneficial tests and resources can be anticipated when optimal palliative care considerations are in place under the guidance of the palliative care consultant.

4. When patients who are terminally ill die well, all parties involved will be satisfied with the care. Observation of, and mentored participation in, the delivery of optimal end-of-life care is an effective training method.

REFERENCES

1. Solomon MZ, O'Donnell LO, Jennings B. Decisions near the end of life: professional views on life-sustaining treatments. Am J Pub Health 1993;83:14–23.
2. Campbell ML, Frank RR. Experience with an end-of-life practice at a university hospital. Crit Care Med 1997;25:197–202.
3. Brody H, Campbell ML, Faber-Langendoen K, Ogle KS. Withdrawing intensive life-sustaining treatment: recommendations for compassionate clinical management. N Engl J Med 1997;336:652–657.
4. Field MJ, Cassel CK. Approaching death: improving care at the end of life. Washington, DC: National Academy Press; 1997.
5. Campbell ML. Forgoing Life-Sustaining Therapy: How to Care for the Patient Who is Near Death. Aliso Viejo, CA: American Association of Critical Care Nurses; 1998.
6. Danis M, Federman D, Fins JJ, et al. Incorporating palliative care into critical care education: principles, challenges and opportunities. Crit Care Med 1999;27:2005–2013.

PATIENT 14

A 75-year-old Aboriginal woman in the ICU with a large, protective family

A 75-year-old Aboriginal woman previously treated for breast cancer widely metastatic to bone and both lungs is admitted to the ICU with a severe pneumonia. During her first day in the ICU, the patient's large extended family visits constantly despite the unit policy of two visitors at a time. When visitors are asked if they are members of the immediate family, they fall silent. The nurses become concerned with the number of visitors. Later in the evening, the family requests permission to perform a ceremony involving chanting and the burning of sweet grass. The nurse manager voices her opinion that such a ceremony would disturb the other patients.

To address the family's request, the physician asks the family to appoint a spokesperson. The family chooses the patient's daughter, who avoids eye contact and appears detached, aloof, and angry. The physician informs the daughter of her mother's poor prognosis and explains that further life-sustaining interventions are futile. The daughter insists that her mother be fully treated with everything that "could save her life." She also demands that her mother not be told about her condition, because "it would kill her spirit." The physician explains that he has a legal and ethical obligation to inform her mother of her prognosis and to seek her agreement with a do-not-resuscitate status. He asks the daughter several times if she knows what her mother would want in this clinical circumstance, but the daughter remains silent.

Question: What cultural factors are influencing this family's behavior? How can the physician and ICU staff most effectively manage these factors and assist the patient and her family?

Diagnosis: Widely metastatic breast cancer in an elderly Aboriginal patient.

Discussion: Profound differences between Western and ethnic cultural world views and values often underlie clinical conflicts and ethical dilemmas in the intensive care of indigenous people. From a Western perspective, the moral reasoning of Aboriginal people may seem difficult to fathom. It derives from the context of the situation at hand, and the logic applied may vary from person to person and from community to community within a single Aboriginal society. In this way, Aboriginal logic differs from Western moral reasoning, which draws from precepts based on scriptures or philosophical tracts, general principles, and guiding rules. Physicians who view Aboriginal end-of-life decision-making from a Western perspective may fail to gain insight into the moral underpinnings of their patients' wishes. Gaining insight into this decision-making process is further complicated by the communication of Aboriginal culture between generations in an oral form.

Western culture and medicine place a high value on truth-telling and encourage physicians to inform patients of their conditions and prognoses. In the face of serious illness, however, many cultures—including many Aboriginal people—believe that the provision of unfavorable information can cause negative outcomes. Members of the Navajo culture, for instance, view medical information as potentially harmful and commonly shield family members from their medical reports.

For patients of Aboriginal heritage, it is important to recognize the limitations of standardized approaches for providing end-of-life care that do not take into account regional and individual perceptual variations. Individualization of care becomes especially important considering the contextual nature of Aboriginal end-of-life decision-making. It is important to acknowledge the centrality of family to health and identity as well as the substantial diversity in beliefs and practices among Aboriginal people.

Developing and maintaining solid and sincere relationships with patients of Aboriginal heritage is of the utmost importance. Health care workers may confuse and alienate their Aboriginal patients by maintaining a professional distance. In offering support, effective clinicians adopt the role of learner and seek to understand how individual factors shape Aboriginal cultural perspectives.

Although certain values—such as respect for dignity, non-interference, sharing of personal concerns, and the importance of family and community—may be common across most cultures, there are nuances as to how these values are perceived and expressed and the importance they are given. Other values, such as truth-telling in providing medical information, may contrast with Western beliefs, yet even these differences may vary among members of a single Aboriginal family.

When caring for patients from other cultures, it is important for the caregiver to consider a patient's view of autonomy. In Western culture, the supremacy of autonomy as the foundation of moral reasoning has deep roots; it forms the foundation for modern health care delivery. Consequently, Western physicians usually assume that the person experiencing the illness is the best person to make their healthcare decisions. Yet for many Aboriginal people, this focus on individuality neglects the vital role of personal interconnectedness and the social and moral meaning of these interrelations. Healthcare providers must discover how to see each person as a unique "cultural being."

To have true respect for a patient of a different culture, caregivers must traverse values alien to their own, different social systems, and alternative decision-making styles. The best way to address cultural differences is to foster open, inquisitive, and balanced communication in the process of making end-of-life decisions. In so doing, one may learn that relatives and clan members wish to be present when a loved one is approaching death. It is not uncommon for a large group to gather. Many Aboriginal people believe that healing, or the passage from life to death, is greatly enhanced by the support and collective energy of the community. Cultural rituals and religious practices hold great importance for many Aboriginal patients and families at times of illness, impending death, and grief. These activities may be essential for families to feel that their loved one is receiving the best care possible. Clinicians can demonstrate genuine caring by allowing and facilitating the performance of important rituals whenever and to the extent possible.

In caring for the present patient, the physician perceived the family's belief that direct communication of the truth about her mother's cancer would contradict their traditional family precepts. He discussed this issue with the daughter and suggested that the patient formally appoint her daughter as proxy decision-maker. He asked the patient, "Would you like to know about your medical condition and how it will affect you, or are you happy for your daughter to make decisions for you?" She affirmed that this was her preference.

Because people of Aboriginal ancestry tend to accept others' choices, the physician retained the obligation to discern if the family's decisions would differ from the patient's wishes. The physician was initially concerned that the daughter's subdued expressions represented anger, but subsequently he recognized her demeanor as an absence of overt emotional expression, which is a cultural characteristic of many Aboriginal people.

The ICU team recognized that the unit's standard visitation policies would restrict the family's ability to participate in the care of a loved one. They extended visitation privileges and also decided to allow the cultural ritual of burning sweet grass by providing a separate room with an open window. After performing these rituals, the daughter withdrew her request "to do everything." Through these culturally sensitive actions and the rituals and interactions they allowed, the patient most likely came to understand the seriousness of her condition and prognosis as she approached her end of life.

Clinical Pearls

1. Aboriginal families place central importance on family and community. Individual experiences and beliefs, however, are also valued, so that caregivers must determine the degree to which individual patients wish to participate in their health decisions.

2. Emotional self-control is common among Aboriginal people. It may be difficult for non-Aboriginal caregivers to understand what is being communicated. Listen carefully and watch for body language.

3. Aboriginal families usually wish to be present during decision-making. Families can assist in understanding a patient's beliefs and wishes. Patients may not strongly differentiate their own best interest from that of their family. "Immediate family" is a culturally relative term.

4. Many Aboriginal people believe that speaking of future illness or consequence may bring it to pass and create unnecessary stress that might further impede one's health. Uncertainty is often easily accepted.

5. Cultural rituals and religious practices hold great importance for many Aboriginal patients and families at times of illness, impending death, and grief. Clinicians can demonstrate genuine caring by allowing and facilitating the performance of important rituals whenever and to the extent possible.

REFERENCES

1. Hultkrantz A. Native Religions of North America: The Power of Visions and Fertility. San Francisco: Harper Collins; 1987: p37–8.
2. Kaufert JM, O'Neil JD. Biomedical Rituals and Informed Consent: Native Canadians and the Negotiation of Clinical Trust. In Weisz G (ed). Social Science Perspectives on Medical Ethics. Philadelphia: University of Pennsylvania Press; 1990: pp 41–63.
4. Muller JH, Desmond B. Ethical dilemmas in a cross-cultural context: a Chinese example. West J Med 1992;157:323–327
5. Caralis PV, Davis B, Wright K, Marcial E. The influence of ethnicity and race on attitudes toward advance directives, life-prolonging treatments, and euthanasia. J Clin Ethics 1993;4:155–165.
6. Blackhall LJ, Murphy ST, Frank G, et al. Ethnicity and attitudes toward patient autonomy. JAMA 1995;274:820–825.
7. Carrese JA, Rhodes LA. Western bioethics on the Navajo reservation: benefit or harm? JAMA 1995;274:826–829.
8. Gilbert CG. End of life issues in Aboriginal North America [occasional paper]. Winnipeg: University of Manitoba; 1999: p 2–3.
9. Ellerby J, Mckenzie J, McKay S, et al. Bioethics for clinicians: Aboriginal bioethics CMAJ 2000;163:845–850.

David M. Poppel, MD
Michael J. Germain, MD

PATIENT 15

A 60-year-old woman on chronic dialysis who cries out "Lord, please take me"

A 60-year-old African-American woman with diabetes and blindness is hospitalized with altered mental status, fever, and gangrene of her lower left leg. She has been managed for 2 years with peritoneal dialysis, supervised by one of her daughters, and has enjoyed a satisfactory quality of life. Three months ago, she underwent an unsuccessful peripheral angioplasty for an ischemic foot that subsequently required a transmetatarsal amputation. Within a month, her condition markedly worsened, and her surgeon recommended a below-knee amputation, which the patient refused. Her competence to make decisions was in doubt, but her family supported her decision. The patient continued to deteriorate, suffering considerable pain despite antibiotics and aggressive analgesia. At times, she would cry out, "Lord, please take me."

During the present admission, the medical team suggests discontinuation of dialysis in view of her poor prognosis without surgery, but the family refuses. The medical team believes that the family does not grasp the severity of the patient's illness, considering their resistance to accepting her prognosis. Increasing tension between the family and staff arises. Despite several meetings of the Ethics Committee with the family, an impasse soon develops.

Question: In what circumstances should discontinuation of dialysis be discussed with a patient and family, and what can they be told to expect if this course is chosen?

Diagnosis: End-stage renal disease, complicated by life-threatening peripheral vascular disease with infection and very poor prognosis for meaningful survival.

Discussion: End stage renal disease (ESRD) affects over 300,000 people in the U.S., with approximately 80,000 incident patients per year. The annual mortality rate is 20% to 25% due to the many comorbid conditions affecting patients with this diagnosis. Cardiac and peripheral vascular diseases account for the vast majority of deaths. Data from the U.S. Renal Data System demonstrate that any patient with ESRD on dialysis has a shortened life expectancy. For example, an African-American woman, aged 60 to 64 years, would normally have an expected remaining lifetime of approximately 21 years; however, this remaining life expectancy drops to 5 years if that person is on dialysis.

Despite technical advances in care, the older age of patients on dialysis, with their attendant comorbidities, has allowed only modest improvements in overall patient survival. Scoring systems can estimate prognosis for a specific patient starting dialysis. For example, based on the Charlson Comorbidity Index, the cohort of 60-year-old patients with ESRD, diabetes, and peripheral vascular disease has a 27% annual mortality rate. Adding any of several other comorbid conditions, such as congestive heart failure or advanced age, places the patient in the "very high" risk cohort, with a 47% annual mortality rate. If requested, prognostic information may be useful to the patient and family in the context of advance care planning that focuses on patient goals. This process properly includes discussion of palliative and end-of-life care when the patient's clinical condition and the patient and family needs warrant such services.

In view of such data, the Renal Physicians Association and the American Society of Nephrology have published guidelines for withholding and withdrawing dialysis. For certain patients with newly diagnosed ESRD complicated by significant comorbidities, dialysis may not be recommended. For other patients, a reasonable "trial period" on dialysis may be proposed, with clear goals defined prospectively, during which the benefit of this treatment may be evaluated. Assessment of the efficacy and value of continued treatment should occur at planned intervals and at times of complications or significant change in clinical status. When the potential failure of dialysis to improve a patient's quality of life is anticipated, expectant discussions concerning discontinuation are warranted at the outset of a trial period. Development of an acute complication, even in a previously stable patient, may highlight the limitations of dialysis as a chronic "life-support" therapy when the reversal of a nonrenal complication is doubtful. As the prognosis for an acceptable quality of life diminishes, a patient and family may wish to review options and focus more on achieving comfort and preparation for life closure than on further attempts at prolonging life.

There is an increasing literature on dialysis discontinuation and palliative care for patients with ESRD. Thirty percent of dialysis discontinuations occur because of a patient's chronic "failure to thrive," whereas 25% follow an acute medical complication. No data are available in a third of reported cases, and a variety of causes explain the remainder. One in five dialysis patients withdraw from dialysis before death. However, it is likely that many of these "discontinuations" occur in the midst of a medical crisis, often only hours before the patient's death. Such instances may not allow sufficient application of palliative care and may not represent optimum practice. An increasing level of awareness by both the public and physicians has led to more timely review of end-of-life planning before crises, allowing greater control and comfort for patients and families. Though initially time-consuming, advance care planning is an essential component of the care of patients with renal failure. It is as integral to the role of the physician as are effort to diagnose and treat disease. By avoiding crises and preventing potential treatment decision-related conflicts, this approach may also save time over the course of a patient's care.

There is a considerable body of literature on the ethical and legal issues of dialysis discontinuation. Withdrawal may be justified on the bases of patient self-determination and the concepts of beneficence and nonmaleficence, principles similar to those applied to competent patients declining other potentially "life-saving" therapies. Such decisions do not constitute suicide. Survey studies confirm that most patients with chronic renal failure support the right of fellow patients to decline dialysis and/or request DNR status, even if the surveyed patient chooses otherwise.

The likelihood of withdrawal from dialysis increases among older patients with more severe comorbid conditions. Whites tend to withdraw from dialysis two to three times more frequently than African-Americans. Women withdraw slightly more often than men. The reasons for racial differences are not well understood, but a general sense of distrust of the medical establishment by minority groups plays a role. Clinicians must remain sensitive to differences in the understanding of end-of-life issues among different racial, religious, and cultural groups. Internal family dynamics may also obstruct development of consensus over how to serve the best interests of the patient. Sensitivity, candor, and flexibility are required in facing such conflicts. As in any other clinical task, skills in discussing prognosis and developing advance directives can be learned from mentors and direct experience. Such communication should receive greater emphasis in medical training programs.

Another barrier to optimum advanced care planning in ESRD patients is a lack of awareness on the part of patients and families concerning the relatively high morbidity and mortality among ESRD patients. Clinicians may be reluctant to share such information or may not be aware of the true extent of mortality in ESRD patients, and they may fear generating an existential crisis or other untoward effects in the patient or family. The patient and family may silently harbor fears that a decision to limit therapy will decrease the attention they subsequently receive from clinicians. Correspondingly, clinicians may avoid such discussions for fear of appearing as if they are "giving up" on the care of the patient.

Too often, clinicians, patients and families assume that "curative" care and "palliative" care are mutually exclusive. When forced to choose between these two approaches to care, patients and families often choose to prolong life. Integration of the services of local hospice organizations and palliative care programs into care can ease the transition to end-of-life care sought by many patients. Renal clinicians need to understand the existing criteria for hospice care under Medicare, Medicaid, and private insurance. If a coexisting nonrenal illness has a prognosis that meets hospice criteria, hospice care will be covered by Medicare, even when dialysis is continued. The benefits of hospice will not only be apparent in the short run, but also help the patient and family come to terms with withdrawal of dialysis when appropriate.

In the present case, the woman's primary nephrologist, who had not been directly involved in her current admission, meets for 1 hour with the family at the request of the inpatient team. As he reviews the facts of the case, he allows the family to express their concerns. The family has heard that death after discontinuing dialysis is painful and accompanied by respiratory distress. They wonder if dialysis discontinuation constitutes suicide. The nephrologist describes the typical pattern of uremic symptoms that follow dialysis discontinuation. As a caucasian, he acknowledges the potential barriers of communication posed by the racial and socioeconomic differences between the family and the medical team. He emphasizes the value of his involvement with the patient and her family over the past year as a basis for rendering advice for the best medical and humane care.

The primary doctor tells the family that he believes their mother when she said she was "ready to go" and did not want treatments to prolong her life. He emphasizes that their mother's illnesses are taking her life, and that the dialysis and even the antibiotics are artificially prolonging it. He recommends that the patient should not undergo cardiopulmonary resuscitation, that she should receive maximum palliative care, and that the medical team should discontinue dialysis. He also explores the rationale for accepting these suggestions based on the primacy of the family's love for the patient and their concern for her well-being and dignity.

After the family discusses these recommendations among themselves, they requested a DNR status and optimum symptom relief, but cannot yet accept withdrawal of dialysis. One daughter notes concern that an out-of-state brother would blame the rest of the family for "letting Mother die."

What can a patient and family expect when dialysis is discontinued? First, death will not be painful. Progressive uremia causes progressive obtundation. Symptoms of distress should be manageable by applying modern principles of palliative care. Though the potential for volume overload with symptomatic pulmonary edema has been noted, it is unlikely to occur, since patients rarely take in enough fluids. On rare occasions, ultrafiltration treatments alone can be applied to control volume without blocking the progression of uremia. Most patients who withdraw from dialysis quietly slip into a state of nonresponsiveness and die in comfort. Death can be expected in 3 to 10 days. This interval may allow culmination of the "work" of a lifetime, offering opportunities for the patient, family, and friends to acknowledge the depth of their relationships, the significance of the patient's life, the challenges of his or her illness, and the courage and grace with which it was faced. It also serves as a time for the family to take comfort in acknowledging the love with which they have cared for the patient.

The next day, after conferring with the out-of-town brother, the family decides to withdraw dialysis. The patient receives a morphine drip for control of her leg pain. She spends the next day in comfort and is able to communicate with her family despite her drowsiness. The family shares a sense of relief in seeing her at peace. On the following day, the patient's 61st birthday, the family gathers at the bedside. While they sing "Happy Birthday" to the patient, she peacefully passes away.

Clinical Pearls

1. A high incidence of comorbid conditions, largely cardiovascular disease and advancing age, contributes to the high annual mortality rate of patients on dialysis (20%–25%). This rate may exceed the mortality rate of many malignancies or HIV infection.

2. Even when technically "successful," dialysis may not afford protection from this rate of mortality, nor does dialysis alone provide adequate palliation of the symptoms that diminish patients' quality of life.

3. From the initial diagnosis of ESRD, the general principles and techniques of palliative care should become a part of the care of the ESRD patient.

4. Advance care planning entails a candid review of a patient's prognosis, as well as anticipatory discussions of care in the setting of future medical crises or gradual failure to thrive. Such discussions should include review of the option for withdrawal from dialysis, the circumstances in which the patient might elect such a course, and, as appropriate, descriptions that anticipate the process of death.

5. Special attention must be paid to racial, religious, and regional ethnic differences that may create barriers to communication about the sensitive area of end-of-life care.

6. A great deal of comfort can be provided patients and families by the assurance that a decision to discontinue dialysis or other forms of supportive care will not diminish the overall level of care given the patient. They can also be assured that palliative care does not signal a withdrawal of concern on the part of the care team for the well-being of the patient and family.

7. Death after withdrawal from dialysis should proceed without substantial discomfort, given application of appropriate palliative care, and should occur in 3 to 10 days. If suitable preparation and planning has occurred, discontinuation of dialysis may allow a peaceful and satisfying closure to a life and bring a degree of solace to a family in a time of grief.

REFERENCES

1. Kjellstrand CM, Dosseter JB: Ethical Problems in Dialysis and Transplantation. Boston, Kluwer Academic Publishers, 1992.
2. Renal Physicians Association, American Society of Nephrology: Shared Decision-Making in the Appropriate Initiation of and Withdrawal from Dialysis (Clinical Practice Guideline. No. 2).Washington, D.C., RPA/ASN, 1999.
3. United States Renal Data System: 2000 Annual Data Report.Bethesda, MD, NIDDKD, June 2000. [www.usrds.org/atlas_2000.htm.]
4. Beddhu S, Bruns FJ, Saul M, et al: A simple comorbidity scale predicts clinical outcomes and costs in dialysis patients. Am J Med 2000:108:609–613.
5. Cohen LM, Germain M, Poppel DM, et al: Dialysis discontinuation and palliative care. Am J Kidney Dis 2000;36:140–144.
6. Cohen LM, Germain MJ, Poppel, DM, et al: Dying well after discontinuing the life-support treatment of dialysis. Arch Intern Med 2000:160:2513–2518.
7. Cohen, LM, Germain MJ, Poppel DM, Rieter G: Renal Palliative Care. In Addington E, Hall J (eds): Palliative Care for Non-Cancer Patients. London, Oxford Press, 2001.
8. Moss AH, Hozayen O, King K, et al: Attitudes of patients toward cardiopulmonary resuscitation in the dialysis unit. Am J Kidney Dis 2001;38(4):847–852.

Kenneth Doka, PhD

PATIENT 16

A 44-year-old woman who is coping with the death of
her husband from pancreatic cancer

A 44-year-old woman is caring for her 47-year-old husband, who is in the late stages of pancreatic cancer. He is now in hospice care, being treated at home. The wife is the primary caregiver, although she does receive some assistance from a daughter who lives in the area. Her other child, a 19-year-old son with cognitive and motor developmental disabilities, lives in a group home in the community. The wife has always played an important role in the son's life. Although the son tries to provide some support, he is grieving the impending loss of his father, and his mother needs to support him.

The woman's relationship with her husband has generally been good. There was a period when her husband was an active alcoholic. He has been in recovery for the past 7 years. The woman claims to be doing reasonably well "given the circumstances," but she does complain of severe neck and shoulder pain. She also expresses ambivalence about her husband, expressing a wish that his suffering end, while at the same point adding "but I do not wish anyone dead."

The hospice nurse-case manager for the family seeks the physician's consultation. She wonders how best to assist this woman as she copes with the impending death of her husband.

Question: What intervention strategies would assist the woman in her role of mother, wife, and caregiver now and facilitate subsequent healthy grieving?

Assessment: The woman is coping with the stress of caregiving and anticipatory grief.

Discussion: It is not unusual for individuals struggling with life-threatening illness, either their own or in a loved one, to experience anticipatory grief. The term *anticipatory grief* refers to the emotional impact of the losses that accompany a progressive debilitating illness—of expectations, roles, abilities, patterns of interactions—and the anticipated final, total loss of a loved one through death. Caregivers may experience their own losses, such as the loss of independence as they are compelled by a loved one's needs to take on additional, unaccustomed responsibilities.

As with any grief, anticipatory grief can be manifested in many ways. These reactions are highly individual, influenced by factors such as the individual's temperament, the nature of the illness, the availability of support, relationships with others (including the dying person), and other psychological, social, cultural, medical, and spiritual variables. Physical reactions such as pain or other physical complaints are not uncommon. Each deserves to be medically evaluated. There may be cognitive manifestations as well, as individuals may find it difficult to concentrate or they may continually review the illness. Grief responses may include a range of emotions including anger, guilt, sadness, and jealousy. In the present patient's case, the wife has feelings of guilt about her wish for her husband to die soon. Such ambivalence is common in instances of extended illness. There may also be spiritual reactions to grief. The onset of a terminal illness at a comparatively young age or the rapid progression of illness can seem profoundly unfair and may cause people to question their faith in God.

The outward manifestations of grief are widely varied as well. We think of the typical face of grief as sad and withdrawn; however, some people react to grief by becoming engaged in activity at a manic pace.

Intervention strategies for anticipatory grief are numerous and must be individualized. First, given the care-giving responsibilities that often accompany the terminal phase of an illness, a caregiver assessment is useful, examining the ways that the illness are not only affecting the patient but also those offering care. In caregivers who have physical complaints, a medical examination is required. Although such symptoms can result from grief and stress, other factors should be ruled out. Anticipatory grief obviously can coexist with medical problems that must be excluded or considered for treatment.

Second, hospice clinicians can help a grieving family member find effective ways to manage stress. It might involve helping the person examine both her support system and the ways she uses that support. In the present case, staff from the group home in which the son lives can be recruited to help explain his father's illness and prognosis and to support him in coping. Stress reduction techniques, such as breathing and relaxation exercises or imaging, may be useful. Caregivers may need to identify formal sources of assistance such as hospice or home-based assistance. As caregivers begin to trust the care their loved one is receiving, they can be encouraged to seek respite and attend to their own needs and quality of life.

One simple way that clinicians can help is to validate and "normalize" grief. People in such situations often benefit from being reassured that grief is a natural aspect of life-threatening illness. Listening in a nonjudgmental manner, clinicians can assist caregivers in exploring their relationship and recognizing how the relationship is affected by the illness. Caregivers also need assistance in examining their reactions and feelings and in exploring their coping techniques. Support or self-help groups can represent a helpful strategy by bringing together individuals all coping with a family member's life-threatening illness. Group activities can help validate grief, assist in problem-solving, and sometimes provide pragmatic assistance for tasks such as transportation, yard work, and household repairs.

Third, clinicians can assist family members in their interaction with the dying person. Informal care-giving, when performed with sufficient support to avoid strain and utter exhaustion on the part of the family member, often facilitates subsequent grief. Life review and reminiscence with the dying person can support the ill person in finding meaning. Care-giving and reminiscence can help survivors as well, enabling them to express the love and appreciation they feel for their ill loved one. In the midst of grief, the process of caregiving can become a time of celebration of life and relationship.

At the time of death, the hospice worker can do a number of things. The worker can allow time with the deceased before the body is removed, inviting the family to participate in ritual, pray, light a candle, or anoint the body prior to removal. Expressions of grief at this time are natural and healthy. Clinicians can assist the family too with necessary but stressful details, such as deciding on rituals, removing the body, and reviewing legal and financial steps they should take. If appropriate, hospice clinicians may encourage the family to plan funeral arrangements, considering rituals, readings, and songs that may have meaning. Rituals that are personal and participatory can facilitate grief. After the death, the grieving family may need to review the illness, the care-giving experience, and the treatment decisions that were made as part of the grieving process.

Although these actions facilitate the grieving process, they will not eliminate subsequent grief. The actual death of a person, however foreseen, anticipated, or even welcomed, still generates grief. The fact that the death was hoped for as a final relief to the person's suffering and the stress of care-giving can be a source of guilt exacerbating grief. Following the death, the hospice clinicians can continue to validate grief and assist the family in finding and effectively utilizing appropriate resources. These may include their intimate network of friends and family, and social support systems, such as their faith communities, self-help, and support groups. Self-help books or grief counselors may also be valuable resources in aiding people in their adaptation to the loss.

Clinical Pearls

1. Anticipatory grief is a normal component of life-threatening illness. Anticipatory grief is not only grief that develops from an anticipated death, but also a reaction to the many losses already experienced in the course of a progressive, debilitating, and ultimately life-limiting illness.

2. Caregiver assessment is an inherent part of holistic family-centered care. Such assessment evaluates how family members and other members of the intimate network are responding to the stress of caring for a person with life-threatening illness.

3. Critical intervention strategies include assisting family members in obtaining effective support from both their informal networks and formal systems of care and teaching stress management.

4. Effective grief counseling during the illness and after the death entails validating grief and assisting people in drawing on ritual and prayer for comfort as well as making use of their own support systems. When indicated, people can also be guided toward appropriate self-help and support groups, self-help books, and grief counselors.

REFERENCES
1. Hamovich M. The Family and the Fatally Ill Child. Los Angeles: Delmar; 1964.
2. Doka KJ. Expectation of death, participation in funeral arrangements, and grief adjustment. Omega 1984;15:119–130.
3. Rando TA. Clinical Dimensions of Anticipatory Mourning: Theory and Practice in Working with the Dying, Their Loved Ones and Their Caregivers. Champaign, IL: Research Press; 2000.

Joshua O. Benditt, MD

PATIENT 17

A 54-year-old man with amyotrophic lateral sclerosis
and progressive shortness of breath

A 54-year-old man presents to your office with progressive dyspnea as well as waking frequently at night and some morning headaches. He was diagnosed with amyotrophic lateral sclerosis (ALS, Lou Gehrig's disease) 2 years ago. The initial symptoms were clumsiness of his hands, but weakness has progressed. He now uses a wheelchair with assistance, although he can stand and transfer himself. He has had no problems with swallowing or episodes of aspiration and denies change in voice quality.

The patient is unequivocally clear that he does not wish to undergo tracheostomy and long-term ventilation. He is interested in learning about any other therapies that might relieve his symptoms.

Physical Examination: General: thin, no distress. Mouth: good palatal elevation, minimal fasciculations of tongue, no secretion pooling. Chest: decreased excursion of diaphragms, clear but diminished breath sounds. Cardiac: normal. Abdomen: normal. Extremities: wasting and fasciculations. Neurologic: upper and lower motor neuron signs, upper greater than lower extremity weakness.

Laboratory Findings: Forced vital capacity (FVC) 2.1 (48% predicted).

Question: In the absence of a tracheostomy, how can this patient's progressive respiratory distress be managed?

Diagnosis: ALS with significant respiratory muscle involvement resulting in dyspnea and nocturnal hypoventilation.

Discussion: ALS is a disease of unknown etiology that causes destruction of upper and lower motor neurons and leads to progressive loss of skeletal muscle function. Ultimately, the respiratory muscles become involved, leading to respiratory failure as the most frequent cause of death. Impairment of ventilatory function can be particularly distressing in causing dyspnea, air hunger, and a sense of "suffocating from within."

In individuals with a variety of neuromuscular diseases, including ALS, ventilatory impairment frequently presents initially with sleep-related symptoms. Neural output to the respiratory muscles decreases during sleep, particularly during rapid eye movement (REM) stages of the sleep cycle. Muscle weakness coupled with decreased neural drive can result in significant hypoventilation, hypercarbia, and even obstructive and central sleep apnea.

It is important to search for the symptoms of sleep disturbance, which may be subtle and include nocturnal awakenings, nocturia, vivid nightmares, night sweats, apneas witnessed by a significant other, daytime hypersomnolence, and a sense of "not having gotten a good night's rest." Signs and symptoms of hypercarbia include morning headaches, "fuzzy thinking," and even altered mental status when the condition is severe. In patients with ALS, a FVC < 50% of predicted is associated with a significant increase in sleep-disturbed breathing and nocturnal hypoventilation. It is reasonable to routinely obtain FVC measures on clinic visits at approximately 3-month intervals for patients with ALS.

Therapy for sleep-disturbed breathing can be initiated when there is significant hypoventilation or central or obstructive sleep apnea documented by sleep studies. Other indications include arterial blood gas measurements showing a $PCO_2 > 45$ or an FVC < 50% predicted. Many ALS clinicians will treat on the basis of a decreased FVC alone, recognizing that the incidence of sleep disturbance in these patients is very high. A formal sleep study can be a very difficult experience for the patient with ALS because of the many physical needs and special equipment that they often require. Arterial blood gases are frequently normal until the disease is very advanced, and because of the discomfort associated with the procedure, ABGs are rarely obtained.

Treatment for sleep-disturbed breathing and hypoventilation in ALS, as in other neuromuscular disorders, involves supporting ventilation during sleep. In almost all cases, clinicians can initiate a trial of noninvasive positive pressure ventilation (NPPV) with a nasal-mask interface. To find the proper fit, a number of different masks may be tried in the office until an appropriate fit is obtained. A noninvasive ventilator, usually a portable pressure-support device, is employed. Therapy is initiated with low inspiratory positive airway pressure (IPAP) of approximately 7 to 8 cm H_2O and an expiratory positive airway pressure (EPAP) of 4 cm H_2O. The IPAP is then titrated to obtain a tidal volume of approximately 8 to 10 ml/kg ideal body weight. Further titration can be accomplished at home using patient symptoms as a guide to therapeutic efficacy.

Careful symptom follow-up in the home through home health, hospice, or a homecare medical equipment company is arranged. Improvement in symptoms is almost always reported in those who are able to tolerate the device. Patients with significant bulbar involvement tend to be less able to tolerate noninvasive ventilation because of air leaks that occur through the mouth or an inability to manage secretions while the ventilator is functioning. Despite these potential problems, a trial of NPPV is warranted in those patients who meet the criteria noted above.

Respiratory insufficiency is progressive in ALS. Despite all known interventions, including NPPV, respiratory failure eventually occurs. Many patients who begin using NPPV only at night progress to use it during daytime up to and including continuous, 24-hour ventilation. Patients accept this therapy in order to reduce dyspnea and air hunger. There is also evidence to indicate that survival may be prolonged in ALS patients who tolerate NPPV. Thus, a device used for symptom palliation may have the added benefit of prolonging life.

However, NPPV cannot support ventilation indefinitely. Therefore, discussions regarding patient preference concerning long-term mechanical ventilation via tracheostomy must take place. Preferably, these discussions should occur early in the course of the disease, when a thorough prospective discussion of the topic can be held, rather than during an emergency. If a patient decides to use NPPV but declines long-term invasive ventilation, careful preparations need to be made for the time when the patient wishes to withdraw NPPV. Home-hospice care with a carefully prepared strategy for the use of anxiolytics and judicious doses of opioids and other dyspnea-reducing agents can be invaluable in this situation. Home visits by the physician are often of great help to both patient and family.

In the present patient, NPPV was initiated with immediate alleviation of symptoms of nocturnal hypoventilation. The patient initially used NPPV only at night, but over the last 6 months, he began using the therapy nearly 24 hours a day. During this period, he was able to complete life-closure tasks without experiencing significant dyspnea. NPPV was removed at the patient's request after adequate anxiolytic and small does of morphine to alleviate dyspnea were given to ensure patient comfort. He died peacefully at home with his family present.

Clinical Pearls

1. ALS is a progressive neuromuscular disorder that mandates the early discussion of advance care planning.

2. Some patients may elect to undergo tracheotomy and initiation of ventilatory support.

3. Patients who decline a tracheotomy may benefit symptomatically with NPPV, which can serve as a palliative intervention at the end of life.

4. Patients who stabilize with NPPV should be invited to discuss with their physician preparations for the time when they may wish to withdraw ventilatory support.

REFERENCES

1. Tidwell J. Pulmonary management of the ALS patient. J Neurosci Nurs 1993;25:337–342.
2. Ferguson KA, Strong MJ, Ahmad D, George CF. Sleep-disordered breathing in amyotrophic lateral sclerosis. Chest 1996;110:664–669.
3. Hopkins LC, Tatarian GT, Pianta TF. Management of ALS: respiratory care. Neurology 1996;47:S123-S125.
4. Cazzolli PA, Oppenheimer EA. Home mechanical ventilation for amyotrophic lateral sclerosis: nasal compared to tracheostomy-intermittent positive pressure ventilation. J Neurol Sci 1996;139:123–183.
5. Smyth A, Riedl M, Kimura R, et al. End of life decisions in amyotrophic lateral sclerosis: a cross- cultural perspective. J Neurol Sci 1997;152:S93-S96.
6. Aboussouan LS, Khan SU, Meeker DP, et al. Effect of noninvasive positive-pressure ventilation on survival in amyotrophic lateral sclerosis. Ann Intern Med 1997;127:450–453.
7. Carter GT, Miller RG. Comprehensive management of amyotrophic lateral sclerosis. Phys Med Rehabil Clin N Am 1998;9:271–84, viii-ix.

Timothy E. Quill, MD
Bradford Priddy, MD

PATIENT 18

A 32-year-old male medical resident with a large yolk sac tumor in his chest requests assistance in dying if his suffering becomes unbearable in the future

A 32-year-old medical resident, 3 weeks before completion of his residency, develops right shoulder pain secondary to a large mediastinal mass that is diagnosed as a yolk sac tumor. His prognosis is uncertain because of the rareness of the cancer, but long-term survival estimates with aggressive chemotherapy and possibly surgery range from 25% to 50%. He is aware of the converse of these statistics—that there is a 50% to 75% chance he will die over the next several months. Despite skillful efforts to palliate his symptoms during the first week of treatment, he has intractable nausea and vomiting from the chemotherapy as well as cellulitis from an indwelling catheter.

Before the resident can throw himself wholeheartedly into continuing his treatment, he feels a compelling need to prepare himself and his wife for the possibility of his death. This includes traditional advance care planning (a health care proxy, living will, and financial will) and also includes contemplating the circumstances of his own death. He knows he would want a peaceful, relatively quick death, and he fears severe physical symptoms, prolonged dependency on others, loss of control of his mind and body, and having his wishes ignored if he becomes ready to die.

He requests access to the means for a hastened death from his physician as a way of reassuring himself that if it becomes clear that his treatment is failing and his suffering becomes unbearable, he will be empowered to make the choice about whether to continue living or end his life. He understands the potential of palliative care and hospice to relieve suffering, but he also knows from first-hand experience that its success is not 100% and that some of the things he fears most can occur in even the most vigilant palliative care program. "One of my biggest fears is that I will be talking earnestly about my life being not worth living, and someone will come up, pat me on the back, and tell me to 'hang in there'."

Question: How should his physician respond to his concerns?

Diagnosis: Yolk sac tumor in a patient with uncertain curative potential who fears progressive disease and an unbearable death.

Discussion: Many terminally ill patients and other individuals, especially those who have witnessed the end-of-life suffering of someone they care about, fear that their deaths will be filled with physical suffering and indignity. Fortunately, most patients will talk about their concerns if prompted in a setting that encourages honesty and openness. Questions the health care provider can ask to facilitate these discussions include, "As you look toward the end of your life, what are your biggest worries?" and "Are there circumstances where you would find life not worth living?" Many patients will tell stories of someone in their lives who experienced severe suffering prior to death, and sometimes the story will reveal the absence of a meaningful physician presence toward the end of life. Such inquiries can often lead to important discussions about the effectiveness of modern pain management or the widespread availability of hospice programs to support patients and their families. These discussions can also create an opportunity for health care providers to reaffirm their commitment to working with the patient and family throughout the dying process no matter where it goes.

A smaller group of patients, if they feel secure in the patient-physician relationship, may explore the physician's commitment further, even to the point of asking "If my suffering becomes unbearable to me and cannot be adequately relieved with usual palliative measures, will you help me to die?" Such patients may have a strong need to maintain control at the end of life and may be as afraid of prolonged dependency as they are of severe physical suffering. Because the current legal environment passively discourages this inquiry into physician-assisted suicide, many patients may feel too timid to raise the question, while those who do raise the question may appear to be overly assertive. Health care professionals should not view such inquiries as pathological but rather should respond to them first by eliciting the full story of the patient's hopes and fears to clarify exactly what they are requesting. Then, the clinician should make sure the patient and family understand the potential effectiveness of modern palliative measures.

Palliative care and hospice are today's standards of care for the dying. When the patient's fears stem from previous substandard care, then the promise of palliative care and hospice will be reassuring. Yet some patients, including the medical resident in this case, have extensive experience with hospice but find it only partially reassuring because they have witnessed in hospice programs what to them would be unacceptable deaths. Most studies suggest that hospice care is highly effective. However, there remain exceptional cases in which suffering becomes severe despite excellent care. For example, 5% to 35% of hospice patients report their pain as moderate to severe 1 week prior to death, and about 25% of such patients report their dyspnea as "unbearable." Moreover, about 25% to 75% of hospice patient develop at least mild delirium before death, and a small but troubling percentage experience terminal agitated delirium. These outcomes or other sources of potential suffering frighten some patients and may stimulate their exploration of the potential for a hastened death in the future.

Inquiries about the potential of a hastened death are relatively common if the doctor-patient relationship is receptive to them. The best data on this subject come from the Netherlands, where physician-assisted suicide and voluntary active euthanasia have been permitted for years in terminally ill patients with severe suffering. Each year, 25,000 individuals (about one-fourth of people who die each year in the Netherlands) inquire about the receptivity of the physician to physician-assisted suicide or euthanasia, compared with 9,000 explicit requests and approximately 3,000 acts. Thus, there are about 8 inquiries for every act. These data suggest that many patients are reassured by the availability of a hastened death that in reality they may never need.

Both the Dutch data and the first few years of data from Oregon (where physician-assisted suicide has been legally available since 1997) suggest that genuine requests and subsequent life-ending acts are rarely due to unrelieved pain, but rather due to a combination of physical symptoms, debility, fatigue, growing weary of dying, and dependence on others. In Oregon, those patients eventually requesting assistance with suicide invariably had access to health care, including hospice, but distinguish themselves by having a strong sense of autonomy and an intense desire to maintain personal control over their own dying. Patients inquiring about potential future assistance with dying would probably have similar characteristics.

The present patient needed to anticipate and address, as best he could, the potential permutations of his dying. For him, this included not only advance care planning but also the possibility of hastening his death if his natural mode of dying became unbearable. As he examined the "last-resort" options that might be possible if palliative measures were insufficient to relieve his suffering, the two that most appealed to him were terminal sedation and physician-assisted suicide. Although terminal sedation is legal and physician-assisted suicide is not (outside of Oregon), the resident feared that the sedation could be incomplete, that he could linger in a twilight state for days or even weeks before death while his wife and loved ones had to endure more prolonged anticipatory grief, and that he might not be empowered to decide when to initiate the process himself. Although he understood the potential pitfalls of physician-assisted suicide—that it might not work, that he might be unable to swallow or digest sufficient medication, or that he might lose capacity before initiating it—the thought of having access to a hastened death in his own hands appealed to him. The freedom to talk about and explore the possibility of both options reassured him that he could retain some choice and control at the end of life should his suffering become unbearable and unrelenting.

Armed with the reassurance that there could be an escape from end-stage suffering, feeling that he had adequately prepared for the possibility of his death, and having the support of a physician who was committed to seeing the process through with him no matter where it went, the resident was able to devote himself more wholeheartedly to treatment. Because he had prepared himself for the worst-case scenario, he was now able to apply the energy liberated toward weathering difficult treatment and achieving the best possible medical outcome. Clearly, this patient needed to settle end-of-life issues at the outset of his disease, before he could move on and fully engage in treatment. Health care providers need to remain receptive to patients who hold this perspective and should support their need to be involved and, indeed, to be in control of their own dying. As this resident put it, "As much as possible, I want to be in the driver's seat of this body!"

After a combination of four cycles of intensive and difficult chemotherapy, followed by surgery to remove a residual teratoma, the resident now appears to be cured 1 year later. Whether settling the early inquiry about his end-of-life options had any bearing on his eventual recovery is only a matter of speculation, but it is clear that the knowledge that there could be an escape freed him to spend his precious energy on other more important matters.

Clinical Pearls

1. Many terminally ill patients and others who have witnessed harsh deaths fear unbearable suffering in their future, and they are willing to talk about it if asked.

2. Palliative care and hospice programs are the standards of care toward the end of life and are able to address most, but not all, severe terminal suffering.

3. The possibility of a hastened death is important to many patients. Having some choice and the potential for escape from suffering can sometimes liberate energy for the fight against disease.

4. Health care providers must learn how to talk about "last-resort" options so that they can support patients and families who are concerned about unbearable end-of-life suffering.

5. Relatively few patients will actually need access to these "last-resort" options if they receive adequate palliative care.

6. Health care providers' explicit commitments to care for their patients and families throughout their final illness to their deaths are fundamental to quality end-of-life care.

REFERENCES

1. Coyle N, Adelhardt J, Foley KM, Portenoy RK. Character of terminal illness in the advanced cancer patient: pain and other symptoms during the last four weeks of life. J Pain Symptom Manage 1990;5:83–93.
2. van der Maas PJ, van Delden JJM, Pijnenborg L. Euthanasia and Other Medical Decisions Concerning the End of Life. Amsterdam: Elsevier Science Publishing 1992, Vol. 22/1–2 (special issue).
4. Block SD, Billings JA. Patient requests to hasten death: evaluation and management in terminal care. Arch Intern Med 1994;154:2039–2047.
5. Quill TE, Cassel CK. Nonabandonment: a central obligation for physicians. Ann Intern Med 1995;122:368–374.
6. Quill TE, Lo, Brock DW. Palliative options of last resort: a comparison of voluntarily stopping eating and drinking, terminal sedation, physician-assisted suicide, and voluntary active euthanasia. JAMA 1997;278:1099–2104.
7. Chin AE, Hedberg K, Higginson GK, Fleming DW. Legalized physician-assisted suicide in Oregon—the first year's experience. N Engl J Med 1999;340:577–583.
8. Lo B, Quill TE, Tulsky J. End-of-life care consensus panel: discussing palliative care with patients. Ann Intern Med 1999;130:744–749.
9. Quill TE. Initiating end of life discussions with severely ill patients: addressing the elephant in the room. JAMA 2000;284:2502–2507.
10. Sullivan AD, Hedberg K, Fleming DW. Legalized physician-assisted suicide in Oregon—the second year. N Engl J Med 2000;342:598–604.
11. Quill TE, Coombs-Lee B, Nunn S. Palliative options of last resort: finding the least harmful alternative. Ann Intern Med 2000;133:563.

Kathleen Puntillo, RN, DNSc

PATIENT 19

A 28-year-old woman dying with acute respiratory distress syndrome who needs palliative care in the ICU

A 28-year-old unmarried woman is admitted to the ICU in acute respiratory distress with a chest radiograph that shows right middle lobe and bibasilar infiltrates. She had been discharged from the hospital just 2 days earlier after having received an allogenic bone marrow transplant for chronic myelogenous leukemia. That hospitalization had been prolonged and marked by multiple complications.

The patient is intubated and placed on mechanical ventilation. She is extubated 4 days later. During the following 5 days, her respiratory condition worsens, and she develops acute respiratory distress syndrome (ARDS). Because she remains alert, she is placed on noninvasive positive pressure ventilation (NPPV) in lieu of intubation. She receives aggressive care with antibiotics, intravenous fentanyl for pain, and lorazepam for anxiety and agitation. She remains oriented and writes notes requesting that she wants to be informed about her condition, treatments, and prognosis. She resists reintubation despite her increasing respiratory distress. Her fiancé, parents, and friends are frequently present, and although distressed about her condition, they honor her care wishes.

Her respiratory condition progressively worsens, and she agrees to reintubation. Despite mechanical ventilation, her oxygenation continues to deteriorate. She requires continuous intravenous infusions of midazolam and fentanyl for sedation and comfort. She continues to receive aggressive life-support efforts, but her general condition fails. After extensive discussions with her family, life-sustaining treatments are withdrawn, and she dies 7 days after admission in comfort with her family present.

Question: What role does the critical care nurse play in supporting patients at end of life and their families?

Diagnosis: Overwhelming respiratory failure from diffuse alveolar hemorrhage after bone marrow transplantation.

Discussion: Of all of the health professionals that comprise the critical care team, only the patient's nurse is present at the bedside 8 to 12 hours each day. Critical care nurses fulfill a multifaceted role in the ICU. This role includes physical and psychological monitoring, titration of medications in response to changing conditions, provision of comfort and hygiene measures, institution of emergency interventions by pre-established protocols, and family support. Nurses also plan and institute changes in care according to goals agreed upon by the health care team, patient, and family.

Critical care nurses recognize that the primary goals of critical care focus on patient resuscitation, stabilization, and recovery from the acute phase of illness or injury. An experienced ICU nurse, however, also recognizes when a patient becomes at high risk of not surviving the ICU stay. For such patients, a nurse can assume an important role in advocating for a multidisciplinary team approach to decision-making in order to formulate appropriate patient treatment goals.

For the present patient, it was important that team members placed the patient's deteriorating condition within the context of her expressed wishes. This required clear and frequent communication among the team members ensuring that information being provided to this alert but very ill woman was based on the best medical opinion possible. At the same time, the team members needed to be sensitive to the patient's understanding and choices. The patient's nurse is in a position to orchestrate the communication of information among the patient, family members, physicians on the various clinical services involved in care, respiratory therapists, social worker, and other care providers.

Truth-telling is an essential component of open communication and compassionate care. The nurse answered the patient's and family's questions about her condition in terms that they could understand without minimizing the seriousness of her condition. When she required reintubation, the patient accepted this intervention knowing that her chances of survival were low. Indeed, the patient did not respond to therapy. In situations in which a patient's condition deteriorates, the critical care nurse can help navigate a peaceful dying for the patient by having all involved consider interventions that emphasize patient comfort rather than aggressive life-promoting treatments. It is important for professionals to realize that a patient's death is not necessarily an indication of imperfect care; sometimes, even in

ICUs, the most appropriate care is directed at achieving comfort and quality of life.

Nurses have a major responsibility to improve the provision of comfort care in the ICU considering that recent studies indicate that many patients die in moderate to severe pain and experience other troubling symptoms. Pain needs to be routinely and systematically assessed and treated in *all* ICU patients, because many patients with pain have conditions, such as chronic obstructive pulmonary disease or congestive heart failure, that health care providers may not associate with pain. The young woman presented here did not have an operative or traumatic source of pain, yet there were many potential sources of extreme discomfort. Like most critically ill patients, she underwent numerous diagnostic and treatment procedures that can cause both pain and anxiety. Even frequent and necessary turning of patients has been shown to sometimes cause substantial pain. Nurses can evaluate the appropriateness of procedures being planned for patients and, as goals shift to comfort with acknowledgment of impending death, advocate for the omission of unnecessary interventions. The most important procedures for patients at end of life are those that promote comfort.

The present patient was frequently dyspneic and anxious. When on NPPV, she struggled to accept the discomfort from the facemask. When she had reprieves from the facemask, the patient would struggle to communicate verbally. Her need to communicate required her nurse to titrate pharmacologic interventions to balance the patient's need for comfort and cardiopulmonary stability with her wish to maintain cognition and communication.

Nurses can also use nonpharmacologic measures to promote patient comfort, such as a bedside fan to promote convection across the patient's face, which has been shown to decrease dyspnea. Positioning the patient in the high Fowler's position also lessens shortness of breath. Repeated reassurances, soothing personal contact, gentle communication including updates of clinical information, and the "therapeutic presence" of the nurse and family decrease anxiety. Frequent mouth care to alleviate thirst and moisten a dry mouth may at times be the most important source of patient comfort. Many nursing activities, such as these, may be "invisible" among the myriad high-tech ICU interventions. Yet they may be the most important measures in promoting comfort and peace as death approaches.

A primary nursing focus of care before, during, and after the patient's death is the patient's family. Nurses can prepare the family for the death, encourage their presence and involvement as death approaches, and support them in their grief and bereavement. Caring for families encompasses three major aspects: access, involvement in caregiving activities, and information and support. Visiting hours should be liberalized for the families of all ICU patients, but this is critically important when a patient is dying. Nurses can support family members who want to participate in the patient's physical care. Nurses can also assist families in performing rituals consistent with their culture or religion. When a patient dies, there is still much that nurses can offer family members. Nurses can provide them information about community grief and bereavement resources. When possible, they are valued attendees at funeral or memorial services of patients for whom they cared. Intermittent contact with family members during the first year after the patient's death is meaningful to the bereaved.

The present patient's family, while grief-stricken, responded well to the nurse's actions on their behalf and appeared to find comfort despite the tragedy of losing their loved one at such a young age.

Clinical Pearls

1. Nurses can advocate for a multidisciplinary team approach to decision-making regarding treatment goals for the dying patient. They can help to negotiate a peaceful dying for the patient by helping professionals, patients, and the patient's family to consider the use of interventions that emphasize patient comfort rather than aggressive therapies.

2. An essential nursing focus during ICU end-of-life care is the assessment and management of pain and other symptoms that may be distressing to the patient.

3. A primary focus of care for nursing before, during, and after the patient's death is the patient's family. Nurses can prepare the family for the patient's death, encourage their presence and involvement up to and during death, and support their grief and bereavement afterward.

REFERENCES

1. Desbiens NA, Wu AW, Broste SK, et al: Pain and satisfaction with pain control in seriously ill hospitalized adults: findings from the SUPPORT research investigations. Crit Care Med 1996;24:1953–1961.
2. Campbell ML: Forgoing Life-Sustaining Therapy. Aliso Viejo, CA, AACN Critical Care Publication, 1998.
3. Chapple HS: Changing the game in the intensive care unit: letting nature take its course. Crit Care Nurse 1999;19(3):25–34.
4. Kaplow R: Use of nursing resources and comfort of cancer patients with and without do-not-resuscitate orders in the intensive care unit. Am J Crit Care 2000;9(2): 87–95.
5. Puntillo KA: The role of critical care nurses in providing and managing end-of-life care. In Curtis JR, Rubenfeld GD (eds): Managing Death in the Intensive Care Unit: The Transition from Cure to Comfort. New York, Oxford University Press, 2000.
6. Nelson JE, Meier DE, Oei EJ, et al: Self-reported symptom experience of critically ill cancer patients receiving intensive care. Crit Care Med 2001;29(2):277–282.
7. Puntillo, KA, Stannard D: The intensive care unit. In Ferrell B, Coyle N (eds): Palliative Nursing. New York, Oxford University Press. 2001.
8. Puntillo, KA, White C, Morris A, et al: Patients' perceptions and responses to procedural pain: results from Thunder II Project. Am J Crit Care 2001;10(4):238–251.

Robin L. Fainsinger, MD

PATIENT 20 ʹ

A 65-year-old man with metastatic lung cancer and decreasing oral fluid intake during home hospice care

A 65-year-old man with non-small cell lung cancer has developed metastases to the liver, thoracolumbar spine, and right femur. After receiving radiotherapy to the chest and bones, he has decided to discontinue further oncologic treatment and enter home care by the local hospice organization. He lives in a single-level house with his wife. They have further support from two daughters and their respective families who live locally. The visiting hospice nurse and physician have extensively discussed the goals of care with the patient and his family. The patient has indicated a desire to die at home, which his family supports. Both he and his family indicate that in keeping him comfortable they are willing to accept the advice of the hospice team.

The main problem has been pain management, which had been well controlled with a long-acting morphine dose of 150 mg twice a day. Other medications have included a regular laxative and an occasional antiemetic. The patient has become increasingly cachetic and asthenic, resulting in decreased mobility with the ability to spend only short periods of time sitting in a bedside chair. His oral intake has decreased due to difficulty swallowing and necessitating a switch of his oral morphine to a continuous subcutaneous infusion of 100 mg in 24 hrs (4 mg/hr) using a pain pump. The patient is able to give himself subcutaneous breakthrough doses of 10 mg, which he uses one to three times per day.

One week after the pain pump was started, the hospice physician makes a home visit. The patient is drowsy, but he is still able to discuss his care. His oral intake of fluids has decreased to a few sips a day. He describes increasing visual hallucinations and intermittent confusion. He reports frequent jerking of his arms and legs, which disturbs him during the day and sometimes awakens him at night. He complains of a dry mouth that is relieved by sucking ice cubes. His urine output has decreased simultaneously with his decreased fluid intake.

During the visit, the two daughters arrive. The family is increasingly concerned about their ability to look after their husband and father at home if the myoclonus, hallucinations, and confusion increase in severity. One of the daughters has found information on an internet site that suggests parenteral hydration can be given at home using a technique called hypodermoclysis. The other daughter is concerned that the description of this technique sounds overly complex for home use, and wonders if there is an alternative approach.

Question: What would be appropriate information regarding different management approaches to suggest to this patient and his family?

Diagnosis: Metastatic lung cancer with risks for progressive dehydration.

Discussion: The circumstances described in this patient and family situation highlight some of the complexities that surround the controversial and widely debated topic of hydration at end of life. At the core of the debate is a common desire to keep patients as comfortable as possible while avoiding unnecessary interventions. As we attempt to make these decisions, we need to evaluate expressions of opinion, information on pathophysiology and biochemical changes, research that looks at a variety of outcomes, family and cultural expectations, as well as reviews and consensus statements that have been published on this topic. We then have to take this diverse and sometimes conflicting information and attempt to apply it to the specific circumstances, location, and cultural backgrounds of our patients.

There is no controversy that terminally ill patients should be encouraged to maintain adequate oral hydration. The controversy revolves around the use of supplemental parenteral hydration. Although there are many published reports illustrating opposing perspectives, arguments for and against parenteral hydration in advanced illness have been summarized. The arguments for avoiding parenteral hydration include assertions that dehydration is a natural process at the end of life and does not cause symptom distress. It may actually contribute to the release of endogenous anesthetics. Dehydration also decreases urine output and lessens the need for bladder catheters, decreases gastrointestinal fluid, and lessens nausea and vomiting. Dehydration also alleviates respiratory problems, such as cough and pulmonary edema, and attenuates peripheral edema and ascites. Efforts to prevent dehydration by the administration of parenteral hydration may prolong the dying process and contribute to discomforts related to decreased mobility due to intravenous or alimentary catheters.

Arguments favoring parenteral hydration include assertions that patients are more comfortable when dehydration is alleviated. Purported benefits include fewer complaints of dry mouth and thirst and diminished confusion and restlessness. Proponents of parenteral hydration contend that no evidence exists to suggest that fluids prolong the dying process and that it represents a minimum standard of care. They voice concerns that withholding parenteral hydration to dying patients may detract from efforts to improve patient comfort and life quality and may be a dangerous precedent, leading to withholding therapies to other compromised patient groups.

Most terminally ill patients dying in hospitals worldwide have an intravenous line in place at the time of death, unless they have experienced a rapid deterioration or unexpected demise. This intravenous access presents a risk for excessive infusions of fluids by unthinking policies of intravenous hydration for cachectic cancer patients. Associated complications include respiratory and gastrointestinal distress, whose occurrence enters the arguments against parenteral hydration. Health care professionals looking after terminally ill patients have reacted to the generalized use of intravenous fluids and perceived negative effects of this management strategy by reporting their observations that avoiding parenteral hydration has not been noted to cause symptom distress in these patients.

However, we also need to recognize that dehydration causes confusion and restlessness in nonterminal patients and that problems of delirium and agitation are often reported in terminally ill patients. Moreover, reduced intravascular volume and associated decreases in glomerular filtration rates can precipitate pre-renal azotemia. Opioid metabolites can then accumulate in the setting of reduced renal excretion, which causes patient confusion, myoclonus, and seizures. These observations have supported the argument that dehydration is a potentially reversible component of these symptoms. Failure to address hydration may contribute to a misguided use of drug therapy to manage symptoms associated with dehydration. It could be considered illogical for a patient to receive medications for myoclonus, seizures, and agitated delirium when these problems could be prevented or resolved with parenteral hydration.

Research into the use of hydration in palliative care settings has tended to focus on three dimensions: 1) the association between biochemical findings and hydration status; 2) biochemical findings and clinical symptoms; and 3) hydration status and clinical symptoms. Research evidence to date has not shown an association between levels of dehydration and symptoms such as dry mouth or thirst. However, there is evidence suggesting that rehydration with 1 to 1.5 liters/day may improve renal function at the end of life, and some evidence indicates that providing parenteral hydration may play a part in the reversal of delirium.

Many articles critical of parenteral hydration in terminally ill patients have only referred to the use of the intravenous route. The use of subcutaneous infusion, commonly called hypodermoclysis, has been well documented and reported in both cancer and non-cancer populations. Reports have recommended the use of solutions with electrolytes, because nonelectrolyte solutions may draw fluid into the interstitial space. Continuous infusions up to 100 mL/hr and bolus infusions of up to 500 mL/hr two to three times per day are well tolerated. Some have recommended the addition of hyaluronidase to these fluids; however, a recent report suggests that hypodermoclysis without hyaluronidase is well tolerated in most patients.

Considering the situation of the present patient, we can anticipate that the manner in which information will be presented to him and his family remains open to the interpretation of the literature and the biases of the health care providers. It would seem reasonable to state that dehydration is a recognized cause of renal failure and that hypodermoclysis is a safe, effective, and well-tolerated way of providing parenteral hydration to him in the home. We could anticipate that by providing hypodermoclysis to the present patient, he may achieve better urine output and an improvement in his renal function, with the result that the opioids accumulating in his system might decrease. This could then result in improvement of his myoclonus, hallucinations, and perhaps the maintenance of better cognition for a limited period of time. The alternative would be to point out that by providing parenteral hydration, we may increase the complexity of care that his family has to provide and that any benefits will likely be short-lived. We could recommend that every effort be made to encourage oral fluid intake, while the opioid dose is decreased. The patient's complaints of pain, as well as problems related to myoclonus, hallucinations, and confusion can be carefully monitored with appropriate further decreases of the opioid dose for the duration of the patient's illness. Whereas the conflicting reviews and consensus statements in this area highlight the unresolved debate, careful individual assessment of the relevance of dehydration to each clinical situation is required.

After a full discussion of the management options, the patient and family requested the initiation of parenteral hydration with hypodermoclysis at 60 ml/hr and a decrease in the morphine infusion to 60 mg in 24 hrs. If the patient's pain returned, it was planned to rotate the patient to a different opioid drug to decrease side effects.

Clinical Pearls

1. Hallucinations, altered sensorium, and myoclonus are common in dying patients, especially those receiving opiates.

2. Dehydration is a cause of delirium and renal failure, while opioid metabolites accumulating in the presence of renal failure are known to cause significant side effects.

3. Parenteral hydration may be helpful for some dying patients. Although there remains controversy surrounding the role of parenteral hydration in terminally ill patients, hypodermoclysis is safe, easy to administer, and well tolerated by many patients.

4. Individual assessment is required in deciding to provide parenteral hydration and/or decreased medications to avoid unnecessary and problematic side effects.

REFERENCES

1. Fainsinger RL, Bruera E. Hypodermoclysis for symptom control vs the Edmonton injector. J Palliat Care 1991;7:5–8.
2. Fainsinger RL, Bruera E. The management of dehydration in terminally ill patients. J Palliat Care 1994;10:55–59.
3. Dunphy K, Finlay I, Rathbone G, et al. Rehydration in palliative and terminal care: if not, why not? Palliat Med 1995;9:221–228.
4. Amadori D, Bruera E, Cozagloi L, et al. Guidelines on artificial nutrition versus hydration in terminal cancer patients. Nutrition 1996;12(3):163–167.
5. Fainsinger RL, Bruera E. When to treat dehydration in a terminally ill patient? Support Care Cancer 1997;5:205–211.
6. National Council for Hospice and Specialist Palliative Care Services. Artificial hydration (AH) for people who are terminally ill. Eur J Palliat Care 1997;4(4):124.
7. Steiner N, Bruera E. Methods of hydration in palliative care patients. J Palliat Care 1998;14(2):6–13.
8. Centeno C, Bruera E. Subcutaneous hydration with no hyaluronidase in patients with advanced cancer. J Pain Symptom Manage 1999;17(5):305–306.
9. Morita T, Ichiki T, Tsunoda J, et al.Three dimensions of the rehydration—dehydration problem in a palliative care setting. J Palliat Care 1999;15(2):60–61.
10. Lawlor PG, Gagnon B, Mancini IL, et al. Occurrence, causes, and outcome of delirium in patients with advanced cancer. Arch Intern Med 2000;160:786–794.

Michael W. Rabow, MD

PATIENT 21

A 73-year-old woman with ovarian cancer who asks "Why me?"

A 73-year-old woman with well-controlled hypertension and hypercholesterolemia complains to her long-standing primary care physician of fatigue and abdominal fullness over the prior 3 weeks. Previously well and actively involved with her five grandchildren, she has been married for 49 years and shares many hobbies with her husband. She is a clarinetist and played for many years in an internationally acclaimed orchestra. A Catholic by birth, she has not attended church since getting married.

Physical Examination: Vital signs normal. General: somewhat fatigued elderly woman. Chest: clear. Cardiac: regular rhythm, no gallop. Abdomen: distended, nontender, with shifting dullness. Pelvic: right adnexal fullness.

Laboratory Findings: Hematocrit 30%, WBC 7,200/μl. Ultrasound pelvis and abdomen: right adnexal mass and moderate ascites. Paracentesis: large numbers of malignant-appearing cells in the peritoneal fluid.

Clinical Course: The patient consults an oncologist and undergoes a complete diagnostic and staging work-up that reveals widely metastatic ovarian cancer. The patient returns to her primary care physician for follow-up in obvious emotional distress, exclaiming that "now there is no hope." She continues, "How could this happen to me, after living such a good life? Who will take care of my husband? My youngest grandchildren won't even remember me when I'm gone."

Question: Can her primary care physician help relieve the patient's suffering and even promote her well-being at the end of life?

Diagnosis: Existential and spiritual suffering at the end of life.

Discussion: Spiritual or existential suffering often occurs when disease or death threatens a person's sense of integrity. The looming threat of mortality may profoundly challenge a patient's sense of meaning in the universe. Although physicians cannot "fix" their patients' existential crises, there is much that can be done to help alleviate suffering. Dying may even present certain emotional and existential opportunities to patients. Ultimately, even in the context of profound loss, physicians may be able to catalyze hope and promote existential growth at the end of life.

The physician's ability to help patients who are suffering is linked to the strength of the patient-physician therapeutic alliance. Addressing the existential pain and emotional vulnerability commonly experienced at the end of life requires a safe and trusting relationship. An explicit confirmation of the alliance is the physician's spoken **promise of non-abandonment**: "No matter what happens, I will be here to help in any way that I can."

Simple listening, reflection, and validation can be powerful interventions for suffering patients. Sharing a few moments in **silence** is a potent expression of the physician's empathy and willingness to bear witness to the reality and intensity of the patient's distress. To best be of service, physicians must **understand the individual patient's unique experience** of illness and suffering. It is usually helpful to ask patients open-ended questions about their understanding of their illness and the feelings it engenders. An invitation to, "Tell me more about what this is like for you," may prompt patients to articulate their personal experience, priorities, and values.

At the end of life, many patients describe a "good death" as one that includes maintaining personal continuity, enhancing relationships, finding meaning, achieving a sense of control, and confronting and preparing for death. It may not be possible for patients to wholly resolve existential suffering; however, gentle guidance and attention to six specific strategies may allow physicians to help alleviate it:

1. **Finding Strength:** Physicians can help patients identify sustaining personal strengths and social supports. Together, physician and patient can explore successful coping strategies from prior experiences. Physicians can help arrange specific resources, including physician follow-up, social work, support groups, and reading material, that bolster a patient's strengths or compensate for weaknesses.
2. **Enhancing Growth:** Patients may be able to compensate for real or anticipated losses. Questions such as "Even though there are some things you can no longer do, what activities can you still enjoy?" or "What else is possible here?" may expand a patient's sense of limitation.
3. **Embracing the Moment:** Some suffering is due to the sense of a limited and unbearable future. Focusing on the present moment may preempt that suffering. Setting priorities is important ("Is there something you've always wished you could do? Why not do it now?"). Encouraging meditation may be helpful as a means of developing a sense of personal well-being in the present moment and as an internal resource for personal comfort in difficult times. Clinical interventions can be planned around a patient's personal needs.
4. **Searching for Meaning:** Suffering may be transformed if the patient grasps from it a sense of transpersonal meaning. As the psychiatrist Viktor Frankl said, "In some way, suffering ceases to be suffering at the moment it finds a meaning." Physicians may ask, "How have you made sense of what is happening here?" or "What would allow you to find a purpose in this?" Life review, journal writing, and revisiting the past through photos and stories may help patients understand the meaning of illness in their life and their concept of the universe. The opportunity to contribute to others or leave a legacy may become profoundly important to patients at the end of life.
5. **Seeking Acceptance and Reconciliation:** For some, accepting suffering may be the first step in overcoming it. Acceptance may allow a change of focus to the tasks of completion and closure at the end of life. As life ends, some patients may seek reconciliation with estranged love ones and find in these reunions unexpected benefits, despite the tragedy of illness. Gently exploring regret, guilt, and shame may help patients identify the sources of estrangement in their lives: "Is there someone you really want to talk to before you die?"
6. **Achieving Transformation:** For some patients, facing death and exploring previously unanalyzed, unresolved conflict may actually lead to a deep sense of peace, completion, or spiritual transformation. Physicians may encourage emotional and spiritual activities (such as art, prayer, visits with loved ones, and spiritual mentoring) to help patients open themselves to these possibilities.

Invariably, serious illness raises the question of hope for both patients and physicians. While false or unrealistic hopes may be counterproductive, **hope may be defined as** *what is still possible.*

Framed this way, there is always hope and physicians can help patients search for what is still possible for them. Hopes may change as clinical conditions develop. The hope to be able to live many more years may transition to the hope to enjoy an upcoming wedding anniversary or to see a lifelong friend one last time.

The present patient consulted an oncologist but decided not to pursue attempts to reverse her illness, focusing instead on symptom management alone. In seeking palliative care, the patient realistically understood her illness and had begun the process of accepting what was possible medically.

Existentially however, the patient expressed significant distress, including confusion about the meaning of her illness and her place in the universe ("Why me?"). She also described a sense of unfinished business with those she loves. Her physician did not attempt to answer her questions, but rather responded to them with expressions of support and empathy ("How painful to have lived a good life and still get such a terrible illness. I am so sorry this has happened to you."). The physician prescribed Dr. Frankl's book, *Man's Search for Meaning,* which the patient read. She talked openly with her husband about her fears and received his reassurance about how much he had learned from her. In her last months, the patient began to focus on saying goodbye and considered her physician's suggestion about leaving a tangible legacy. The patient decided that she wished to leave each grandchild a gift of her recorded music. In revisiting her old symphony recordings, she experienced a profound sense of accomplishment and was enlivened by the opportunity to share her love of music in a lasting way.

Clinical Pearls

1. Patients may be deeply reassured by a physician's promise of non-abandonment.

2. Physicians can bear witness with simple listening and offer empathetic silence to patients who are suffering.

3. Helping patients find strength, enhance growth, embrace the moment, search for meaning, seek acceptance and reconciliation, and achieve transformation may help alleviate suffering.

4. In the face of existential suffering, hope for *what is still possible* always remains.

5. Growth is possible at the end of life, and physicians can help catalyze it.

REFERENCES
1. Frankl VE. Man's Search for Meaning. Boston: Beacon Press; 1959.
2. Cassell EJ. The nature of suffering and the goals of medicine. N Engl J Med 1982;306:639–645.
3. Quill TE, Cassel CK. Nonabandonment: a central obligation for physicians. Ann Intern Med 1995;122:368–374.
4. Byock I. Dying Well: The Prospect for Growth at the End of Life. New York: Riverhead Books; 1997.
5. Rabow MW, McPhee SJ. Beyond breaking bad news: how to help patients who suffer. West J Med 1999;171:260–263.
6. Block SD. Perspectives on care at the close of life: psychological considerations, growth, and transcendence at the end of life: the art of the possible. JAMA 2001;285:2898–2905.

Jerome Kurent, MD
Rosalyn DeWitt-Marshall, MD

PATIENT 22

A 78-year-old African-American man who is experiencing uncontrolled pain at the end of life

A 78-year-old man of African-American heritage is being evaluated for home hospice care. Eighteen months earlier, he was diagnosed with metastatic colon cancer and underwent a course of poorly tolerated chemotherapy. He has subsequently experienced persistent bone pain and recurrent abdominal discomfort. Both the patient and his wife have strong spiritual beliefs and prefer to leave his medical future "in God's hands." They have maintained limited contact with the patient's primary care physician, who had started long-acting opioid analgesics and nonsteroidal anti-inflammatory drugs for the patient's pain. Recently, the patient has been taking these medications only intermittently.

As the patient experiences more frequent and severe pain as well as emotional distress associated with functional decline, his physician recommends hospice referral. The patient's wife states that she did not want hospice to replace her role as family caregiver. She considers hospice care as an expression of "giving up." The patient also declines to complete a formal written advance directive. The primary care physician suggests that the patient have a do-not-resuscitate status, but the patient requests that "everything be done" to prolong his life.

With continued functional decline, the patient and his wife eventually agree to enroll in home hospice on a trial basis. The hospice nursing staff evaluates the patient and suspects that he is experiencing more pain than he is willing to acknowledge. Although there are nonverbal indications of ongoing pain, such as grimacing and agitation, the patient does not wish to describe his discomfort to the nurse or request additional pain medications.

Question: What factors should the hospice nurse consider in formulating a treatment plan?

Diagnosis: Persistent pain at the end of life with ethnic and cultural barriers to effective pain control.

Discussion: Ethnicity and cultural diversity have an important impact on the needs of patient and family caregivers during terminal illness. Problems with access to care and knowledge of services available at the end-of-life often plague poor, medically underserved and economically disadvantaged minority communities.

Hospice is greatly underutilized in African-American communities. African-American patients represent only 8% to 10% of all hospice enrollees. This low participation reflects limited knowledge of the role of hospice in end-of-life care. Consequently, they fail to receive adequate pain and symptom control during the terminal phases of disease.

Members of the African-American community also frequently indicate a reluctance to complete formal written advance directives. Underutilization of advance directives by this community appears to be based on several factors, which include mistrust of the medical establishment, taboos about death and dying, and strongly held religious views. Low socioeconomic conditions among some African-American communities also contribute to the underutilization of advance directives, as in other ethnic groups. The hopes for divine intervention or a miracle often influence treatment decisions by terminally ill patients and family caregivers.

Studies indicate that African-American patients often express strong preferences to undergo life-prolonging procedures and to "do everything" to prolong life. If the issue of withdrawing life support is raised by the physician, the reply sometimes is "it should be left in God's hands." Some family members may express concerns that completing a written advance directive may provide a reason to limit care at the end-of-life.

Although 80% to 90% of the American population select home as the preferred place of death, significantly fewer African-Americans express this preference. Up to one-third of African-American patients may not wish to die at home and prefer that death occurs in an institutional setting. This preference should be considered when caring for terminally ill patients. When death becomes imminent, hospice agencies should consider admittance to a health care facility to honor the patient's as well as the family's wishes.

Reduced expectations for pain and symptom control are especially evident in the geriatric African-American population. These lower expectations may arise from past experiences with dying family members and friends who had unrelieved pain and other symptoms. Some patients and families assume that pain is an inevitable and necessary part of the dying process. Patients and family caregivers also express the belief that God may be testing the patient's faith. Consequently, the patient may be reluctant to request and accept adequate pain control interventions. In contrast, younger African-Americans express a much stronger desire for adequate pain control as compared with older numbers of their community. These lowered expectations also exist within other minority groups as well.

Physicians should actively inquire whether pain is present and evaluate its severity because approximately 90% of pain at the end of life can be adequately managed. Active efforts focusing on pain assessment and management are an obligation of the physician caring for terminally ill patients, who may otherwise choose to suffer in silence.

The present patient exemplifies several aspects of the influence of African-American ethnicity and culture on end-of-life care. The patient and his wife were initially reluctant to accept hospice service, which was equated with "giving up." Additionally, the wife wished to remain her husband's primary source of support and care. The patient and family also show that reassurance and education by the physician can alleviate these concerns and encourage patients to accept effective end-of-life care.

The patient enrolled in a hospice home-care program that provided a comprehensive regimen for symptom control. The patient still only intermittently requested pain medications and died 6 weeks later in his sleep. After his death, his wife acknowledged that he had experienced considerable pain during his last days of life. Despite this pain, she emphasized that both she and her husband were very satisfied with the care they received. She indicated that his strong faith had helped him endure the pain, which he interpreted as God's way of testing his faith. She also considered pain to be a normal part of the dying process.

Clinical Pearls

1. Hospice is greatly underutilized by terminally ill African-American patients. Physicians should explain to patients and their families that the role of hospice is to provide comfort care and to maximize quality of remaining life, and not to replace the role of family caregiver.

2. Spirituality plays a powerful role in the African-American community and may influence a patient's acceptance of end-of-life care interventions. Pain is sometimes interpreted as a test of one's faith. In a manner that respects African-American values and within the context of their spiritual world view, patients and their families should be encouraged to accept pain control interventions.

3. Geriatric patients often accept untreated pain as an inevitable part of growing old and the dying process. These cultural issues and resistance to routine symptom treatments require skillful communication and a proactive approach by the physician utilizing pain assessment instruments and appropriate therapeutic interventions.

4. Advance care planning and decision-making is often a family decision. Although reluctance to complete written advance directives often exists, the physician should encourage patient and family discussions regarding advance care planning.

REFERENCES

1. Caralis PV, Davis B, Wright K, Marcial E. The influence of ethnicity and race on attitudes toward advance directives, life-prolonging treatments, and euthanasia. J Clin Ethics 1993;4:155–165.
2. Kumasaka L, Miles A. "My pain is God's will." Am J Nurs 1996;96:45–47.
3. McKinley ED, Garrett JM, Evans AT, Davis M. Differences in end-of-life decision-making among black and white ambulatory cancer patients. J Gen Intern Med 1996;11:651–656.
4. Hospice Care: A Physician's Guide. National Hospice Organization, 1998.
5. Blackhall LJ, Frank G, Murphy ST, et al. Ethnicity and attitudes towards life sustaining technology. Soc Sci Med 1999;48:1779–1789.
6. Mebane EW, Oman RF, Kroonen LT, Goldstein MK. The influence of physician race, age, and gender on physician attitudes toward advance care directives and preferences for end-of-life decision-making. J Am Geriatr Soc 1999;47:579–591.
7. Reese DJ, Ahern RE, Nair S, et al. Hospice access and use by African-Americans: addressing cultural and institutional barriers through participatory action research. Soc Work 1999;44:549–559.
8. Crawley L, Payne R, Bolden J, et al. Palliative and end-of-life care in the African-American community. JAMA 2000;284:2518–2521.
9. Schmidt LM. Why cultural issues must be recognized at the end-of-life. Last Acts 2001:(winter).

John E. Heffner, MD

PATIENT 23

A 75-year-old man with a DNR order who requires transport to the radiology department for a procedure

A 75-year-old man with a history of pancreatic cancer is hospitalized because of nausea, vomiting, and painless jaundice. He had developed abdominal pain 5 months ago and underwent an abdominal CT scan that demonstrated a 5-cm mass in the midportion of his pancreas. Because of his advanced age and coexisting severe emphysema, with his family's agreement, the patient requested no further evaluation or treatment and entered home hospice care. His pain was treated successfully with oral analgesics. He had remained homebound but able to eat until the onset of his present symptoms.

Physical Examination: Vital signs: normal. General: thin appearing male with jaundice. Skin: decreased turgor. Neck: elevated neck veins. Chest: decreased breath sounds, hyper-resonant to percussion. Cardiac: parasternal lift, right-sided S3. Abdomen: tender in the epigastrium. Extremities: 2+ ankle pitting edema. Neurologic: alert.

Laboratory findings: Hct 28%, WBC 8,000/μl. Bilirubin 5 mg/dl. BUN 35 mg/dl, creatinine 2.5 mg/dl. Chest radiograph: hyperinflated lung fields with flat diaphragms.

Course: The physicians consider that the patient's symptoms are due to tumor extension with obstruction of the common bile duct. They order an abdominal CT scan in preparation for placement of a palliative stent. A do-not-resuscitate (DNR) status is ordered in compliance with the patient's and family's wishes. As the patient is being prepared for transfer to the radiology department, the family asks the nurse how personnel in radiology would be aware of the patient's DNR status and what safeguards against unwanted resuscitation would be in place.

Question: How should the nurse respond to the family? What safeguards are warranted in this setting?

Diagnosis: Pancreatic cancer with biliary obstruction in a patient who refuses resuscitation in all clinical circumstances.

Discussion: Because the default response of caregivers to patients who develop cardiopulmonary arrest includes the initiation of advanced cardiopulmonary life support, patients who do not desire life supportive interventions must communicate their wishes to their physicians. Physicians then communicate the patient's wishes to other healthcare providers who may be called upon to evaluate and treat the patient if a sudden life-threatening event occurs. DNR orders are intended to communicate these wishes to all caregivers and to implement the wishes of patients to refuse life-sustaining interventions.

Unfortunately, DNR orders often fail in their purpose of safeguarding patients against undesired life-prolonging interventions. In some hospitals, DNR orders have become complex, allowing some but not all life-supportive interventions for patients in certain clinical circumstances. For instance, some patients may accept electrical cardioversion for a cardiac arrhythmia but refuse intubation and mechanical ventilation. Because of these complexities, bedside caregivers may differ in their understanding of a patient's specific wishes. For instance, several studies have demonstrated that housestaff, nurses, and attending physicians often have differing interpretations of the implications of DNR orders with regard to the events that would trigger specific components of advanced life support. Additionally, attending physicians often exercise license in interpreting whether patients with a DNR order would still desire life-supportive interventions in certain circumstances. Many physicians, for example, do not believe that a DNR order encompasses a life-threatening condition that arises from an iatrogenic event.

Procedures for implementing DNR orders for hospitalized patients have traditionally focused on caregivers who provide bedside care and do not include hospital employees and caregivers who interact with patients during transfer for surgery or other procedures. Consequently, some physicians have argued that DNR orders should be routinely suspended for patients who choose to undergo surgical procedures. Although controversy still exists regarding DNR orders in the operating room, recent guidelines emphasize the importance of honoring patients' DNR wishes. If surgeons or anesthesiologists want to abridge a DNR order, ethical consensus emphasizes the importance of discussing treatment options with the patient and clearly establishing a mutually agreeable planned response to life-threatening events before transfer to the operating room.

Safeguards for patients with DNR orders who wish to avoid CPR and who are transported away from their ward or ICU beds for nonoperative procedures are less well developed, compared with procedures for honoring DNR status in the operating room. A recent study, for example, demonstrated that 80% of radiology departments in acute care hospitals do not have written protocols describing their responses to patients with DNR orders who develop cardiopulmonary arrest while in radiology. Consequently, the radiology departments surveyed in the study reflected varying responses to life-threatening events in such patients. Nearly 25% of departments routinely initiate CPR for patients with DNR orders, and 40% have resuscitated patients despite a DNR order being in place.

These observations indicate a need for procedures to safeguard patients' wishes when they choose to avoid resuscitation attempts during an admission to an acute care hospital. Such policies should inform patients as to the response of caregivers if a patient with a DNR order develops a cardiopulmonary arrest during transport. Policies should also specify the need for negotiating DNR status with patients in special circumstances in which caregivers would consider a DNR order inappropriate during transport. A central principle is full disclosure to the patient regarding what they should expect to experience while being transported for procedures.

The nurse for the present patient could not address the family's concerns. She had never before been asked these questions and simply did not know if policies existed or what directions they might contain. She contacted the attending physician, who called the radiologist scheduled to supervise the CT scan. Having communicated the patient's DNR status and having received reassurance that it would be honored in the radiology department, the attending physician instructed the nurse to inform the patient. The nurse called the radiology supervisor to inform him of the patient's DNR status. This event stimulated the hospital to develop a policy that communicated patients' DNR orders during transport and ensured their end-of-life wishes.

Clinical Pearls

1. A DNR order is intended to safeguard a patient's end-of-life wishes in all circumstances intended by the patient.

2. Hospitalized patients may be at risk of undergoing undesired resuscitation during an operative procedure or during transport away from their bedside unless their DNR status is understood and honored by all caregivers and hospital personnel.

3. The response of radiology department personnel to patients with DNR orders who develop a cardiopulmonary event serves as a model for understanding the risk of unwanted resuscitation. Radiology department directors have indicated in survey studies that they would disregard a patient's DNR status in nearly 25% of instances if resuscitation appeared necessary. Nearly 40% of departments have resuscitated patients despite a DNR order being in place.

4. Hospitals can safeguard patients' end-of-life wishes by developing policies for implementing DNR orders during patient transport away from their hospital beds.

REFERENCES

1. La Puma J, Silverstein MD, Stocking CB, et al. Life-sustaining treatment: a prospective study of patients with DNR orders in a teaching hospital. Arch Intern Med 1988;148:2193–2195.
2. Committee on Ethics American College of Surgeons. Statement of advance directives by patients: do not resuscitate in the operating room. Am Coll Surg Bull 1994;79:29.
3. Ethical guidelines for the anesthesia care of patients with do not resuscitate orders or other directives that limit treatment. In American Society of Anesthesiologists 1994 Directory of Members, 59th ed. Park Ridge, IL: American Society of Anesthesiologists; 1994: pp 746–747.
4. Heffner JE, Barbieri C, Casey K. Procedure-specific do-not-resuscitate orders: effect on communication of treatment limitations. Arch Intern Med 1996;156(7):793–797.
5. Jacobson JA, Gully JE, Mann H. "Do not resuscitate" orders in the radiology department: an interpretation. Radiology 1996;198:21–24.
6. Terry PB. Resuscitation and radiology [editorial, comment]. Radiology 1996;198(1):17–8.
7. Casarett D, Ross LF. Overriding a patient's refusal of treatment after an iatrogenic complication. N Engl J Med 1997;336:1908–1910.
8. Heffner JE, Barbieri C. Compliance with do-not-resuscitate orders for hospitalized patients transported to radiology departments. Ann Intern Med 1998;129:801–805.
9. Truog RD, Waisel DB, Burns JP. DNR in the OR: a goal-directed approach. Anesthesiology 1999;90:289–295.

Bonnie F. Fahy, RN, MN

PATIENT 24

A 64-year-old man with COPD and disabling dyspnea enters pulmonary rehabilitation contemplating euthanasia

A 64-year-old man with chronic obstructive pulmonary disease (COPD) is referred to outpatient pulmonary rehabilitation because of profound exertional dyspnea that limits his ability to perform simple activities of daily living. He had worked as a mechanic until 6 months ago, when he stopped working because of intolerable dyspnea. He has never been hospitalized and has not received any information on symptom management other than instruction in the use of an albuterol metered-dose inhaler. Because of profound dyspnea and an inability to work, he describes his quality of life as unacceptable.

During the initial assessment by the pulmonary rehab coordinator, he describes having watched his father slowly smother as he died from COPD. The patient states that he does not want to experience the same death. He further asserts he does not understand what is wrong with his lungs or what his medications are supposed to do. Because he can see no alternative to spending his remaining years in "misery," he is interested in looking into euthanasia. He also thinks that enrollment in pulmonary rehabilitation is futile and will not improve his condition.

The patient has not discussed his prognosis or end-of-life concerns with his physician because his physician was always "too busy." He has not executed a durable power of attorney for health care and is unaware of its purpose. For the last several months, he has contemplated completing a living will that states he would approve of no life support under any circumstances; as of yet, however, he has not obtained a living will form. He agrees to complete the entire pulmonary rehabilitation program before pursuing any other options to end his discomfort.

Question: Does pulmonary rehabilitation have a role in education about advance care planning?

Diagnosis: Patient with far-advanced COPD in need of symptom management and assistance with end-of-life planning.

Discussion: The circumstances of this frustrated patient are representative of many patients entering an outpatient pulmonary rehabilitation program. Most newly enrolled patients have little to no understanding of their lung disease or therapies, fear the progression of their pulmonary disease and associated symptoms, and have limited insight into advance care planning and who can advise them on end-of-life care. Consequently, many patients with moderate to severe lung disease experience persistent dyspnea that they assume will progress at the end of life, causing them to "suffocate to death." This concern is a central fear considering that freedom from shortness of breath is ranked high among respiratory patients who describe what they would wish to experience at the end of life.

Pulmonary rehabilitation provides multiple benefits for such patients. The primary goal of pulmonary rehab is to restore the patient to the highest possible level of independent function. Patients and their families learn about their disease, therapeutic options, and strategies to assist in coping with their respiratory conditions. Patients also gain insights into becoming more actively involved in managing their own health care and less dependent on health care providers and expensive medical interventions. Pulmonary rehabilitation focuses less on reversing the disease process and more on improving the patient's disability. In so doing, patients experience less ungrounded fears and anxieties and gain an ability to take more charge of their lives.

Fortunately, most patients with chronic lung disease experience improvement in their shortness of breath when they receive instruction in breathing strategies during enrollment in pulmonary rehabilitation. The instruction of pursed lip and abdominal breathing and the application of these techniques to panic control are essential and effective components of pulmonary rehabilitation. Assessments of a patient's respiratory status and resulting global functional limitations and capacity are incorporated within individualized care planning for each patient. This knowledge and process can correct misconceptions, allay many needless fears, and establish a base upon which the rationale for therapeutic interventions for ongoing care and end-of-life planning can be applied. The realization that the diagnosis of a chronic lung disease alone does not imply imminent death is a comfort to many patients. Gaining this knowledge is frequently said to "lift a burden of the unknown" and allow patients to go forward with future planning that includes end-of-life decision-making.

Another essential component of a pulmonary rehabilitation program is exercise training. Improved exercise tolerance teamed with panic control techniques gives patients a sense of control over their lung disease and a lessened degree of disability and handicap. Improved activity levels allow patients to formulate comprehensive advance care planning with an enhanced sense of well-being, rather than from circumstances of dependency and "misery" that influence the end-of-life choices of some patients.

In the pulmonary rehabilitation curriculum, comprehensive therapeutic interventions are discussed, in addition to the proper technique of using an inhaled bronchodilator. Supplemental oxygen, noninvasive ventilation, and airway intubation with mechanical ventilation are reviewed. The implications of mechanical ventilation are frequently misunderstood and inappropriately feared. Educational sessions on the nature and outcomes of life-supportive care are considered valuable and are well received by the majority of patients with chronic disease. Many patients otherwise carry a misperception that once they are intubated, they will never again have the ability to breathe on their own. Also, many patients think that they do not have the right to request the removal of an endotracheal tube if extubation would result in their death. Educational curricula can provide information on the indications for use and the mechanics of assisted ventilation.

Educators within rehabilitation programs can also effectively present the ethical and legal considerations surrounding decisions to undergo ventilatory support and to request the withholding and withdrawal of life-supportive care. Patients and families are encouraged to discuss the patient's life values and goals, not only with each other but also with the patient's physician. Without knowledge of assisted ventilation and likely outcomes of life-supportive care, patients with lung disease cannot provide truly informed consent when faced with end-of-life decisions during critical illnesses.

The psychosocial component of a pulmonary rehabilitation curriculum not only deals with stress reduction techniques and the importance of communication in general, but also further prepares the patient to engage in the discussion of end-of-life issues with their family and physician. Building on the information discussed in the educational sessions that address pathophysiology and therapeutic interventions, information related to advance directives and hospice care is introduced. The differences between a durable power of attorney for health care and a living will are discussed, with sample forms available for patients and family members.

With an enhanced understanding of their lung disease gained through pulmonary rehabilitation, many patients who previously thought they would not want life support under any circumstances may accept such care in certain circumstances. Hospice care is also included in the discussion of end-of-life issues. Patients commonly think that hospice services are appropriate only when death is imminent, and that physicians should determine when hospice services should be initiated. Learning that patients or their families can introduce discussions of hospice care, that someone receiving hospice services can "graduate" from hospice without dying, and that services can be reinstituted at a later date can be very reassuring.

The present patient was receptive to the inclusion of advance planning education in his pulmonary rehabilitation curriculum. Before enrolling in pulmonary rehabilitation, he thought he had no other alternative than to seek information on euthanasia. After instruction in the proper use of his medications, coupled with the use of breathing strategies and individualized exercise training, he increased his exercise capacity, experienced an enhanced performance of activities of daily living, and ultimately returned to work. The knowledge of advance directives gained from the educational sessions resulted in the patient initiating a conversation with his wife and physician that discussed his prognosis and therapeutic alternatives for end-of-life care. The patient and his wife each completed a durable power of attorney for health care as well as a living will.

At the completion of the pulmonary rehabilitation program, the patient was only mildly limited by dyspnea and became aware that most patients with COPD who require hospitalization for respiratory failure recover after a short course of mechanical ventilation. He decided to accept life-supportive care in some clinical circumstances, which he discussed with his physician and wife.

Clinical Pearls

1. Most patients entering pulmonary rehabilitation desire a greater understanding of end-of-life care, and they consider nonphysician educators within pulmonary rehabilitation to be as acceptable as physicians for this information.

2. Pulmonary rehabilitation programs assist patients in the self-management of their disease and promote their ability to cope with their respiratory disabilities. They are valuable sites for educating patients about advanced directives and encouraging patient-physician discussions of end-of-life care.

3. Patients who have been educated as to the importance of advance care planning are more likely to complete written advance directives and to discuss their end-of-life wishes with their health care providers.

4. Goals of care can be clarified and all involved can be assured that treatment remains consistent with patients' and families' values and preferences. Alleviation of dyspnea and anxiety and professional attention to issues of life completion can enhance quality of life for those facing life's end.

REFERENCES

1. Heffner JE, Fahy B, Hilling, L, Barbieri C: Attitudes regarding advance directives among patients in pulmonary rehabilitation. Am J Respir Crit Care Med 1996;154:1735–1740.
2. Heffner JE, Fahy B, Hilling, L, Barbieri C: Outcomes of advance directive education of pulmonary rehabilitation patients. Am J Respir Crit Care Med 1997;155:1055–1059.
3. American Thoracic Society: ATS statement: pulmonary rehabilitation 1999. Am J Respir Crit Care Med 1999;159:1666–1682.
4. Larson DG, Tobin DR: End-of-life conversations: evolving practice and theory. JAMA 2000;284:1573–1578.
5. Steinhauser KE, Christakis NA, Clipp EC, et al: Factors considered important at the end of life by patients, family, physicians, and other care providers. JAMA 2000;284:2476–2482.

Joseph W. Shega, MD
Greg A. Sachs, MD

PATIENT 25

An 89-year-old woman with advanced dementia, recurrent aspiration pneumonia, and weight loss needs a feeding tube?

An 89-year-old woman who was diagnosed with Alzheimer's disease about 8 years ago presents to the hospital with aspiration pneumonia. This is one of several admissions for her for pneumonia in the past year. The patient needs assistance with feeding and all other activities of daily living. Before this admission, she spent her days in bed or sitting in a chair in the kitchen surrounded by family. She is nonambulatory, does not convey intelligible vocabulary, and is only intermittently oriented to herself. Additionally, she has lost about 10% of her body weight over the past year, although a complete evaluation did not reveal other conditions that might be contributing to her weight loss, such as medication side effects, depression, or malignancy.

Physical Examination: Blood pressure 100/60, pulse 110, respirations 32, temperature 38.8° C, transcutaneous oxygen saturation 87% on room air. General: confused, muttering incomprehensibly, agitated, occasionally striking out when approached. Oropharynx: teeth chipped, coated with tartar, and mucous membranes dry. Chest: crackles left lower lobe with dullness to percussion and tactile fremitus. Cardiac: tachycardic; no murmurs, rubs, or gallops. Abdomen: soft normoactive bowel sounds, no masses or tenderness. Skin: stage 3, clean, poorly granulating sacral ulcer; size 5 cm $\times$ 3cm $\times$ 1 cm deep.

Laboratory Findings: WBC 13,000/μl with left shift, BUN 62 mg/dl, creatinine 1.6 mg/dl, electrolytes normal. Chest radiograph: left lower lobe pneumonia.

Hospital Course: The patient receives intravenous fluids, oxygen, and antibiotics. Her pneumonia improves within 2 days and her fever, agitation, hypoxia, and elevated white count resolve. Despite this, she continues to have poor caloric intake. Optimal modification of food texture, color, flavor, and preferences has not increased intake. Furthermore, encouragement and slow hand-feeding by staff and family members have not boosted the number of calories consumed.

A speech therapist conducts a swallowing evaluation, which demonstrates moderate dysphagia consistent with her advanced dementia. The speech therapist notes in the patient's record, "The patient is at significant risk of recurrent aspiration, and a feeding tube should be considered." A routine nutritional assessment documents inadequate caloric intake. The patient's family asks whether a feeding tube should be placed, because mom is not eating and they worry about "her starving to death."

Question: Should a feeding tube be placed in this patient?

Diagnosis: Patient dying from the complications of dementia.

Discussion: Dementia is characterized by an impairment of memory, plus impairment in at least one other of the following cognitive domains: language, abstract thinking, judgment, planning, or visual-spatial skills. Diagnostic criteria also require loss of function at work, in a social setting, or at home. Dementia increases in prevalence with age. By age 65, about 10% of community-dwelling older adults are affected, and this proportion increases to almost 50% by age 85. It is projected that, as our society ages, the number of persons suffering with dementia will grow from the approximately 4 million today to 14 million by 2050.

Despite being so common among older adults, dementia is often not recognized as a terminal illness. Instead, dementia is frequently described as a disease that people die *with*, rather than something they die *from*. Yet, studies show persons with advanced dementia have a much higher mortality than those without cognitive impairment. For instance, hospitalized acutely ill patients with advanced dementia have a fourfold increase in 6-month mortality when admitted with a diagnosis of pneumonia or hip fracture compared to age-matched, cognitively intact patients with the same diagnosis.

Thus, patients with advanced dementia can either die from the dementia, or the dementia may be a major contributor to the cause of an acute event that leads to death. Common impairments in this latter group include immobility, inability to provide self-care, loss of interest in food or things that previously provided pleasure, and a decline of coordinated tasks such as swallowing, gait, or continence. These impairments predispose patients to decreased oral intake, aspiration of materials, skin breakdown, and infections (pneumonia and urinary tract infection most commonly). Undoubtedly, the combination of neurocognitive decline and the predisposition to many illnesses lead to a high mortality. Indeed, when physicians, other health care providers, and relatives of persons with dementia were surveyed, a majority in each group favored a palliative care approach for persons with advanced dementia.

The current patient seems to be an ideal candidate for palliative care. She presented to the emergency room with recurrent aspiration pneumonia. Advanced dementia patients are at higher risk for aspiration pneumonia for a multitude of reasons, including cricopharyngeal incoordination, decreased esophageal motility, altered lower esophageal sphincter tone exacerbated by an array of medications, and impaired gastric emptying. Usual measures of elevating the head of the bed lack effectiveness, as patients frequently assume a fetal position. Despite this, physicians, nurses, dieticians, and speech therapists often recommend placing a feeding tube to decrease aspiration. However, studies do not support the efficacy of tube placement. In fact, some studies indicate patients might aspirate more frequently after placement of a feeding tube. This increased risk may be due to lowered esophageal sphincter pressure after feeding tube placement and an altered gastroesophageal angle. Finally, feeding tube placement does not decrease the aspiration of oropharyngeal secretions.

In addition to the lack of impact on the risk of aspiration pneumonia, artificial nutrition and hydration may not extend life to a significant extent. The mortality rate among patients over age 60 receiving feeding tubes is very high. A recent prospective community-based study recruited all patients over age 60 referred for feeding tube placement. In that study, the 60-day mortality was 37% and the 1-year mortality approximated 70%. Moreover, those individuals who did survive suffered from an array of complications, including obstruction of the tube (10%), infection at the tube site (8.7%), and irritation around the tube (8.7%). The high mortality rate found in this study was similar to that found in a study using Medicare claims data, which showed 30-day and 1-year mortalities being 24% and 63%, respectively. Finally, in a study comparing survival of nursing home residents who had chewing and swallowing difficulties, those individuals who were tube-fed had an increased mortality compared to those who were not tube-fed.

In the present patient, both family and medical professionals inquired about the appropriateness of placing a feeding tube to alleviate potential hunger and/or thirst. Because this patient is not able to communicate her feelings of hunger or thirst, one must extrapolate from the experiences of others. For instance, it is common for patients dying of malignancy to progressively lose interest in eating and drinking. These patients typically deny any hunger or sensation of thirst except for a dry mouth and throat. Similarly, those who participate in hunger strikes deny significant discomfort after a few days of abstinence. Despite this empiric evidence, many health care providers are intent on placing a feeding tube to prevent presumed suffering associated with caloric deprivation. Partly as a result, advanced dementia patients often receive substandard oral care. Focus is moved from the oropharynx to the feeding tube site. Patients with feeding tubes frequently develop exquisitely painful oral ulcers and fissures on the lips or oral mucosa from inattentive care.

Conversely, when family members move beyond a sole focus on enteral nutrition, healthcare professional can assist them in nurturing their loved ones through frequent and comprehensive oral care. Additionally, slow hand-feeding can be attempted; this may provide the patient and caregivers with intimate contact during a nurturing act and can benefit the patient with pleasure from both food taste and texture. Other benefits of not placing a feeding tube in such patients include less choking on oral secretions, less irritation of skin breakdown, and fewer diaper changes.

Patients' families are understandably concerned about malnutrition and added suffering. However, available evidence strongly suggests that artificial nutrition and hydration do not improve nutritional status. A well-designed study following neurologically impaired individuals who had feeding tubes and were given adequate formula still exhibited signs of malnutrition 1 year later. In fact, there was no change in the number of pressure ulcers among patients with adequate calories over the year follow-up. Similarly, in a prospective community-based study of patients receiving percutaneous enteral tube feeding, nutritional parameters did not show improvement.

Whether or not a percutaneous tube is placed for artificial nutrition and hydration, the present patient is dying from complications of dementia. She cannot be expected to benefit from placement of an artificial feeding tube for the indications described. Surgically placed gastrostomy tubes do not decrease the risk of aspiration, significantly improve nutritional parameters, or decrease pressure ulcer rates. Patients such as the one presented die despite such medical interventions and are probably best served by good oral care and slow hand-feeding, as well as other palliative care approaches including treatment of pain and other symptoms. The physicians caring for the present patient recommended that the feeding tube not be placed. The patient was discharged back to the care of her family, who were instructed on methods of slow hand-feeding.

Clinical Pearls

1. Dementia is a terminal illness.

2. Feeding tubes, including percutaneous enterogastrostomy tubes, have not been shown to decrease the risk of recurrent aspiration pneumonia or to improve nutritional parameters in advanced dementia.

3. Mortality in this population is high and may be higher after a feeding tube is placed. In general, the mortality rate is 24% at 30 days and 63% at 1 year after tube placement.

4. Patients with advanced dementia who stop eating apparently do not suffer from hunger and thirst.

5. Patients with advanced dementia who develop difficulties eating should be offered slow hand-feeding and nurturing care which is consistent with a palliative focus.

REFERENCES
1. Billings JA: Comfort measures for the terminally ill is dehydration painful? J Am Geriatr Soc 1985:33:808–810.
2. Grant M, Rudberg M, Jacobs B: Gastrostomy placement and mortality among hospitalized Medicare beneficiaries. JAMA 1998;279:1973–1976.
3. Mitchell S, Kiely D, Lipitz, L: Does artificial nutrition prolong the survival of institutionalized elders with chewing and swallowing problems? J Gerontol 1998:53A:M207-M213.
4. Finucane T, Christmas C, Travis K: Tube feeding in patients with advanced dementia a review of the evidence. JAMA 1999:282:1365–1370.
5. Gillick M: Rethinking the role of tube feeding in patients with advanced dementia. N Engl J Med 2000:342:206–210.
6. Callahan C, Haag K, Nisi R, et al: Outcomes of percutaneous endoscopic gastrostomy among older adults in a community setting. J Am Geriatr Soc 2000:48:1048–1054.
7. Morrison RS, Siu AL: Survival in end-stage dementia following acute illness. JAMA 2000:284:47–87.

Scott Lorin, MD
Judith Nelson, MD, JD

PATIENT 26

A very elderly woman with acute respiratory failure

An 89-year-old woman is brought to the hospital with severe pneumonia. She has a past medical history of non-insulin-dependent diabetes mellitus, mild ischemic cardiomyopathy, osteoarthritis, and hearing impairment. Since her husband's death 2 years ago, she has lived with her daughter at home, where she ambulated slowly and with some difficulty but handled most of her daily activities without assistance. The day before admission, she developed chills and a productive cough, with increasing shortness of breath. Her daughter contacted their primary care physician, who arranged to evaluate the patient in the Emergency Department and then decided to admit her to a general medical unit in the hospital.

Physical Examination: Blood pressure 90/50, pulse 130, temperature 38.6° C, respirations 28. General: alert and oriented, diaphoretic with labored breathing. Cardiac: tachycardic, + S3 gallop, without murmur. Chest: bilateral basilar crackles, bronchial breath sounds and egophony in the left upper and lower fields, posteriorly. Extremities: deformity and decreased joint motion of the left knee, mild pitting edema to both ankles.

Laboratory Findings: WBC 18,600/μl with 92% neutrophils, BUN 54 mg/dl, creatinine 1.8 mg/dl. Arterial blood gas (room air): pH 7.48, PCO_2 30 mm Hg, PO_2 65 mm Hg. Chest radiograph: dense consolidation in the left upper and lower lobes.

Hospital Course: Despite broad-spectrum antibiotic treatment, the patient deteriorates over the first day in the hospital, with worsening gas exchange, confusion, and development of bilateral infiltrates on the chest radiograph. The patient is intubated and mechanical ventilation is initiated on the ward, and the patient is then transferred to the ICU.

Shortly thereafter, the patient's daughter, who is her health care proxy, approaches the critical care team for information and discussion of the treatment plan. Anxious and upset, she notes that she never discussed resuscitation or life-supporting treatments directly with her mother, although there were family discussions during her father's illness in which her mother opposed but her brother favored mechanical ventilation for the father. The primary care physician also had not discussed treatment preferences with the patient. The daughter tells the critical care team that she would consider withdrawal of mechanical ventilation if there is no hope that her mother will recover.

Question: What special considerations are relevant in decision-making about life-supporting treatment for a very elderly, critically ill patient?

Diagnosis: Severe, life-threatening, pneumonia with acute lung injury and respiratory failure in a very old patient.

Discussion: A large and rapidly increasing number of elderly patients, like this one, receive life-supportive treatment and other care in ICUs, where patients aged 65 years or older comprise approximately 60% of all admissions. This group is expected to expand more than any other in the U.S. population in the coming decades, with greatest growth of the "oldest old"—over-85—subgroup. In end-of-life decision-making as well as other aspects of care for very elderly patients during life-threatening illness, we must be attentive to distinctive, difficult issues that may arise.

Informed decision-making by patients, families, and providers requires knowledge of relevant evidence about the effectiveness and burdens of intensive care. Although it is often thought that elderly patients are benefited less and burdened more, existing evidence suggests that after controlling for severity of illness and/or previous health and functional status, age as such is a less important, or even insignificant, predictor of ICU outcome. Studies separately examining outcomes of intensive care for the "oldest old" (at age 89, the present patient falls into this subgroup) support the same general conclusion. A stronger, negative influence of advancing age has been observed in some studies of patients requiring mechanical ventilation, but a recent prospective study found no difference between elderly patients and others in duration of mechanical ventilation, length of stay in the ICU or the hospital, or mortality rate, after adjustment for severity of illness.

The majority of elderly survivors of intensive care, like younger counterparts, return to their previous level of function, with the previous level of function serving as an important determinant of functional recovery. For the present patient, then, outcome will be determined mainly by her acute illness, which is life-threatening but not invariably terminal, and her chronic health state, which is imperfect but reasonably compensated. Decision-making is especially difficult when, as here, the risk of death or disability is high, but recovery to baseline health and function is possible and life-supporting treatment has potential benefit.

This patient's inability to participate in decision-making, unfortunately, is common for critically ill patients generally and for elderly patients in particular. Also common is the absence of an advance directive—although older patients are generally willing to discuss their preferences concerning intensive care and end-of-life care, there is little actual communication with either the family or physician. This is a serious omission because without such discussions, the preferences of elderly patients for life-supporting treatments are only poorly predicted by surrogates, including their closest relatives and long-standing primary doctors. In this case, the patient's reported opposition to mechanical ventilation for her late husband could be explored further, but unless she also expressed that she would not want it for herself, it would not bear directly on decision-making about her own treatment. More useful would be information that the family might provide about the patient's view of acceptable function and quality of life for herself, as that is the appropriate focus for decision-making about life-supporting treatment.

Both the clinical team and the family must strive to avoid inappropriate projection onto the patient of their own beliefs and values, including standards of life quality. In general, the elderly are more satisfied than younger people with the quality of their lives, despite chronic illness or functional impairment. Moreover, as shown in the Hospitalized Elderly Longitudinal Project, elderly patients may value the time spent in their usual state of health, even if they see it as suboptimal, more than they value excellent health if that means a shorter life. Physicians often underestimate the desire of older patients for aggressive care and tend to withhold life-sustaining treatments because of their misperceptions of the elderly's preferences. In fact, even after adjustment for prognoses and preferences for life-extending care, older patient age is associated with a greater tendency on the part of health care providers to withhold aggressive treatments, including ventilator support and other intensive care interventions, dialysis, and surgery.

Elderly individuals interviewed in inpatient and outpatient settings have typically expressed a preference for resuscitation in the event of an arrest and in the absence of severe neurologic impairment, but this desire may reflect poor understanding of CPR and overestimation of the likelihood of a successful outcome. With respect to other interventions, Danis and coworkers found that in the context of a hypothetical terminal illness, 76% of elderly outpatients wanted intensive care, 86% wanted "artificial respiration," and 69% wanted tube-feeding. Among 287 patients with a mean age of 77 years who were interviewed in a recent study during routine geriatric office visits, 88% would opt for mechanical ventilation if the duration were brief (several days to a week), whereas less than 4% wanted "long-term" mechanical ventilation of an unspecified duration. Data like these may help to inform decisions about the patient in this case, who has not made her own preferences clear. However, studies of outpatients and hypothetical situations must be cautiously interpreted and their lessons cautiously applied in specific cases of life-threatening illness or injury in critical care settings.

For this elderly patient, as for many others, regardless of age, the most acceptable approach now may be a time-limited trial of mechanical ventilation and other intensive care, with frequent reassessment of the relative benefits and burdens of ongoing aggressive treatment. Consent for entry of a DNR order at this point would not be inconsistent with such a trial. Her acute illness, although very severe, is not inevitably fatal, and in the absence of contrary evidence, it is fair to assume that she would be satisfied to return to her prior level of function and willing to have at least a short trial of intensive care to achieve that goal. Ideally, consensus favoring this approach could be reached after discussions involving not only the patient's daughter, who as the health care proxy is her legally recognized decision-maker, but also her son and the primary care physician as well as the interdisciplinary ICU team. Because of the earlier disagreement about mechanical ventilation for the father, there is some potential for conflict within the family, which can only deepen the distress that this family must already be experiencing and complicate their grief if the patient dies.

If life-prolonging treatment is continued at this point, it will still be appropriate to attend carefully and aggressively to the patient's comfort. Although data with respect to symptom experience and management for critically ill, elderly patients are scant, existing evidence suggests that unrelieved physical and emotional symptoms are generally prevalent during ICU treatment and underestimated by caregivers. Particularly for patients at high risk of death, as in this case, it is essential that excellent palliative care be provided along with intensive care in an integrated way. Expertise of specialists in geriatric medicine and/or palliative care may be engaged, as needed and available, to titrate symptom treatment appropriately for an elderly patient with multiple organ dysfunction, like this one. There is no evidence, however, that symptom distress is a necessary component of critical illness or its treatment, for elderly or other patients, nor that prevention or palliation of patient suffering would compromise aggressive efforts to save or prolong lives. In fact, an emerging body of evidence suggests that symptom distress is associated with unfavorable outcomes, including higher mortality, and should therefore be a major focus of ICU treatment for patients in all age groups.

For the present patient, the senior ICU physician and nurse held a meeting with the patient's primary physician, the daughter (the health care proxy), and son, at which agreement was reached to maintain life-supporting treatments for an initial period of several days; a DNR order was also entered. The patient's respiratory status failed to improve, and on the third ICU day, she suffered a massive myocardial infarction with significant hemodynamic compromise. At that point, both children, and all of the clinicians, favored withdrawal of life support while continuing comfort-oriented therapy. Mechanical ventilation was discontinued and the patient died quickly thereafter, with no apparent suffering.

Clinical Pearls

1. Even for the "oldest old," patient age is a less important predictor of ICU outcome than severity of illness and baseline health and functional status. Previous function is the strongest determinant of the level of functional recovery.

2. Physicians often underestimate the desire of older patients for aggressive, life-extending care and tend to withhold such care because of their misperceptions of the preferences of the elderly. Older people tend to be more satisfied than younger people with the quality of their lives, notwithstanding chronic illness or functional impairment, and to value longer life more than excellent health.

3. If acceptable (to the patient) functional recovery is a realistic goal, it is reasonable to initiate a time-limited trial of intensive care for a very elderly patient, with frequent reassessment of the relative burdens and benefits and with integration of aggressive symptom management and family support into the overall plan of ICU care.

REFERENCES

1. Uhlmann RF, Pearlman RA, Cain KC. Physicians' and spouses' predictions of elderly patients' resuscitation preferences. J Gerontol 1988;43:M115-M121.
2. Murphy DJ, Murray AM, Robinson BE, Campion EW. Outcomes of cardiopulmonary resuscitation in the elderly. Ann Intern Med 1989;111:199–205.
3. Chelluri L, Pinsky MR, Grenvik A. Outcome of intensive care of the "oldest-old" critically ill patients. Crit Care Med 1992;20:757–761.
4. Danis M, Garrett J, Harris R, Donald LP. Stability of choices about life-sustaining treatments. Ann Intern Med 1994;120:567–573.
5. Murphy DJ, Santilli S. Elderly patients' preferences for long-term life support. Arch Fam Med 1998;7:484–488.
6. Tsevat J, Dawson NV, Wu AW, et al. Health values of hospitalized patients 80 years or older. JAMA 1998;279:371–375.
7. Ely EW, Evans GW, Haponik EF. Mechanical ventilation in a cohort of elderly patients admitted to an intensive care unit. Ann Intern Med 1999;131:96–104.
8. Hamel MB, Teno JM, Goldman L, et al, for the SUPPORT Investigators. Patient age and decisions to withhold life-sustaining treatments from seriously ill, hospitalized adults. Ann Intern Med 1999;130:116–125.
9. Nelson JE, Danis M. End-of-life care in the intensive care unit: where are we now? Crit Care Med 2001;29:N2-N9.
10. Nelson JE, Nierman DM. Special concerns for the very old. In Curtis JR, Rubenfeld GD (eds): The Transition from Cure to Comfort: Managing Death in the Intensive Care Unit. New York, Oxford University Press, 2001, pp 349–367.

PATIENT 27

A 10-year-old boy with unmanageable aqueductal
stenosis and unremitting severe pain

A 10-year-old boy with congenital aqueductal stenosis is seen in the pediatric ICU following his 37th ventriculoperitoneal shunt procedure. His condition was diagnosed at 2 years of age following a febrile illness. Since his initial illness, he has been seen by neurosurgeons in five regional pediatric medical centers. He had a period of relative quiescence with few shunt malfunctions from ages 4 to 8, during which time he attended regular school, read at a level more than 5 years above grade level, and participated in soccer and swimming. During that time, he lived with his mother, father, and two younger siblings.

At 8 years of age, frequent shunt malfunctions and persistent head pain occurred. His vision and fine motor function became increasingly impaired, and many different attempts to relieve his ventriculomegaly were less than optimally successful. At present, he is in pain, is agitated, and frustrated. He describes his pain as 6 on a 10-point scale.

Physical Examination: Blood pressure 130/95, pulse 104, respirations 30, temperature 37.2° C, weight 137 lbs. General: large for age, obese, alert. HEENT: multiple well-healed scalp incisions, internalized shunt with bubble compressible at left parietal region. Eyes: deviated symmetrically inferiorly, with no visual fields, "sunsetting" present. Chest: clear. Cardiac: regular, no murmur. Abdomen: multiple well-healed scars, no masses, nontender. Neurologic: normal mental status, no sight, occasional myoclonus, and hyperreflexia.

Hospital Course: The child states that he will tolerate no further neurosurgical interventions. He experiences two episodes of anaphylaxis that required intubation, circulatory support, and antihistamine therapies associated with newly identified latex allergy. His pain is managed with morphine and lorazepam, but the myoclonus worsens. Morphine is rotated to hydromorphone, with reduction in the myoclonic jerks. His mother is exhausted, frustrated, and teary. The patient tells his mother that he cannot take the pain much longer and he does not want any further surgery.

Question: How do you help the child and family decide on a plan of care?

Diagnosis: Progressive, terminal, unshuntable hydrocephalus and severe cephalgia associated with increased intracranial pressure. Acquired latex allergy.

Discussion: The transition from life-prolonging to palliative therapies is never easy. These decisions are often harder to make when the patient is a child. Families and young patients with life-limiting illness need guidance and support while evaluating options of care. Health care providers must remember that children are their parent's and our society's hopes and dreams for the future, and that this concept for a positive future will affect how parents make decisions regarding their child's care. Anticipatory guidance for decision-making should be extended to the family.

Communication with children and their families is a skill that can be learned. Effective communication with children depends on the developmental level and intellectual capacity of the child as well as their life and illness experience. Children tend to be literal in their understanding of words, can mistake euphemisms, yet have vivid imaginations and magical thinking. It is important to be specific and avoid jargon and euphemisms when speaking to them. Clinicians need to ask them what they think is happening to them and why.

Children are subject to determinism in thinking and believe that bad things happen when people are bad or that being good protects people from harm. We can convey to children overtly and clearly that their diseases are not their fault. In addition, children are egocentric beings who believe that everyone knows what they are thinking and feeling, and that others know their thoughts without having to be told. Children may think we know when they are in pain just because we are adults and their caregivers, and that they should not have to tell us what we already know. It is important to clarify that this is not so, emphasizing that they need to tell us what hurts, what makes them angry, and what they are experiencing in order to get them the help and treatments they need.

A **child's understanding of death** also varies with developmental stage and family culture. Infants lack a sense of time and experience "death" as separation. Toddlers can link time with concrete events and know that dead things disappear, but they think that this disappearance is temporary and that rescue is possible. A child this age does not understand why the grandmother, whose body they see in the casket, won't come out and read a story to them or respond to the child's questions.

By school age, children can tell time, yet tend to think of the future as a long way off. They know that death is selective, that old people and animals die, and that there are physical limitations to

death. By adolescent children have developed formal operational thought, can perceive of the future, and know that death is final and irreversible. Most adolescents, however, think of death as exceedingly unlikely to happen to them. The adolescent who knows of the type of trauma associated with motor vehicle accidents is still unlikely to wear a seat belt in the belief that they will not be affected by such events. In general, children with chronic illness are often more mature with regard to matters of medical treatment, decisions, and prognosis than others their age.

Children also need special consideration in regard to pain and symptom control. In the developed world, most of the pain and physical suffering that dying children experience comes not from the disease process itself, but from the diagnostic and therapeutic procedures associated with the treatment of these life-limiting conditions. In its 1998 guide *Cancer Pain Relief and Palliative Care in Children*, the World Health Organization stated that "unlike adults children cannot independently seek pain relief and are therefore vulnerable, they need adults to recognize their pain before they can receive appropriate treatment." Skills at assessing pain in children can be learned. As in adults, the gold standard is **patient self-report**. Children should simply be asked if, where, and how they hurt. Pain management principles are similar in children and adults, with the exceptions of the very young (< 3 months of age) and premature whose hepatic and renal systems for metabolizing medications are not fully developed.

In regard to **decision-making**, children, as soon as they are developmentally able, should be included in discussions and decisions for end-of-life care. Clearly, the present patient knows the experience of frequent neurosurgeries and symptoms of unrelenting hydrocephalus. His feelings and preferences should be respected in the decision-making process. Children have the right to **assent** to the consent for treatment their parents grant. Their opinions should always be sought and should carry increasing weight in the decision-making process proportionate to their capacity to understand their situation, the treatment options, and implications for their longevity and well-being. All attempts to treat pain and to allow for adequate rest for the patient and their families should be made in order for the patient and family to use their best judgment in making important decisions.

Asking the child and family what they want is always important. Listening to their answers is even more so. Physicians and other health care providers are often quick to offer solutions and spend little time exploring what is really a priority for the dying child. Questions such as "What would success look like?", "What would be left undone if you died today?," and "What first?" help the health care professional safely start the conversations that allow the child and family to explore and tell us what we need to hear to help them plan the important phase of life known as dying.

For the present patient, a relatively manageable condition has become complicated and painful, despite all reasonable efforts for symptom and functional improvement. It is unlikely that further attempts to shunt this child's painful hydrocephalus will be successful, and the child himself appears to be aware of this. The family and the child, once his pain was adequately treated and following a good night's rest by all, sat at the child's bedside with the staff of the pediatric ICU, the neurosurgeon, and pediatrician. He expressed his desire to be pain-free even if it required sedation to do so; he asked to go home, to spend a night eating pizza, playing a game with his family; and he wanted to be able to spend some time with his classmates. He told all present how much he loved his family and he thanked the nurses for all that they had done for him. He was assured by his pediatrician that everything would be done to help him be comfortable at home and to achieve those things he most wanted.

He was discharged to home with his family 2 days later. His pain escalated again 13 days following discharge. It was managed with analgesia and sedation in the home by hospice and his pediatrician. His extended family was present when he died.

Clinical Pearls

1. Communication with children and their families about end-of-life issues is an important skill for the health care professional. Communication skills can be learned and can be taught.

2. Children's understanding of death varies with developmental stage and life experience.

3. Pain and symptom management in children is similar to that in adults with a few exceptions.

4. Children should be involved in decisions about their end-of-life care.

REFERENCES

1. Committee on Bioethics, American Academy of Pediatrics. Guidelines on forgoing life-sustaining medical treatment. Pediatrics 1994;93:532–536.
2. Committee on Bioethics, American Academy of Pediatrics. Informed consent, parental permission, and assent in pediatric practice. Pediatrics 1995;95:314–317.
3. World Health Organization. Cancer Pain Relief and Palliative Care in Children. Geneva, WHO Press, 1998.
4. Committee on Bioethics and Committee on Hospital Care, American Academy of Pediatrics. Palliative care for children. Pediatrics 2000;106:351–357.
5. Compendium of Pediatric Palliative Care. Arlington, VA, National Hospice and Palliative Care Organization, 2000.

Dennis S. Pacl, MD

PATIENT 28

A 72-year-old man with pleural adenocarcinoma whose family requests that "everything be done"

A 72-year-old man is admitted to the hospital for severe dyspnea on exertion and chest pain. He was previously in excellent health without significant medical problems. He and his wife are the owners of an industrial distribution company. He has two adult children from a previous marriage, a fulfilling personal life, and a "vibrant" marriage. An avid jogger, he runs up to 3 miles several times a week. In the previous 2 months, however, he has experienced increasing dyspnea.

The patient is evaluated with a chest CT that reveals a large right pleural effusion. He undergoes diagnostic thoroscopy, which demonstrates a poorly differentiated adenocarcinoma of unknown primary and talc pleurodesis. A medical oncologist recommends an aggressive platinum-based cytotoxic chemotherapy combination. The patient expresses apprehension to his primary care physician about undergoing chemotherapy. He understands that he has advanced cancer with poor clinical prognostic markers. However, he states that he feels guilty that he would be letting his family down if he doesn't choose "to fight this." Indeed, his wife and children, as well as a close family friend, who is a prominent physician in the community, are pushing for him to "try everything" there is to offer.

Rapid titration of morphine by patient-controlled analgesia provides adequate analgesia for his chest pain. His dyspnea worsens and he is admitted to the ICU requiring noninvasive positive pressure ventilation. His mental status remains lucid when stimulated, though he is generally somnolent. In a conference attended by the family, their doctor friend, the thoracic surgeon, and medical oncologist, his wife sums up the situation by saying, "We need to DO something. We have to have something to hope for."

Question: What assistance can be provided by a palliative medicine consultant?

Diagnosis: A patient with advanced cancer who has not been adequately informed about all treatment options including palliative care.

Discussion: All too frequently, in the process of obtaining informed consent in acute care settings, problems arise that complicate patient and family decision-making. Clinicians may present patients and families with treatment choices without fully considering the context of a patient's illness and post-intervention scenarios. Fully informed consent for chemotherapy in the face of advanced disease must take into account the burden of the intervention, the severity of existing symptom burden, as well as the likelihood that the recommended intervention will restore health and vitality. The present patient experienced a rapid decline in functional capacity consistent with his diagnosis. The oncologist was asked to "do something," the assumption and implication being that not offering "aggressive" life-prolonging therapy means "doing nothing."

If treatment options, including palliative care, are explained within the context of the experience of a patient's illness, patients can be provided an opportunity for truly informed consent. Informed consent requires that the context of the illness is well defined for the patient and the family. In cases such as the one presented, having both the oncologist and surgeon discuss the medical condition and treatment options with the ill person and family helps ensure that the their questions will be addressed and that they will understand the risks and potential benefits of life-prolonging interventions.

The present patient felt that chemotherapy might not alter the progression of his illness in a beneficial way. He was worried about suffering he might experience and wanted to preserve the quality of whatever life he had left. His concerns prompted his willingness to discuss the illness and to describe his personal values and fears.

Involvement of the patient is important because family members may not appreciate the burden of illness, much less the burden of "aggressive" interventions. A family conference is a good vehicle to make sure that everyone understands the disease process and how treatment options will impact the patient. As a palliative care consultant, we can emphasize what is important to the patient and present the treatment options within that context, and at the same time redefine hope as that which is reasonable to expect, framed within the context of the disease experience and the patient's values. The palliative care consultant's role is to arm the patient and family with the best information so that they can make choices within context. Our colleagues in the subspecialties generally recommend interventions with which they are comfortable. Recommended interventions are usually those that exist within their armamentarium to "fight" disease. Palliative care or hospice may be an afterthought when there is "nothing else we can do." If palliative care does not exist in a physician's armamentarium, it is not likely to be presented as a viable option that represents "really doing something."

Requests by patients or their families to "do everything" can often be reframed by emphatically stating, "I want to do everything I can to improve both the length and quality of your (loved one's) life. I want to fix everything that can be fixed. When there is balance that must be struck between quality and quantity of life, I'll help you make the choice that fits best for you." Commitment to the patient and family can be emphasized. This includes commitment to treating conditions that will improve the patient's sense of well-being. Hospice chaplains describe the therapeutic value of just being there, to explain what is happening and demonstrate our commitment; they refer to this as "the ministry of presence." This is indeed a powerful tool in our armamentarium as palliative care consultants, one that our colleagues often fail to recognize. It is something that we can offer in any situation. In some situations, it may be that by being there, explaining the disease process and placing the treatment choices into context, we are indeed "doing everything" that will help and result in an improved well-being.

In the present case, the palliative care physician remained silent during the family conference while the thoracic surgeon described the extent of disease that he had visualized by thoracoscopy. It was at this time that the oncologist became truly aware of the extent of this patient's disease, his symptom burden, and debility. When the patient's wife said, "We have to have something to hope for," the palliative care consultant interjected that, perhaps, we can still hope for freedom from pain and quality time spent together as family. He reinforced the importance of quality of life for this patient, having had a robust existence to this point and looking forward to declining health and burdensome treatment that was not likely to produce improved health status. This clearly placed the proposed intervention within the context not just of the illness, but also within the person's and family's life.

In the process of this discussion, the oncologist withdrew his recommendation for chemotherapy, much to the relief of the patient. The patient's anxiety diminished and his opioid requirement went down twofold over the next 24 hours without further intervention. The patient was discharged to home, spent 2 weeks with his family, and died peacefully. Soon after the funeral, the patient's physician friend contacted the palliative doctor and commented on the remarkable passing of his friend and the special role that physicians have in caring for dying patients. A few weeks later, the palliative care consultant received a beautiful card from the patient's wife, thanking him for helping her "with the difficult choices" they had faced.

Clinical Pearls

1. Recommendations for "aggressive" life-prolonging treatments sometimes fail to take into account the context of the patient's illness, symptom burden, and debility.

2. Physicians may not be feel confident in offering palliative care and, therefore, a palliative plan of care may not be presented competently and confidently as a legitimate treatment option. This can reinforce the "do everything" versus "do nothing" misperception of life-prolonging and palliative (including hospice) care.

3. The therapeutic value to the patient and family of a physician's commitment to staying involved and being present deserves recognition as an essential element of advanced illness care.

REFERENCES

1. Maguire P, Walsh S, Jeacock J, Kingston R. Physical and psychological needs of patients dying from colo-rectal cancer. Palliat Med 1999;13:45–50.
2. Wear S. Enhancing clinician provision of informed consent and counseling: some pedagogical strategies. J Med Philos 1999;24:34–42.
3. Tomamichel M, Jaime H, Degrate A, et.al. Proposing phase I studies: patients', relatives', nurses', and specialists' perceptions. Ann Oncol 2000;11:289–294.

Richard Mularski, MD

PATIENT 29

A 49-year-old woman with metastatic breast cancer and acute respiratory distress syndrome who lacks decision-making capacity and a surrogate decision-maker

A 49-year-old woman with a history of breast carcinoma metastatic to the lungs and CNS presents with confusion, dyspnea, and chest pain. She has exhausted available chemotherapy and has been receiving experimental hormonal manipulation. She has a history of coronary artery disease with two previous myocardial infarctions. An MRI done last week demonstrated vertebral abnormalities and impingement at the midthoracic spinal cord. Her family leaves the emergency department after plans for ICU admission are made.

Physical Examination: Blood pressure 84/50, pulse 134, temperature 39.6° C, respirations 28, oxygen saturation 88% on oxygen at 6 liters/hr. General: cachectic, confused, disoriented, and perseverating about getting to a wedding. Chest: diffuse rhonchi with bilateral dullness to percussion. Neurologic: no focal finding. EKG: inferior Q waves with diffuse ST- and T-wave changes. Chest radiograph: small bilateral effusions, patchy consolidation and some nodular opacities.

Laboratory Findings: Blood gases (room air): pH 7.28, $PaCO_2$ 38 mm Hg, PaO_2 48 mm Hg. WBC 19,000/ml with 82% neutrophils and 9% bands, troponin I 2.0 ng/ml, albumin 1.9 g/dl. Electrolytes normal, BUN 48 mg/dl, creatinine 1.5 mg/dl.

Hospital Course: The patient was admitted to the ICU at 2:00 AM and was stabilized with noninvasive positive pressure ventilation by a facemask and high flow oxygen. Serial cardiac enzymes, blood cultures, and sputum culture were obtained. She received volume resuscitation, intravenous antibiotics, high-dose steroids, and an intravenous opiate and benzodiazepine for comfort.

The emergency department physician did not address goals of admission nor patient preferences with the family; they could not be reached at the time of admission. Her oncologist is out of the country, and her internist is not on call. The resident admitting the patient is concerned about the patient's wishes in the event that she suffers a cardiopulmonary arrest or requires endotracheal intubation for ventilatory support. He had been moved by what he describes as "torturing these poor cancer patients at the end of their lives." His attending physician, exhausted by a busy week on call, had just left the hospital an hour ago. The resident contemplates running a "slow code" if anything were to happen overnight, administering intravenous morphine as an alternative to intubation, and readdressing the situation when the attending physician and the family are available.

Question: Should the resident write DNR orders and set limits to the aggressiveness of treatment?

Diagnosis: A critically ill patient with a poor prognosis who lacks both decision-making capacity and a surrogate decision-maker.

Discussion: Unfortunately, many patients with poor prognoses are admitted to the ICU without adequate advance planning because of inadequate discussion, communication, and documentation of end-of-life wishes and goals for medical therapy. The resident, faced with the challenge of uncertainty in code status and preferences for aggressive ICU care, should apply standard medical therapy while placing a high priority on addressing and clarifying care preferences.

Two ethical principles assist the clinician in determining aggressiveness of care. Code status must be differentiated from goals of therapy and desire for treatment. Although in the ICU, such distinctions may become blurred, determination of DNR status does not translate into an order not to aggressively treat illness or administer intensive care. A very poor prognosis for survival to an acceptable quality of life from CPR does not portend or suggest a low chance for successful treatment of reversible conditions or achievement of a patient's goals with aggressive therapy. Limitations of therapy, such as restricting the application of hemodialysis, use of an additional inotropic medication, or intubation, may be appropriate as the trajectory of an illness becomes apparent and prognosis and patient goals are clarified. From an ethical standpoint, withholding (not initiating a therapy) and withdrawing (stopping a therapy that is inconsistent with goals of care) are considered equivalent. For urgent situations in which there is a lack of clarity in prognosis or patient goals, an intervention may be initially applied and later withdrawn as appropriate.

In the United States, ethical and legal standards emphasize autonomy and establish the patient's right to determine his or her own goals for medical care, including the refusal or removal of any intervention. Physicians are obligated to obtain informed consent. An exception is emergencies during which, in absence of definitive information of patient refusal or a physician DNR order, rescue workers and clinicians function under a doctrine of presumed consent. The consent process requires that the physician provides sufficient information about the therapy, determines decisional capacity of the patient, and attempts to exclude coercion from the patient's decision. This equally applies to withholding or withdrawing of treatments and determination of code status, and it requires a high standard, as the outcome of withholding CPR will likely result in the patient's death.

Determination of decision-making capacity can be reduced into four separate criteria:

1. The ability of a patient to understand relevant information regarding a treatment decision;
2. The ability of a patient to appreciate the significance of that information for his or her situation, including the consequences of treatment options as well as no treatment;
3. The ability of a patient to reason with the relevant information, so as to engage in rational deliberation weighing treatment options and deciding on a choice; and
4. The ability of a patient to express that choice.

Decisional capacity is considered specific to the task at hand, determined at any point in time for a specific task, and should be weighted against the consequences of the decision. For example, a patient with dementia faced with the decision to consent to the suturing of a laceration may have the ability to comprehend the options of therapy, including risks and benefits, and can appropriately weigh these to express a choice consistent with the criteria specific to the consequences of that decision. However, decisional capacity may not be present for that same patient at a different time or when faced with a different decision, especially one that has more serious consequences, such as refusing intubation and ventilation for respiratory failure that almost certainly would result in death.

When a patient lacks decisional capacity, a surrogate should be identified to provide consent for procedures, to allow withholding or withdrawing of treatments, or to determine resuscitation status. The principle on which such decisions should be made is **substitutive judgment**, in which a surrogate bases decisions on the wishes the patient expressed in the past or the articulated values of the patient as they may apply to the current situation. When such knowledge is lacking, a surrogate and physician may apply the best interest standard, promoting the welfare of the patient using what a reasonable person might choose as the best option, weighing the benefits and burdens of the treatment, in the absence of the expressed wishes of the patient.

A hierarchy for surrogacy is usually determined by state law. For example, priority may go to a spouse/partner, parent, adult children, sibling, kin, or friend in this order for legally designating a decision-maker in instances of conflict. Most states also allow a designated power of attorney for healthcare to be established a priori by a legal document signed by the patient at a time he or she possessed decisional capacity or as determined by a judge at the request of a surrogate on behalf of an incompetent person. In matters relating to code status, level of aggressive therapy, and determination of surrogate, the clinician should try to honor the most recent articulation by a patient at the time he or she was last felt to have decisional capacity, within the confines of the laws by which the clinician is bound. Advance directives are seldom helpful in specific cases of withholding and withdrawing of therapy but may serve as guidance to the patient's wishes and desires for aggressive treatment. Dilemmas are best mediated by institutional teams with expertise and impartiality, such as ethics committees.

Early determination of the goals of therapy, including addressing issues of end-of-life care preferences and palliative care, can go a long way toward honoring the autonomy of a patient and family and avoiding conflict in the uncertain ICU arena. Patients and their loved ones may approach ICU care very differently along the course of illness. Clarification of short-term and long-term goals may reveal a spectrum from aggressive intervention to comfort care as the nature of an illness and its chance for cure unfold. Communication among healthcare providers, the patient, and his or her loved ones is a cornerstone of success. An example for a checklist that facilitates this process at the time of admission to an ICU follows:

- Discuss and document goals of care, likely outcomes and prognoses, and a reevaluation plan
- Discuss and document advance care planning, DNR orders, decision-making capacity, durable power of attorney for healthcare, and surrogacy
- Identify symptoms and treatment plan for palliation, e.g., pain, dyspnea, anxiety, thirst, etc.
- Address psychosocial and spiritual needs
- Define goals for therapy and outcomes among members of the interdisciplinary care team
- Plan the timing of family conferences and attend to family dynamics and cultural issues

In general, determining and ordering a DNR status for a patient should follow the procedure for informed consent with the patient or their surrogate. In certain circumstances, it is permissible for a physician to make a decision that CPR is not an effective therapy for a particular patient or circumstance. This is not fundamentally different from a surgeon determining that the risk of an operation is too great or the prognosis too bleak to allow an attempt at its performance. As it is a standard of care to attempt resuscitation in the absence of an existing DNR order or person's request to withhold CPR, the patient and family should be informed of a physician's decision to withhold resuscitation.

In cases when a patient or surrogate may demand that "everything be done" despite a determination by the physician that an intervention would be "futile," it is likely that legal and ethical precedence will support the unilateral decision by the physician to order DNR. It should be emphatically noted that **futility** should not be invoked when observers are instead making a subjective interpretation of a patient's current or future quality of life. Futility refers only to a physician's determination that a therapy will be of no physiologic benefit. No universally agreed upon qualitative or quantitative definition of futility exists, and probabilistic estimates of prognosis for most interventions are inadequate to allow the concept of futility to be applied in most cases of conflict. For this reason, it is recommended that a standard approach be justly and uniformly applied to ethical dilemmas that involve futile therapies which conflict with the expressed wishes for therapy, including the effort to transfer the patient to a physician willing to comply with the patient's or family's wishes.

The **"slow code,"** also termed show, light blue, partial, or Hollywood code, is an incomplete resuscitative effort deliberately applied with the goal of failing to bring a patient back to life. This dishonest effort violates professional obligations to patients and their families and circumvents the important ethical norm of truth-telling. Under this practice, healthcare providers use delaying tactics to ensure that any resuscitation effort will fail, yet will relate to survivors that everything had been done to save the patient. The bioethical consideration of this topic is strong and remonstrative. The American College of Physicians *Ethics Manual* considers such half-hearted resuscitation efforts to be unethical, and one author calls the practice "reprehensible . . . a crass dissimulation."

The present patient had a goal of attending her only daughter's wedding in 2 months and would accept aggressive care, even if the chance of recovery to discharge was quite low. A DNR order was written after her family and physicians agreed that the chance of a meaningful survival precluded the burden of CPR. However, her preferences for therapy were honored. She required 10 days of ICU care, including mechanical ventilation for ARDS, and received radiation therapy to her spinal metastases. She survived to attend her daughter's wedding and was later referred to hospice. She died at home nearly 3 months after her admission to the hospital.

Clinical Pearls

1. 1. A "slow code" is an immoral and unethical practice that has no place in medical care.

2. Use of a checklist at the time of ICU admission facilitates end-of-life care and communication.

3. Determination of code status includes establishing a patient's decisional capacity by screening for the following three factors: the patient understands the relevant information, the patient appreciates the context and consequences of a decision, and the patient has reasoning and rational deliberation skills.

4. Surrogate decision-makers should be asked to apply substitutive judgment for a patient, attempting to base decisions on the wishes the patient expressed in the past or articulated values of the patient as they may apply to a current situation.

5. In urgent conditions where there is a lack of clarity in prognosis or patient goals, a default to aggressive life-prolonging care is appropriate, while placing a high priority on clarifying the patient's end-of-life care preferences.

REFERENCES

1. President's Commission for the Study of Ethical Problems in Medicine and Biomedical and Behavioral Research. Deciding to Forgo Life-Sustaining Treatment: A Report on the Ethical, Medical, and Legal Issues in Treatment Decisions. Washington, DC: U.S. Government Printing Office; 1983.
2. ACCP/SCCM Consensus Panel: Ethical and moral guidelines for the initiation, continuation, and withdrawal of intensive care. Chest 1990;97:949–958.
3. American Thoracic Society Bioethics Task Force. Withholding and withdrawing life-sustaining therapy. Ann Intern Med 1991;115:478–485.
4. American College of Physicians Ethics Manual, 3rd ed. Ann Intern Med 1992;117:747–960.
5. Jonsen AR, Siegler M, Winslade WJ. Clinical Ethics: A Practical Approach to Ethical Decisions in Clinical Medicine, 4th ed. New York: McGraw-Hill; 1998.
6. Gazelle G. The slow code—should anyone rush to its defense? N Engl J Med 1998;338:467–469.
7. Grisso T, Appelbaum P.S. Assessing Competence to Consent to Treatment: A Guide for Physicians and Other Health Professionals. New York: Oxford University Press; 1998.
8. Curtis JR, Rubenfeld GD (eds): Managing Death in the Intensive Care Unit: The Transition from Cure to Comfort. New York: Oxford University Press; 2000.
9. Mularski RA, Bascom P, Osborne ML. Compassionate end-of-life care in the ICU: educational agendas for interdisciplinary end-of-life curricula. Crit Care Med 2001;29(suppl 2):N16-N23.

Priscilla D. Kissick, RN, MN

PATIENT 30

A 72-year-old woman with nonresectable lung cancer who is living alone

A 72-year-old African-American woman, who is living alone, is experiencing increasing difficulties with pain management. She was diagnosed with small cell lung cancer 6 months ago. At the time of diagnosis, she had carefully considered treatment options and elected palliative care, with the focus on maintaining her independence and quality of life as long as possible. The patient was told she had less than a year to live. Currently her main symptoms are cough, fatigue, bone pain from metastases, and weight loss. She has a Karnofsky performance score of 60%. Pain is controlled with 30 mg of slow-release morphine twice a day. She has recently experienced episodic anxiety attacks.

The patient is the mother of three grown children, all of whom live out of state. She is a retired government employee with a modest pension in addition to her social security benefits. She owns her single-family row home, has lived independently for the past 20 years, and has an active social life revolving around church and family.

Question: As the patient approaches the end of life, how can she receive effective palliative care yet remain at home?

Diagnosis: Terminal lung cancer in a patient who needs hospice home care.

Discussion: Hospice care at the end of life provides a range of services that includes hospice living-alone support. Initiating living-alone services requires an evaluation to determine if the patient is a suitable candidate. Appropriate patients should still be ambulatory, which allows sufficient time to establish a plan of care and arrange needed resources. The home setting should have adequate resources, which include a functioning phone and fire alarms in working condition. Patients should be willing to accept safety measures, such as a medical alert and a lock box to allow access to the home by caregivers. Patients must have good cognitive capabilities and lack a recent history of drug abuse. Smoking is discouraged. Physicians can call in a hospice living-alone referral for patients who fulfill these criteria.

Often, the initial intake visit has a social worker precede the hospice nurse. Any available family members should participate in the initial visits to provide backup and to receive reassurance that patients can manage their own care with the assistance of the hospice program. In addition to obtaining hospice informed consent and signing hospice election papers, patients in the living-alone program have to complete additional paper work specific to the this program. During the initial visits, hospice workers assist patients in completing a durable power of attorney and a long-term plan of care. Patients are given opportunities to verbalize their wishes to remain at home through the end of life.

The first visit is crucial to the success of the living-alone program. Hospice workers recognize that the program enrolls patients who are frequently fiercely independent. Although they may initially allow the hospice team access to the home, they often become less willing to sacrifice their independence and participate in collaborative problem-solving unless ground rules are immediately established. Hospice clinicians wisely emphasize the patient's goals and focus in the short term on practical ways of meeting those goals.

The hospice social workers develop early plans for care in anticipation of when patients can no longer be left alone. Family members are encouraged to take family medical leave from work when patients become dependent on support around the clock. The hospice program supports medical leave applications with appropriate documentation and explanatory calls or letters. Patients can be supported by companion services if family members experience delays in initiating family medical leaves. An important component of the plan of care is a carefully developed, individualized means for updating family members on the patient's condition and medical needs, so as to facilitate their greater involvement if the patient requires continuous support. A chart that clearly details responsibilities of specific family members is helpful. Ongoing communication with family and friends is valuable to maintain consistency of care and minimize conflict.

Spiritual care is often welcomed by patients and families, even those who do not regularly attend church or formally practice religion. Hospice pastoral contacts patients' pastors, who are typically gratified that hospice has become involved and will be providing spiritual support that will supplement efforts by the patients' church families.

The hospice nurse evaluated the present patient with the daughter in attendance. The patient was found her to be cognitively sound and able to follow safety requirements. A visit schedule was established with a home health aide three times a week to assist with personal care, light housekeeping, and meal preparation. A volunteer was assigned to provide companionship and make weekend telephone calls to ensure that the patient was safe and well. The social worker assumed the responsibility of completing advance planning, reinforcing relaxation technique education, addressing safety concerns, and keeping the family informed. The hospice chaplain assisted the patient with life review and spiritual support.

Within 3 weeks, the patient required an increase in her pain medication dosages. The patient's children alternated in making weekend visits and recognized signs of her increased weakness and fatigue with less interest in family and church. Smoking precautions were reinforced, and the patient agreed to smoke only when others were in the home or in the bathroom if she were alone.

Two weeks later, the patient had a fall at night. The med-alert was called, and a near neighbor was able to respond. No injuries were sustained. It was decided that the patient had become too weak to be alone. The plan of care was put in place with around the clock companions for 2 days until the daughter could finalize her medical leave of absence. The hospice increased their visit patterns. Symptoms were well control. Five days later, the patient died peacefully at home in her own bed with two of her children at the bedside.

Clinical Pearls

1. Hospice services for patients living at home alone are possible and can enable patients to stay at home through the end of life.

2. Long-term planning for living-alone patients who wish to die at home is critical. The "tough questions" must be asked early.

3. Durable power of attorney must be obtained as early as possible, with clear communication among all involved concerning these powers. Ongoing communication and charting of responsibilities for family and friends are valuable in maintaining consistency and minimizing conflict.

4. Hospice must be proactive in all aspects of care; success of the plan of care is predicated on minimizing surprises.

5. Hospice care can enable patients living alone to maintain personal independence yet coordinate and provide adequate support as function declines and death approaches.

REFERENCES

1. Bly JL, Kissick PD. Hospice care for patients living alone: results of a demonstration program. Hospice J 1994;9:9–20.
2. Capossela C, Warnock S, Miller S. —*Share the Care*. New York, Simon and Schuster, 1995.
3. National Family Caregivers Association: *www.nfcacares.org* (multiple resources for family caregivers, including those at a distance from their ill loved ones).
4. Partnership for Caring: *www.partnershipforcaring.org* (multiple resources for patients and families regarding advance care planning and advance directives).

Elizabeth Chaitin, DHCE
Robert M. Arnold, MD

PATIENT 31

A 60-year-old seriously ill man with impaired mentation whose family and physicians disagree over treatment plans

A 60-year-old man is admitted from home with hyperglycemia, dyspnea, cough, and purulent sputum. He has a history of severe hypoxic brain injury resulting from a cardiac arrest and stroke suffered during abdominal surgery 1 year ago. His medical history is also pertinent for diabetes, hypertension, and congestive heart failure. He has been subsequently managed at home with a tracheostomy, gastrostomy tube, and an indwelling Foley catheter. He has severe limitations of mentation and responds only to painful stimuli. His sister is designated as his primary caretaker and power of attorney for health care.

Physical Examination: Temperature 39.3° C, blood pressure 80/50, pulse 116 irregular. General: malnourished. Neck: tracheostomy tube in place with purulent secretions. Chest: coarse bilateral rhonchi. Cardiac: irregular tachycardia. Abdomen: gastrostomy tube, otherwise unremarkable. Skin: stage 4–5 decubital ulcers on sacrum and buttock with tracking to his bone. Neurologic: responds only minimally to painful stimuli; severe contractures of all extremities.

Laboratory Findings: WBC 22,000 μl with a left shift. Sacral wound cultures: *Pseudomonas aeruginosa* and methicillin-resistant *Staphylococcus aureus*. Chest radiograph: three-lobe airspace opacities compatible with pneumonia.

Clinical Course: Considering his poor underlying neurologic status and the severity of his pneumonia and sepsis, the physicians believe that the patient is most likely terminal. When the physicians approach the family to discuss the prognosis and goals of therapy, the patient's sister states that she "does not want to hear anything negative." She and the other family members contend that a miracle will heal their loved one.

The patient is kept at full-code status and continues to receive multiple antibiotics. Despite these measures, he remains febrile to 39°. The housestaff and attending physician tell the family daily about the "futility" of the current plan of action. The family accuses the doctors of not caring about the patient and imply that the physicians' actions may be motivated by financial concerns. The doctors feel that the treatment they are being compelled to provide is inhumane and wonder if they can override the family and change the focus of care to comfort measures only.

Question: How can the physicians resolve this situation?

Diagnosis: Clinical conflict regarding treatment goals and prognosis arising from asymmetric dialogue between physicians and family members.

Discussion: When physicians and families disagree over the goals of care, frustration usually ensues. When the health care team views the state of physiologic care as being nonbeneficial or futile, they often assume that the family has reached the same conclusion. In situations in which the family does not agree with the physicians' assessment, physicians often consider resorting to a judgment of "medical futility." Such a determination might allow the physicians to consider unilaterally overriding the family's decision. The perceived importance of the concept of medical futility has spawned an enormous amount of literature that attempts to define futility and describe how this concept should be applied.

In practice, however, invoking the concept of futility as a medical "trump card" is rarely productive, instead often generating heightened conflict. Resolving such disputes requires better communication. Although frustration with families who, in the judgment of the health care team are demanding treatments that are ineffective and sometimes seem cruel, is understandable, resorting to a judgment of futility is perceived as an exercise of unilateral physician power. When faced with a family that wants treatment the physician believes is unreasonable, a physician might ask the following questions:

1. Am I talking to the appropriate surrogate?
2. Does the surrogate understand even though he or she may not necessarily agree with my interpretation of the medical situation? If not, why?
3. Does the surrogate have a different opinion about treatment, despite agreeing with my interpretation of the patient's diagnosis and prognosis? If yes, why?

The balance in thinking between patient, family, and physician about when care should be limited or discontinued only comes when the family's emotional and intellectual understanding of the care provided and the physician's opinions blend. This symmetry of thought can be achieved only through conversations that discuss the values base of the patient, surrogate, and family, the role of the patient within the family, the understanding of both parties regarding the current illness and its progress, and their psychosocial reaction to the situation. The key strategy is to focus on values. Except in rare circumstances in which the family's motives are suspect, clinicians can affirm that they respect the family's values and caring intention and in this manner approach care planning in a way that advances those values. The critical goal in the interpersonal dynamic and ongoing communication between clinician and family is to shift from being seen by the family as an adversary in the encounter to being an ally and advocate for the patient's and family's well-being.

Usually one family member is chosen to be the primary decision-maker for a patient. This individual, or surrogate, can be chosen formally through an advance directive or identified informally through family process. The surrogate's role is to make the choice she or he thinks the patient would want. The moral criteria for choosing a surrogate focuses on who knows the patient best and who can best represent the patient's desires in the current situation. For example, in certain situations it may be more appropriate to talk with the next-door neighbor who saw the patient every day than with a distant cousin who has not spoken to the patient for years. Putting this principle into practice means asking surrogates what they think their *loved one* would want, rather than asking, "what do *you* think we should do for your loved one?

Often, families disagree with the health care teams' recommendation because they do not understand the medical facts. This disagreement can occur for several reasons:

1. Health care providers have not spoken with the family. More commonly, conversations between physicians and families can appear to take place on different planes, with the doctor's language and medical terms being difficult for the family to understand.
2. Neither the linguistic terms nor the style of the presentation is as important as the meaning each person places upon certain words. For example, doctors talk in probabilistic terms, while many families think in black and white. Vague terms such as "unlikely" may mean the doctor thinks the therapy or course of treatment has a $< 1\%$ chance of success, but the family may think it means a $< 20\%$ chance.
3. When families talk to different doctors, they may hear slightly different stories, leading to confusion. The lack of sufficient time to process information may contribute to family confusion during a crisis. Even under the best of circumstances, people typically retain only 30% to 40% of medical information given them; this percentage is lower when a person is stressed, tired, and emotionally upset.
4. Finally, the family may be unable to process the information because of denial, a psychological defense mechanism that protects one from information that is too traumatic.

The only way to determine which of these factors is influencing the situation is to ask the family to explain what they have been told regarding their loved one's illness and what their understanding is of the prognosis and treatment options. This effort will help the physician distinguish instances in which the family does not understand the information from those in which they do not agree with the physician's assessment.

At times the most frustrating interchange occurs when a family seems to understand and may even agree with the medical opinion provided, but still insists on the current level of care. Again, rather than becoming frustrated, the health care providers should try to understand why the family has made this choice. In some instances, either because of previous personal experience or cultural beliefs, the family may not trust the doctors or the healthcare system. In other situations, the intrafamily dynamics may be influencing the situation. The family may feel guilt for one reason or another or may be worried that they are being asked to "kill" their loved one.

The most difficult situations are those in which the best interests of the patient are not at the core of the family's motivation. At times, family members may be playing out an intrafamily conflict over who "loves their mom the best." Rarely, family members act out of financial incentives or other self-serving motives. More commonly, a family may want to go forward because of their ideas of what is an acceptable chance of therapeutic success. Or they may be hoping for a miracle, based on their strong religious or spiritual beliefs.

Prior to trying to convince the family of one's own view, providers should make certain that they understand the family's thinking. It is often helpful to emphasize, and at intervals remind everyone involved, that it is the illness and its complications, rather than any individuals involved, that are causing the patient's death and that the person is already being kept alive by medical treatment.

To successfully negotiate treatment goals, symmetry must be obtained between the emotional and physiologic aspects of care. This symmetry is obtained through conversation with the primary decision-maker in which consideration is given to the role of family relationships, social factors, cultural factors, and/or spiritual belief structure.

The physicians caring for the present patient requested a consultation from the ethics committee. A physician member of the committee sat with the family for an extended period and discussed their perceptions, understandings, and concerns. The patient's attending physician was brought into this dialogue and helped to promote a mutual understanding of the patient's life values, goals, and prognosis. It was decided to maintain the present level of care and to initiate a DNR status, but to monitor him for signs of improvement over the next 2 days. The family was encouraged to stay close by. The physician and hospital staff helped the family with pragmatic issues of transportation, arrangements for lodging, meals, and calls with family at a distance.

By the next day, the patient was clearly worse. After initiation of palliative care with opiates intended to relieve dyspnea, the patient died peacefully with his family and physicians by his side.

Clinical Pearls

1. The concept of futility is sometimes considered in an effort to override the decision of the surrogate, but it often leads to heightened conflict.

2. Conversations regarding prognosis must be held with the primary decision-maker if mutually acceptable decisions are to be reached.

3. To successfully negotiate end of life issues, some symmetry must be present between the emotional and physiologic aspects of care.

4. This symmetry is obtained by focusing on values and by considering the role of family relationships, social factors, cultural factors, and/or spiritual belief structure when speaking with surrogates about the plan of care. The primary goal of the conversation is to clarify what the family understands and what they believe will happen and why. Except in rare situations, the family can be affirmed in their values and their caring intention. This affirmation can assist clinicians in developing an allied, collaborative relationship with the family in planning care that advances the values they and the patient hold.

REFERENCES

1. Lantos JD, Singer PA, Walker RM, et al. The illusion of futility in clinical practice. Am J Med 1989:87:81–84.
2. Brock D, Buchanan A. Deciding for Others: The Ethics of Surrogate Decision Making. Cambridge: Cambridge University Press; 1990.
3. Tomlinson T, Brody H. Futility and the ethics of resuscitation. JAMA 1990;264:1276–1280.
4. American Thoracic Society. Withholding and withdrawing life-sustaining therapy. Ann Intern Med 1991;115:478–485.
5. Truog RD, Brett AS, Frader J. The problem with futility. N Engl J Med 1992:236:1560–1564.
6. Schneiderman LJ, Jecker NS, Jonson AR. Medical futility: its meaning and ethical implications. Ann Intern Med 1992:112: 949–954.
7. Griener GG. The physician's authority to withhold futile treatment. J Med Philos 1995;20:207–224.
8. Field MJ, Cassel CK (eds). Approaching Death: Improving Care at the End of Life. Washington, DC: Committee on Care at the End of Life, National Academy Press; 1997.
9. Stone D, Patton B, Heen S. Difficult Conversations: How to Discuss What Matters Most. New York: Penguin Group; 1999.
10. Caplan L. Handling conflict in end-of-life care. JAMA 2000;283,3199.
11. Goold SD, Williams B, Arnold RM. Conflict regarding decisions to limit treatment: a differential diagnosis. JAMA 2000;283:909–914.

Eduardo Bruera, MD
Catherine Sweeney, MB

PATIENT 32

A 59-year-old woman with metastatic breast carcinoma complicated by anorexia/cachexia/fatigue syndrome

A 59-year-old woman with advanced carcinoma of the breast comes to the outpatient clinic. She was diagnosed 4 years earlier and underwent surgery, postoperative radiation therapy, and three different types of chemotherapy after experiencing progressive disease. At present, she has multiple bony metastases, lung metastases, locally recurrent disease, and liver metastases.

Symptoms during the last 2 months included profound fatigue (7/10) and pain with an intensity of 4/10, which has been well controlled with sustained-release oral morphine 200 mg/day. During the last 2 weeks, fatigue has become more intense, and she is now spending most of the time at home in bed. She also has profound anorexia (8/10) and weight loss of > 10% body weight. She eats one-half of her breakfast every morning and no other solid food during the remainder of the day. The patient also experiences persistent nausea (6/10) with vomiting once every day.

The patient does not appear to be suffering from depression or anxiety, and her cognitive studies are normal. There is no evidence on physical examination of bowel obstruction. Her blood work reveals no anemia.

Question: What can be done to alleviate this patient's symptoms?

Diagnosis: Advanced breast carcinoma with metastases and anorexia/cachexia/fatigue syndrome.

Discussion: Many patients with terminal cancer progressively develop a syndrome characterized by anorexia, cachexia, and fatigue. These symptoms occur in > 80% of patients with advanced cancer, who also commonly suffer from chronic nausea. Well-performed clinical studies demonstrate that **corticosteroids** can improve appetite, asthenia, chronic nausea, and pain in patients with advanced cancer who do not otherwise develop significant improvement in nutritional status. The best type of corticosteroids and their ideal dose and route of administration have not been conclusively established. Most experts, however, recommend daily doses of approximately 40 mg of prednisone or 10 mg of dexamethasone, given in divided doses two to four times per day, either orally or subcutaneously.

Benefits associated with the use of corticosteroids are usually observed quite rapidly, within 2 to 4 days of treatment. In contrast, the main side effects of therapy occur with prolonged treatment. Major adverse effects include increased frequency of infections, hyperglycemia (particularly in diabetic patients), steroid-induced myopathy, osteoporosis, and occasionally neurotoxicity with agitation, depression, or delirium.

Because most patients tolerate high doses of corticosteroids without difficulty for short periods, it usually a good idea to start the patient on a reasonably high dose (i.e., 20–40 mg of prednisone per day). This approach allows the clinician to rapidly assess the patient for improvement in the treated symptoms of fatigue, anorexia, nau-

sea, and pain. If no improvement occurs, corticosteroids can be discontinued abruptly after 2 to 4 days of therapy. Conversely, if symptoms improve, the steroid dose can be titrated down to the lowest effective dose that controls symptoms.

Megestrol acetate, a progestational agent, is an alternative to corticosteroids for treating anorexia and cachexia. Several randomized controlled trials have demonstrated that this drug improves appetite, produces weight gain, and enhances a feeling of well-being for patients with advanced cancer. There is also evidence to support the use of megestrol acetate to treat cancer fatigue. A beneficial effect occurs within 7 to 10 days and does not depend on weight gain.

The present patient was started on 10 mg of dexamethasone twice a day, and within 48 hours, she experienced appreciable improvement in appetite, asthenia, and chronic nausea. Pain remained in good control. Over the following 3 weeks, her dexamethasone dose was progressively decreased to 4 mg twice a day. Other measures were taken to improve her gastrointestinal function, including enemas and regular laxatives, and metoclopramide 10 mg every 4 hours, was given to control her nausea.

In approximately 4 weeks, the patient experienced progressive delirium and became bedridden. Delirium was controlled with small doses of haloperidol. Opioids were continued parenterally in a dose calculated to replace previous oral doses and titrated for comfort. The patient died 48 hours after admission to the hospital without signs of agitation or physical distress.

Clinical Pearls

1. Cachexia and fatigue occur in > 80% of patients with advanced cancer.

2. There is good evidence that corticosteroids are capable of improving appetite, asthenia, chronic nausea, and pain in patients with advanced cancer.

3. The best type, dose, and route of administration of corticosteroids for this indication have not been conclusively established; usually, approximately 40 mg of prednisone or 10 mg of dexamethasone is given from two to four times daily, orally or subcutaneously.

4. Symptomatic benefits are usually observed within 2 to 4 days of treatment. If benefit is seen, the dose can be titrated down to the minimum effective dose. If benefit is not seen, corticosteroids should be discontinued.

REFERENCES

1. Bruera E, Roca E, Cedaro L, et al. Action of oral methylprednisolone in terminal cancer patients: a prospective randomized double-blind study. Cancer Treat Rep 1985;69:751–754.
2. Bruera E, Neumann C, Brenneis C, Quan H. Frequency of symptom distress and poor prognostic indicators in palliative cancer patients admitted to a tertiary palliative care unit, hospices, and acute care hospitals. J Palliat Care 2000;16:16–21.
3. Bruera E, Sweeney C. Cachexia and asthenia in cancer patients. Lancet Oncol 2000;1:138–147.

Eduardo Bruera, MD
Catherine Sweeney, MB

PATIENT 33

A 48-year-old woman with colon cancer who develops
profound analgesia-induced sedation

A 48-year-old woman comes to the office with advanced colon cancer that was diagnosed 3 years earlier. After initial surgery and adjuvant chemotherapy, she developed both painful local recurrent disease and painful liver metastases. She is currently receiving slow-release morphine 90 mg every 12 hrs for continuous visceral pain. The patient has good pain control but experiences sedation and fatigue most of the time. However, a decrease in the opioid dose results in increased pain intensity.

It is decided to change the type of opioid to hydromorphone in divided doses totaling 36 mg/day orally. After 3 days of therapy, the patient remains in good pain control but overly sedated. She can no longer participate in the care of her two young children, and she becomes concerned that she will be unable to attend a wedding in the family this weekend, which has great meaning to her. She recognizes the need to control her pain but is distraught by the continued sedation.

Question: How can sedation be reduced in this patient?

Diagnosis: Advanced colonic carcinoma, with sedation secondary to opioid medication at doses needed for analgesia.

Discussion: Although titration of opioid drugs can produce good analgesia for patients with visceral pain, sedation is the dose-limiting toxicity. For many patients, despite multiple opioid titrations, clinicians may be unable to find the therapeutic window between a lower threshold that relieves pain and a higher threshold that results in sedation. Approximately 7% to 10% of patients receiving potent opioids for cancer pain fall into this category of a very narrow or nonexisting therapeutic window. For the present patient, the dose capable of achieving good analgesia overlaps with the dose capable of causing sedation and fatigue, and the sedation did not decrease over time, as occurs in most patients.

Methylphenidate is a mild psychostimulant used successfully in the management of attention deficit hyperactivity disorder in both children and adults and in the management of depression in geriatric populations. Several randomized, controlled trials provide evidence demonstrating that methylphenidate is capable of reducing opioid-induced sedation while maintaining or enhancing analgesia. For patients with severe incidental pain, methylphenidate often allows major increases in opioid doses that would otherwise result in severe sedation.

The usual starting dose of methylphenidate is 10 mg with breakfast and 5 mg with lunch. The present patient was started at this dose and was able to remain alert and active in the care of her children. During the day of the wedding, she was encouraged to take an extra 5 mg dose at 4 PM in order to be more alert and able to socialize during the festivities.

Occasional patients develop tolerance to the psychostimulant effects of methylphenidate. These patients require frequent increases of dose up to a maximum of 30 to 40 mg/day.

The main side effects of methylphenidate include cardiovascular toxicity in those patients with previous arrhythmias, ischemic heart disease, or severe arterial hypertension, and neurologic side effects including anxiety or aggravation of mild preexisting delirium. A detailed medical history and physical examination, with close attention to the cardiovascular system and assessment of baseline cognitive function, should be undertaken before commencing therapy with methylphenidate. Contraindications include any evidence of hyperactive or mixed delirium with psychomotor agitation, increased arousal, hallucinations, or paranoid ideation. The patient's history should also be reviewed for previous episodes of paranoid ideation.

The present patient required a mild increase in the dose of methylphenidate to 20 mg in the morning and 10 mg at noon 3 weeks after its initiation. Home hospice care was arranged, and the patient died without apparent distress in the company of her family at home 4 weeks later.

Clinical Pearls

1. In 7% to 10% of patients, the opioid dose capable of achieving good analgesia overlaps with the dose capable of causing sedation and fatigue, and the sedation does not decrease over time.

2. Psychostimulants such as methylphenidate can reduce opioid-induced sedation while maintaining or enhancing analgesia.

3. Psychostimulants should not be prescribed in patients with features of hyperactive delirium, a history of paranoid episodes, or cardiovascular disease.

REFERENCES

1. Bruera E, Brenneis C, Chadwick S, et al. Methylphenidate associated with narcotics for the treatment of cancer pain. Cancer Treat Rep 1987;71:67–70.
2. Bruera E, Fainsinger R, MacEachern T, Hanson J. The use of methylphenidate in patients with incident cancer pain receiving regular opiates: a preliminary report. Pain 1992;50:75–77.
3. Fainsinger R, Schoeller T, Bruera E. Methadone in the management of cancer pain: a review. Pain 1993;52:137–147.
4. Bruera E, Watanabe S. Psychostimulants as adjuvant analgesics. J Pain Symptom Manage 1994;9:412–415.
5. Bruera E, Neumann CM. The uses of psychotropics in symptom management in advanced cancer. Psychooncology 1998;7:346–358.

Ronald J. Crossno, MD

PATIENT 34

A 64-year-old rural rancher with end-stage lung cancer and painful metastases

A 64-year-old man with widely metastatic lung cancer returns home from an urban cancer center after failure of aggressive treatment. His discharge instructions were to call his local doctor for symptom management. He has pain in multiple sites and nausea that limits oral intake and the use of oral medications. When contacted, his physician first advises him to come to the nearest hospital for care. However, the patient's primary wish is to remain at home, and he asks his doctor to refer him for hospice.

Physical Findings: On the initial hospice clinical visit, the patient was sitting up in bed, awake but with impaired concentration. Mild tachycardia and tachypnea. General: grimacing with any movement. Chest: diminished breath sounds, central venous portal in place. Abdomen: tender, nodular liver-edge. Extremities: multiple tender long-bone deformities. Neurologic: awake and alert.

Social History: He had retired several years ago to become a rancher. He and his wife retired to this rural community. The wife is his primary care provider, and all other family are out of state. Their ranch is 150 miles from the closest tertiary care center with oncology services, where he was treated. Travel there was exhausting, even before his pain became incapacitating. The nearest medical facility is 45 miles away; the closest hospice nurse lives 40 miles away. Indeed, the closest store of any kind is 14 miles away.

Hospice Admission: His analgesic regimen includes oral nonsteroidal anti-inflammatory agents, fentanyl 25-μg transdermal patches, and oxycodone (Percocet) for breakthrough pain. He rates his pain as 8 on a 10-point visual analog scale. His wife is visibly exhausted, but voices determination to keep him at home.

Question: How does one provide end-of-life services when access to care is so limited?

Diagnosis: Terminal metastatic lung cancer with severe pain.

Discussion: When given the choice, most Americans wish to die at home. This opinion also holds true for rural residents. Home hospice has made delivery on this desire the expected standard. Unfortunately, health care, including hospice care, is often limited in remote areas. Many hospices focus their admissions on urban or suburban areas. Hospices that provide rural care often limit the range of services they can provide. There are numerous anecdotal reports of families learning about end-of-life care from one or two nurse visits and then doing everything else themselves.

As in any end-of-life situation, clinicians caring for terminally ill patients in rural areas must determine what the patient and family know and understand about the disease process and what they believe is going to happen. What are their goals and how do they prioritize them? How might these priorities change as death approaches? How comfortable are the patient and family with the process? What support systems are in place? How will living in a remote area impact care?

Most long-time rural inhabitants tend to be self-reliant individualists who understand what is and is not available. Unfortunately, many people who move to the country are not aware of limitations of health services, including home health and hospice care. Such rural realities include a lack of immediate conveniences. Although electricity and telephones are almost universal in rural communities, many rural residents maintain their own water and septic systems. The nearest pharmacy, grocery store, or even convenience store may be many miles away, with limited business hours. Urban family members who come to help a loved one living in a rural setting may need to be educated about these limitations of rural life. Sometimes families make the decision to relocate the ill family member to a more urban setting for palliative and end-of-life care.

Health care for residents of isolated communities usually involves significant travel time. Transfer to an inpatient facility for acute pain or end-of-life care may be impractical. Yet not every patient and family cared for by hospice is accepting of a home death. In those cases, in which the actual death is not desired to occur in the home, the hospice team must work carefully with the patient and family to develop alternative plans. Special planning for death pronouncement and certification is required for a home death. Even with preplanning, removal of the body may take several hours.

Therefore, rural hospices must carefully plan for all contingencies. A major portion of these preparations involves ensuring that the in-home medications for symptom relief are adequate, even if not currently needed. Some hospices have developed a contingency packet of emergency medications that is routinely left in the home. Medications that can be given by non-oral routes when the patient can no longer swallow should be included in these preparations. An example would be rectal diazepam to control status epilepticus. Careful education on why these medications are ordered prepares the patient and family, who may become anxious at the thought of possibly needing to administer all of them when these medications arrive. Fortunately, the telephone triage nurse can often talk families through emergencies, as long as the medications are on site.

The provision of rural end-of-life care usually requires innovation and creative planning. Involvement of trained hospice volunteers, and of non-hospice volunteers, is essential. Neighbors, coworkers, members of the family's religious community, and service groups may all be of help. Most rural residents know and are familiar with everyone who lives "just down the road." Being aware of the potential isolation of rural life, these neighbors usually show a unique increased willingness to help out. With appropriate patient consent, informing neighbors or church-members of the need for their help often generates a wellspring of efforts, practical and emotional.

With careful patient and family consent, provision of care in nonstandard ways may be acceptable. This includes compounding medications for nontraditional routes of administration, such as gels or suppositories. Someone managing their own home water system easily learns to supervise medication pumps and proper administration of parenteral medications.

In the present case, the patient was unable to tolerate oral medication, and the fentanyl patches were not adhering well to his skin. A morphine infusion was begun, using his permanent venous access. (A subcutaneous infusion would have been used if access were absent.) His spouse readily learned to manage the IV line. The hospice nurse changed the med bag during scheduled visits, every 1 to 2 days. Care was taken to ensure that adequate supplies of medications were maintained in the home. Neighbors were enlisted to provide meals and rest breaks for the wife.

After the infusion was begun according to opioid conversion calculations, the morphine required titration over several days to 150 mg/hr with 50-mg boluses via a patient-controlled analgesia device for breakthrough pain. The patient reported his best night's sleep in months after achieving this level. For the first time in 2 weeks, he enjoyed visiting with his wife and friends. After several weeks at this level, he experienced a pain crisis, which was managed with the as-needed boluses. When increased infusion and bolus doses depleted his bag early, a frantic call from his wife found the on-call nurse 90 miles away on another call. The triage nurse contacted emergency medical services. The paramedic, who was a personal friend of the family, responded to change the bag with the full understanding of "no resuscitation" and "no transport." The patient experienced no interruption in his pain management, which was again increased with good effect. The next day he became less responsive. He died peacefully 3 days later, his wish to do so at home fulfilled.

Clinical Pearls

1. A rural setting can challenge, but need not interfere with, excellent end-of-life care and state-of-the-art palliative care techniques. Out-of-home backup is limited, so careful planning is necessary to ensure appropriate preparation for emergencies and crises as they arise. Palliative care in rural settings demands creativity and innovation.

2. Be creative in utilizing nontraditional opportunities to provide care that is unique to each particular setting. Becoming familiar with and enlisting local resources in advance can be invaluable.

3. Neighbors, friends, hospice volunteers, and members of the patient or family's workplace or faith community may be a valuable resource.

REFERENCES

1. Gallup Organization: Knowledge and Attitudes Relating to Hospice Care: Survey conducted for the National Hospice Organization. Princeton, NJ: The Gallup Organization; Sep 1996.
2. Tyler BA, Perry, MA, Lofton TC, Millar F. The Quest to Die With Dignity: An Analysis of Americans' Values, Opinions and Attitudes Concerning End-of-Life Care. Appleton, WI: American Health Decisions; 1997.
3. Farrell MJ. National palliative care education and training needs analysis. Contemp Nurs 1998;7(2):60–67.
4. Issues for palliative care in rural Australia. Collegian 1998;4(3):22–27, 41.
5. Kirby J. Rural patients miss out of palliative care option. The Edmonton Journal 1999;Sep 22.

PATIENT 35

A 64-year-old man admitted to a CCU with an acute myocardial infarction and multiple end-stage medical conditions

A 64-year-old man with chronic renal insufficiency, severe peripheral vascular disease, coronary artery disease, and congestive heart failure is admitted to the cardiac care unit (CCU) for shortness of breath. Significant medical history includes three myocardial infarctions, an ejection fraction of 19%, several strokes resulting in right-sided hemiparesis, and a left below-knee amputation from an old war injury. He is accompanied by his caregivers, a daughter and a son, who are devoted to him. The family reports that he has been bedridden for several months, has not had "sufficient" food or water in the past several days, and is now unable to swallow pills. His mental status is described as "going in and out of the picture." The daughter and son are exhausted and frightened by the "sudden decline" and believe that they are no longer able to care for their father. They are especially concerned that with each setback, the patient's functional and mental capacities are further reduced. The patient and family have not previously discussed the terminal nature of his condition, the patient's preferences for life support, including CPR, or the appropriate goals of care.

Physical Examination: Heart rate variable 40–116, blood pressure from 70/40 to 110/60 depending on cardiac rhythm, respirations 32. General: 130 lbs, diaphoretic, dyspneic, with an irregular thready pulse. Rubs his chest and grimaces. Skin: dusky with markedly slow capillary refill. Abdomen: soft, no peripheral edema, no jaundice. Neurologic: mumbling incoherently, intermittently agitated but not combative, responds to verbal stimuli, but does not follow commands.

Laboratory Findings: Blood tests: consistent with chronic renal failure, dehydration, and acute myocardial infarction. Cardiac monitor: sinus rhythm with multi-focal ventricular and atrial contractions with intermittent periods of a junctional rhythm. SpO_2 (2 liters/min nasal cannula O_2) 90%.

Hospital Course: The patient is considered high risk for any heart catheterization interventions, and he does not appear to be a cardiac surgical candidate. The CCU team concludes that the patient is not imminently dying but is in the terminal phases of his disease and will benefit most from a treatment plan that integrates palliative care into the standard medical regimen in the CCU.

Question: How does the CCU team introduce a palliative care plan into the dominant medical culture of the acute care setting?

Diagnosis: Acute myocardial infarction in a patient with advanced disease and multiple comorbidities who would benefit from palliative care.

Discussion: From a theoretical perspective, formulating a palliative care plan is a dynamic, integrative, and collaborative process between an interdisciplinary team, a patient (or surrogate), and the patient's family. The primary goal of palliative care planning is to implement therapies that relieve pain and suffering so as to maximize quality of life. Pain, suffering, and quality of life are often described as multidimensional, subjective constructs that are framed by a person's experiences. Therefore, communication is a critical skill for clinicians involved with palliative care teams.

However, improved communication and provision of information to physicians regarding patient preferences for treatment may not improve outcomes at the end of life. Alternatively, interdisciplinary collaborative teams that actively promote enhanced communication with patient and family *and* direct patient care do change outcomes at the end of life.

Palliative care plans are put into operation by exquisite attention to the patient's expressed physical, psychosocial, and spiritual care needs. This caveat holds true for a patient in the intensive care unit, the general hospital ward, outpatient clinic, or at home. Ideally, an interdisciplinary team will respond to the complex constructs of pain and suffering to improve the quality of life remaining and allow the patient to die in comfort. Care of the terminally ill requires an emphasis on the patient's responses to illness over and above the usual responses directed toward the underlying disease. Rarely is physiologic pain the sole source of suffering for terminally ill patients. Clinicians must not only be effective communicators, but they must also be competent in diagnosis and treatment. Dyspnea or nausea can be as devastating as pain. Delirium can cripple a family's hopes for closure. Depression, caregiver exhaustion, spiritual pain, or intolerable regret can paralyze attempts to improve quality of life.

Clearly, existential suffering cannot be relieved without the control of pain and other troubling physical symptoms. At the same time, in order to comprehensively relieve suffering of a dying person, the health care team must not limit itself to responding only to physiologic imbalances. The primary advantage of an interdisciplinary team is its ability to integrate evidence and expertise from medicine, nursing, pharmacology, psychology, social work, chaplaincy, and other complementary therapeutic disciplines.

One serious misconception is that palliative care plans cannot employ "technical," "aggressive," or "life-prolonging" traditional medical therapies. Technological advances offer unique strategies for pain and symptom control. Application of these types of therapies must be congruent and offer a promise for outcomes that can realistically improve patients' subjective quality of life. Central venous access catheters should not be ruled out simply because "the patient is dying." These catheters may be the only option for intravenous access.

Another misconception is that patients requiring palliative care are "easy to care for." Most dying patients in the ICU face a loss of identity and self, may feel their spirituality being tested, and grieve the loss of their relationships and futures. These issues transpire in a context of ongoing multisystem failure and profound alterations of physiologic function. Families may suffer with the stresses of caregiving and the losses that advanced illness in a loved one brings, as well as with the pain of anticipatory grief. ICU caregivers must not only address all of these matters, but also focus attention to the family. All of these challenges promote end-of-life care in the ICU as a fertile area for patient care research.

Lastly, uncertainty is a silent partner in the palliative care plan. Accurate prognostication of the time of death remains elusive. Research in palliative care is in its infancy. The best palliative care plan may still fail to relieve pain and suffering, improve quality of life, or orchestrate the "good death." We must become familiar with the feeling of uncertainty and be willing to share this elusive concept with our patients and families.

On admission to the CCU, the present patient received supportive care to manage his arrhythmias and reverse cardiac ischemia. Pain and dyspnea were controlled by titrating doses of intravenous morphine. Haloperidol was chosen to control delirium. Nursing care included strict attention to hygiene, positioning (semi-Fowler's and with arms raised on pillows), strict control of the environment (reduce noise, optimal warmth, natural light), and open visitation for the caregivers. Nurses quietly placed the external pacemaker in his room. Within 2 hours, the patient's hemodynamic and respiratory profile stabilized; however, his cardiac rhythm remained ominous with persisting fluctuations of ST elevations, QRS segments were widening, and urine output falling. He continued to manifest signs of delirium and remained agitated and in obvious discomfort.

At this point, the nurses and physicians begin to discuss additional treatment options, such as placing an intravenous pacemaker to stabilize the cardiac rhythm. One cardiology fellow is uncomfortable at not placing the pacemaker; the nursing staff are certain that to insert the pacemaker, the patient will have to be intubated; and another physician feels that any additional therapies are futile given the ominous cardiac rhythm. The clinical team decides that a family meeting is needed to develop a patient-centered plan of care in which goals can be identified that are congruent with the patient's preferences and achievable quality of life.

The charge nurse organizes the patient care conference with the family and interdisciplinary team. The nurse introduces the concept of a palliative care plan, and the team asks the family to express the patient's preexisting preferences. The physician presents the treatment options that are most likely to meet the goals of care. The patient had expressed wishes not to be placed on a "breathing machine" and did not want artificial feeding or hydration if the outlook was grim. The patient had avoided advance directives in the past, because the assumption was that DNR meant no care at all. The team assures the family that DNR means only "do not perform CPR" and does not imply an abandonment of the patient's palliative care goals or other needs. The family conveyed the patient's feelings and preferences. He was not afraid to die. His biggest fear was of physical pain—as physical pain reminded him of war and dying alone. He did not have a preference to die at home or in the hospital.

The goals of care are established. The family was exceptionally relieved that the team included them, as they considered themselves his only support system. They expressed a desire to be with him when he died. The palliative care plan was straightforward and included several elements:

1. Physical Care: Continue to support cardiovascular system with inotropic agents, continue the morphine drip to relieve pain and dyspnea, continue to manage delirium with haloperidol. No additional drug agents unless required for the management of distressing symptoms. If inotropic agents are successfully weaned to off, they are not to be reintroduced. A DNR order was established.

2. Psychosocial Care: Family is to visit frequently and speak to patient and to participate with simple care tasks that they otherwise would have completed at home. For the patient's sake and their own, they decided to engage in life-review, reminiscing and telling stories in his presence about his and the family's life. The Bereavement services office of the medical center and the patient's community church were notified for future support. Social services assistance with urgent financial planning related to this hospitalization and possible placement was arranged. The social worker also began preliminary discussions regarding home hospice.

3. Spiritual Care: Family was supported with chaplain visits and with calls to local and distant friends. Patient had not followed a specific denomination.

Three days later, the patient was transferred to the general cardiology floor with symptoms of pain, dyspnea and delirium controlled with a morphine drip and low doses of haloperidol. Vital signs, cardiac monitoring, lab work, and radiology exams were all discontinued. Nursing care remained the same. He died 4 days later with his family present.

Clinical Pearls

1. Communication, interdisciplinary collaboration, mutual goal-setting (establishing goals of care), and shared accountability are the four cornerstones of a successful palliative care plan.

2. Palliative care plans must address the personal physical, psychological, social, and spiritual domains of pain, suffering, and quality of life.

3. The implementation of a palliative care plan demands time, integrity, compassion, and competence.

4. Palliative care is hard work and often qualifies as "intensive care."

5. Uncertainty is an inevitable aspect of planning in advanced incurable illness.

REFERENCES

1. Cassel EJ. The nature of suffering and the goals of medicine. N Engl J Med 1982;36:639–646.
2. SUPPORT Principal Investigators. A controlled trial to improve care for seriously ill hospitalized patients: the study to understand prognoses and preferences for outcomes and risks of treatments (SUPPORT). JAMA 1995;274:1591–1598.
3. Cherny NI, Coyle N, Foley K. Guidelines in the care of the dying patient. Hematol Oncol Clin North Am 1996;10:261–285.
4. Campbell M, Frank R. Experience with an end-of-life practice at a university hospital. Crit Care Med 1997;25:197–202.
5. Brant J. The art of palliative care: living with hope, dying with dignity. Oncol Nurs For 1998;25:995–1004.
6. McCaffery M, Pasero C. Pain: Clinical Manual. St. Louis: Mosby; 1999.
7. Stewart AL, Teno J, Patrick DL, Lynn J. The concept of quality of life of dying persons in the context of health care. J Pain Symptom Manage 1999;17:93–107.
8. Foley KM. Pain and symptom control in the dying ICU patient. In Curtis JR, Rubenfeld GD (eds). Managing Death in the Intensive Care Unit. New York: Oxford University Press; 2001: pp 103–125.

Marshall B. Kapp, JD, MPH

PATIENT 36

A 65-year-old man with end-stage metastatic cancer who requests discontinuation of life-sustaining medical interventions

A 65-year-old man with metastatic lung cancer is admitted to the ICU because of severe shortness of breath. He was treated 6 months earlier with chemotherapy and radiotherapy, but his cancer failed to respond. During the last 2 months, he was managed at home with narcotic analgesics for severe back pain related to bony metastases. During the last 3 days, he noted progressive shortness of breath, cough with purulent sputum, and fevers.

Physical Examination: General: marked shortness of breath. Skin: decreased turgor. Chest: decreased breath sounds over the right hemithorax. Neurologic: alert and responsive.

Laboratory Findings: WBC 18,000/μl with a left shift, BUN 40 mg/dl, creatinine 2.1 mg/dl. Chest radiograph: dense airspace opacities involving the entire right lung.

Hospital Course: The patient undergoes intubation and mechanical ventilation for a diagnosis of pneumonia. He remains awake but is only intermittently lucid. Because of progressive renal failure, hemodialysis is initiated. On the fourth hospital day, the patient writes on a pad, "Please let me die," and hands the pad to the attending physician, who had never met the patient before the current admission. The physician recommends to the patient's wife of 40 years and his two adult children, who have kept a vigil by the bedside, that palliative care be initiated and the ventilator discontinued. The family and the rest of the ICU team agree with this recommendation, but some of the team members are anxious about potential legal exposure connected with this course of action.

Question: What are the legal liability implications associated with withholding dialysis and withdrawing a ventilator from a dying patient in an ICU when the patient, family, and health care team all agree with this course of action?

Answer: There is little risk of adverse legal consequences for members of the ICU team for withholding or withdrawing life-sustaining medical treatments from a dying adult patient when the patient, family, and professional team are in agreement with this course of action.

Discussion: It is common for health care professionals to have anxiety about being exposed to potential legal action as a result of their decisions to withhold or withdraw life-sustaining medical treatments, such as ventilators and dialysis, from critically ill patients. Specific fears range from being targeted in civil malpractice litigation brought by family members or others on behalf of a deceased patient, to being the focus of criminal investigations and prosecutions charging homicide and/or patient abuse or neglect, to being the object of licensure proceedings initiated by state administrative boards that regulate professions. It is well established in the United States as a matter of both constitutional and common (case) law, however, that any **mentally capable adult patient** has the fundamental right to make personal medical choices, including a decision to refuse or discontinue life-sustaining medical treatments so long as the decision is made voluntarily and after relevant information has been shared with the patient.

The patient's mental capacity needed to exercise this right is a threshold issue in the decision-making process. Therefore, it is incumbent on the physicians and other members of the ICU team to conduct a timely, conscientious assessment of the patient's current cognitive and emotional abilities and deficits. The importance of this requirement is further emphasized by the observation that the courts, in the context of a guardianship proceeding, have not yet formally resolved this issue.

The ICU team must determine as a working, clinical matter whether the patient now possesses sufficient ability to rationally understand and manipulate pertinent information in order to make and express a decision about treatment, and to adequately appreciate the consequences of that decision. This evaluation is especially important for the present patient whose degree of lucidity is questionable and appears to fluctuate.

If the clinical evaluation concludes that the patient presently is adequately capable of deciding about life-sustaining medical treatments, the patient's decision to refuse further life-sustaining medical treatments and to accept palliative care instead is legally entitled to respect. Such respect does not expose members of the ICU team to legal repercussions. Indeed, in a few jurisdictions, their failure to respect the wishes of a competent patient, especially when the family is in agreement with those wishes, might expose the ICU team to civil litigation based on a theory of medical assault and battery.

If the patient lacks sufficient present capacity to make his own autonomous treatment decisions, decision-making authority would devolve to a surrogate. Such devolution of authority may occur formally through a court's guardianship (conservatorship) order or a written durable power of attorney instrument, naming the patient's desired agent, executed by the patient earlier while still capable of doing so. In the case of the present patient, there is neither a guardianship order nor a durable power of attorney for health care. In more than 30 states, statutes have been enacted that establish a priority order of individuals who are empowered to make medical decisions for an incapacitated patient in the absence of a formal grant of authority by a court or the patient. Even if there is no applicable statute in a particular jurisdiction, the longstanding custom has been for health care professionals to turn to available, interested "next of kin" for medical decisions when the patient cannot personally speak autonomously. When the immediate family is involved, informed, in agreement with each other, and appears to be acting in the patient's best interests, reliance on the family as decision-maker—even in the absence of officially conferred legal authority—is legally proper.

There are several facets of an effective **risk management strategy** to reduce the likelihood of adverse legal repercussions resulting from discontinuation of life-sustaining treatment. As a primary matter, honest, empathetic, continuing dialogue among members of the ICU team, the patient, and family is important in fostering the kind of positive relationship that avoids subsequent legal activity. Families generally seek legal redress when they have been surprised by an unanticipated bad result and good relations with the providers have not been cultivated. Second, the ICU team must document in the patient's medical record their process for making and implementing their decisions about life-sustaining medical treatments. This documentation must be timely, accurate, and complete. It is necessary to document who was involved in making particular choices and the rationale for recommendations and decisions made. Third, in especially unclear and uncomfortable situations, members of the ICU team should consider seeking consultation with the hospital's risk management department and/or its institutional ethics committee.

In caring for the present patient, the ICU team ascertained that the patient and family were properly informed about available options and their foreseeable consequences. It was also established that the family agreed with the recommendations for discontinuation of life-sustaining treatments and the provision of palliative care. The ICU team initiated comfort measures to relieve the patient's anxiety and dyspnea and subsequently discon- nected the ventilator. The attending physician carefully documented these actions and the ratio- nale for them in the patient's medical chart. The patient died peacefully, surrounded by his family, several hours later. The family expressed appreci- ation for the care he received.

Clinical Pearls

1. Because a mentally capable patient has the legal right to accept or reject medical interventions, including life-sustaining medical treatments, it is essential for the health care team to conscientiously assess in an ongoing fashion the patient's capacity to make medical decisions.

2. Surrogate decisions for the withdrawal or withholding of life-sustaining medical treatments from a patient with impaired decision-making capacity are ordinarily legally valid when: (1) family members or other surrogate decision-makers are in agreement among themselves, and (2) decisions are consistent with the patient's known or inferred own wishes (substituted judgment) or the surrogate's appraisal of the patient's best in- terests.

3. Key elements of effective legal risk management in withholding or withdrawing life-sustaining medical treatments include:
- excellent communication among the relevant parties,
- thorough documentation in the medical record of decisions including how and by whom they were reached, and
- consultation with the hospital's risk manager and/or institutional ethics committee in appropriate circumstances.

REFERENCES

1. Dubler NN: Balancing life and death—proceed with caution. Am J Public Health 1993;83:23–25.
2. Meisel A: The Right to Die, 2nd ed. New York, John Wiley & Sons, 1995.
3. Meisel A: The 'right to die': a case study in American lawmaking. Eur J Health Law 1996;3:49–74.
4. Kapp MB: Legal issues in critical care. In Hall JB, Schmidt GA, Wood LGH (eds): Principles of Critical Care, 2nd ed. New York, McGraw-Hill, 1998.
5. Meisel A, Jernigan JC, Youngner SJ: Prosecutors and end-of-life decision making. Arch Intern Med 1999;159:1089–1095.
6. Luce JM, Alpers A: Legal aspects of withholding and withdrawing life support from critically ill patients in the United States and providing palliative care to them. Am J Respir Crit Care Med 2000;162:2029–2032.
7. Meisel A, Snyder L, Quill T: Seven legal barriers to end-of-life care: myths, realities, and grains of truth. JAMA 2000;284:2495–2501.
8. Kapp MB: Legal liability anxieties in the ICU. In Curtis JR, Rubenfeld GD (eds): Managing Death in the Intensive Care Unit: The Transition from Cure to Comfort. New York, Oxford University Press, 2001.

John M. Luce, MD

PATIENT 37

A 64-year-old man with COPD who accepts intubation and mechanical ventilation, but not indefinitely

A 64-year-old man is admitted to the ICU for an exacerbation of chronic obstructive pulmonary disease (COPD). He was admitted to the same ICU 7 months earlier with a similar exacerbation that required 3 weeks of endotracheal intubation and mechanical ventilation.

Physical Examination:　Blood pressure 117/75, pulse 123, respirations 37, temperature 38.5° C. General: thin, lethargic, tachypneic. Chest: decreased breath sounds, ronchi at right base. Cardiac: increased S2.

Laboratory Findings:　Electrolytes normal except for total CO_2 of 37 meq/l. Arterial blood gas on 2 liters/min of oxygen: pH 7.34, $PaCO_2$ 65 mm Hg, PaO_2 52 mm Hg. Chest radiograph: hyperinflation with possible right lower lobe infiltrate.

Hospital Course:　The patient is treated with supplemental oxygen at 2 liters/min, aerosolized bronchodilators, and intravenous antibiotics and corticosteroids. His $PaCO_2$ subsequently rises to 75 mm Hg and his PaO_2 falls to 45 mm Hg. He is administered bilevel positive airway pressure via facemask, but he becomes even more dyspneic. The patient agrees that he is willing to receive intubation and mechanical ventilation at this point, but he and his wife both state that they are unwilling to have him "left on the ventilator like a vegetable."

Question:　What should the patient and his wife be told?

Answer: Therapies that do not benefit patients are not continued indefinitely in most American ICUs today.

Discussion: Two or three decades ago in the United States, patients requiring life-sustaining treatment for exacerbations of COPD and other illnesses might well have feared being intubated and mechanically ventilated beyond the point that they could benefit from these therapies. In fact, those patients and families who asked that life support be withheld and withdrawn frequently found that physicians and hospitals were unwilling to do so because they considered these actions illegal and unethical. Because of this belief, the perception that intensive care promised to improve most clinical outcomes, the silence of professional societies on the issue of patient autonomy, and the lack of legal mechanisms whereby patients and their families could define the circumstances under which autonomy can be exercised, many if not most patients who died in the ICU did so while receiving life-prolonging rather than palliative care.

In the past 20 to 30 years, however, a number of factors have contributed to marked changes in the nature of death in the ICU. For example, legal cases such as *Bartling* and *Bouvia* in California established that competent patients can refuse any and all therapies, including those that are life-saving, under the legal principles of informed consent and informed refusal. Similarly, in the *Quinlan* case in New Jersey and the *Barber* case in California, the courts applied the principles of informed consent and informed refusal to the care of incompetent patients, ruling that the patients' family members could act as surrogates and make "substituted judgments" for them. In the *Cruzan* case, the U.S. Supreme Court accepted the viewpoint that a competent person's right to forgo treatment is a liberty interest, although it allowed the states to set their own standards, enabling the state of Missouri to require "clear and convincing evidence" of incompetent patients' wishes before surrogates were permitted to have life-sustaining therapy forgone.

In parallel with these court decisions, research studies have revealed that not all patients benefit from care in the ICU. During the same period of time, professional societies such as the Society of Critical Care Medicine have issued position papers emphasizing the ethical propriety of patients or their surrogates making decisions regarding the withholding and withdrawal of life support. The federal Patient Self-Determination Act of 1991 requires that caregivers at health care facilities ask patients if they have advance directives and help them prepare such directives if they do not. Living wills and other declarations of patient intent have become increasingly common, and many states allow patients to formally appoint surrogates using the durable power of attorney for health care.

The impact of these and other historical developments on the nature of dying in America has been amply documented. For example, in studies conducted in two medical-surgical ICUs at hospitals affiliated with the University of California, San Francisco (UCSF), we demonstrated that in 1987–1988, 50% of patients who died in the ICUs did so during the withholding and withdrawal of life support. During 1992–1993, 90% of patients died in this fashion. Similarly, in a national study of end-of-life care involving 131 ICUs in 38 states, we found that during a 6-month study period, only 20% of patients who died in the ICUs did so after receiving full life support, including attempted CPR. In contrast, 24% died after receiving full life support but not attempted CPR; 14% had life support withheld; 36% had life support withdrawn; and 6% were brain-dead.

While life-prolonging care increasingly is being limited in patients who do not benefit from it, more attention is being given to administering palliative therapy. In a study in the two ICUs in UCSF-affiliated hospitals, we showed that all patients who were considered capable of experiencing pain received sedatives and analgesics during the withholding and withdrawal of life support. Since then, position papers, journal articles, and textbook chapters have outlined the appropriate use of these agents and other treatments in dying patients, including those with COPD. The U.S. Supreme Court, in its recent *Glucksberg* and *Vacco* decisions, has sanctioned the giving of drugs, even to the point of "terminal sedation," provided that physicians intend to relieve suffering and not hasten death.

In keeping with this progress, most patients and family members, including those in the present case, can be assured that intubation, mechanical ventilation, and other kinds of life support are not continued indefinitely in most American ICUs. This is not to say that all ICUs follow this approach or that palliative care is perfect. Patients concerned about protecting their autonomy should still articulate their wishes in advance of critical illness and incompetence and designate durable power of attorney. Patients, their designated proxies, or family members should insist that caregivers include them in devising treatment plans. Furthermore, all parties should regard the ICU as a therapeutic trial in which life-prolonging interventions should give way to palliative measures if the trial fails.

Fortunately, the present patient, his wife, and

physicians all agreed that he should be given a trial of mechanical ventilation for his exacerbation of COPD. They set a limit of 1 week on the ventilator. He responded to treatment and was extubated within 5 days. On discharge, he said that he would be willing to be intubated and ventilated again on a trial basis if he experienced yet another COPD exacerbation.

Clinical Pearls

1. In contrast to the situation 20 to 30 years ago, most patients who die in ICUs in the United States today do so during the withholding and withdrawal of life support.

2. The changing nature of death in the ICU is attributable to state and federal court decisions affirming the right of patients to refuse treatments, including those that are life-sustaining; the demonstration that not all patients benefit from intensive care; the promotion of patient autonomy by ethicists and professional societies; and the development of mechanisms, such as the durable power of attorney, to protect patient autonomy.

3. Patients and their families should be assured that therapies that do not provide benefit are not continued indefinitely in most American ICUs.

4. Nevertheless, patients and surrogates should insist that patient autonomy be respected by physicians and that palliative care be provided them.

REFERENCES

1. Wilson WD, Smedira NG, Fink C, et al. Ordering and administration of sedatives during the withholding and withdrawal of life support. JAMA 1992;267:949–953.
2. Desbiens NA, Wu AK, Bloste SK, et al, for the SUPPORT investigators. Pain and satisfaction with pain control in seriously ill hospitalized patients: findings from the SUPPORT research investigation. Crit Care Med 1996;24:1953–1961.
3. Luce JM, Prendergast TJ. The changing nature of death in the ICU. In Curtis JR, Rubenfeld GD (eds): Managing Death in the Intensive Care Unit: The Transition from Cure to Comfort. New York, Oxford University Press, 2001.
4. Heffner JE. Chronic obstructive pulmonary disease. In Curtis JR, Rubenfeld GD (eds): Managing Death in the Intensive Care Unit: The Transition from Cure to Comfort. New York,, Oxford University Press, 2001.
5. Luce JM, Luce JA. Management of dyspnea in patients with far-advanced lung disease. JAMA 2001;285:1331–1337.
6. Luce JM, Alpers A. End-of-life care: what do the American courts say? Crit Care Med 2001;29:N40-N45.

Lisa Krammer, RN
Cameron Muir, MD

PATIENT 38

A 65-year-old man with advanced cancer with nausea, vomiting, dyspnea, and dysphagia who desires home care

A 65-year-old man with advanced colorectal cancer metastatic to lung and liver has been hospitalized several times recently for antitumor treatment of abdominal carcinomatosis and pulmonary lymphangitic spread. Symptom management was initiated during these hospitalizations. He has been monitored at home by home health since his discharge from the hospital. For the past 2 days, he has experienced nausea and vomiting, worsening dyspnea, progressive dysphagia, and anxiety. He has become progressively weaker with a gradual loss of appetite, and rapidly declining functional status. Recently, he expressed to his physician his decision to forgo anticancer therapy.

Currently, he takes ondansatron 8 mg every 4 to 6 hours as needed for nausea and vomiting and oxygen at 3 liters by nasal cannula for dyspnea. He has declined intravenous access. He is married with no children, and has a very supportive extended family nearby. He strongly desires to spend the remainder of his life at home with his symptoms controlled. His wife is committed to uphold his wish.

Physical Examination: HEENT: dry mucosal membranes with white plaques across buccal mucosa and posterior pharynx. Cardiac: tachycardia. Chest: poor inspiratory effort, bibasilar crackles, no wheezing. Abdomen: large, nontender, hypoactive bowel sounds, hepatomegaly, no ascites. Extremities: +3 pitting edema.

Question: Can these symptoms of advanced disease be relieved efficiently and effectively at home?

Diagnosis: Advanced colorectal cancer, nausea, vomiting, dyspnea, and dysphagia with a desire to remain at home.

Discussion: During advanced stages of illness, specifically in end-of-life care, patients are likely to suffer from a number of complex and distressing symptoms. Nausea, vomiting, dyspnea, and dysphagia are a few of the symptoms encountered and, if unrelieved, preclude a patient and family from achieving an optimal quality of life and a peaceful death.

The incidence of nausea and vomiting at the end of life is estimated to be between 40% and 70%. **Emesis** due to cortical stimulation (anxiety, anticipatory) is alleviated by corticosteroids, anxiolytics, and cannabinoids. Vomiting induced by stimulation of the chemoreceptor trigger zone (drugs, toxins, metabolic derangement, other) can be treated with dopamine antagonists, antihistamines, anticholinergics, and selective serotonin antagonists. Nausea and vomiting associated with stimulation of the vestibular apparatus (movement associated) is managed with antihistamines and anticholinergics. Emesis associated with vagally mediated peripheral afferents (distortion/irritation of GI tract, gastric stasis, other) is alleviated with dopamine antagonists, serotonin antagonists, and prokinetic agents. Antacids, H_1 blockers, and proton pump inhibitors may also be indicated. Nonpharmacologic measures of massage, relaxation strategies, biofeedback, guided imagery, and acupuncture/acupressure are also beneficial in alleviating nausea and vomiting.

In the present case, the patient's emetogenetic process is triggered by a combination of stimulation of the cortical pathway, as evidence by his anxiety, and the vagally mediated peripheral afferents as a result of his abdominal carcinomatosis and hypokinetic intestine.

Dyspnea, or the subjective experience of labored or difficult breathing, occurs in 21% to 75% of patients in the days to weeks before death. Either separately or in combination, the stimulation of the cortex (anxiety or somatization), lung mechanoreceptors (edema, tumor, other), and lung chemoreceptors (abnormal serum gases) trigger the respiratory center of the medulla to affect respiratory drive and produce the sensation of breathlessness. Management consists of pharmacologic therapy with oxygen, opioids, and anxiolytics, while corticosteroids and bronchodilators may be helpful in some patients. Nonpharmacologic measures are also beneficial (see above). In this case, the patient's anxiety invokes the cortex, and his lung metastasis and lymphangitic carcinomatosis stimulate the mechanoreceptors to collectively activate the respiratory center and produce a sense of dyspnea.

Dysphagia, in the absence of head and neck cancer and motoneuron disease, is reported to occur in 23% of patients at the end of life. Mechanical obstruction (tumor), functional disturbance (fibrosis, disinterest, weakness, nerve damage, other), and mucosal inflammation (infection, other) disrupt the normal anatomy and physiology, resulting in swallowing difficulties. The incidence increases as patients become unable to swallow because of weakness or impaired consciousness. Evaluation and management include consideration of artificial feeding and/or hydration (parenteral nutrition is generally not beneficial in patients with advanced disease); investigation of possible obstruction and suitability for interventions (surgical, stent placement, pharmacologic management); treatment of any mucosal infection; prescribing opioids for pain; evaluating medications that exacerbate swallowing difficulties (anticholinergics); ensuring safety measures if aspiration is occurring (proper consistency of food preparations, suitable positioning, and Pace while swallowing); and addressing the psychological impact of dysphagia.

The present patient was believed to be suffering from dysphagia because his oropharyngeal mucosal lining was inflamed with oral candidiasis and because of a functional disturbance associated with his progressive, generalized weakness.

With the progression of disease in the end of life, one of the challenges in effectively maintaining optimal symptom management in the home is developing alternative treatment strategies for medication administration. Sublingual, buccal, rectal, and subcutaneous administrations are useful avenues to deliver medications. An advantage of using the **sublingual or buccal route** includes a very rapid action. The first-pass effect is bypassed because the drug is absorbed directly into the systemic circulation. Sublingual and buccal administration requires very little expertise, preparation or supervision. However, there are also disadvantages of using this approach. Sublingual formulations of many medications are lacking, high doses cannot be easily administered, and sublingual absorption is poor.

Rectal medications often offer an effective, but often overlooked, alternative. They are ideal when chronic administration is not anticipated and when an alternative to both oral medication and injections is desired. When placed in the lower part of the rectum, extensive hepatic metabolism can be avoided because the drug bypasses the portal circulation. A significant number of medications are available in suppository form (or can be compounded). The major disadvantage is that many patients find rectal administration objectionable, especially if family members administer the medication. Also, the condition of the rectal mucosa, blood flow to the rectal area, use of lubricants, dehydration, and presence of feces influence the rectal absorption of drugs.

An additional alternative treatment strategy for medication administration is the **subcutaneous (SC) route**. It is an appealing alternative because peak plasma concentrations are achieved within 15 to 30 minutes, and intermittent or continuous infusion of medications can be delivered. The only device required is a portable syringe driver with a 25- to 27-gauge needle that can be changed as infrequently as once a week. One major disadvantage is that there are limitations to the volume injected. The maximum average rate is 5 ml/hr. However, when necessary, the rate may be increased to 8 ml/hr if the patient is comfortable at the infusion site. Limited data are available as to what medications can be delivered subcutaneously. The most frequently utilized drug classes are opioid analgesics, antiemetics, anxiolytic sedatives, corticosteroids, and anticholinergic drugs (see Table 1). Often, end-of-life symptoms necessitate a combination of medications in order to achieve effective symptom management.

Table 1. Medications That Have Been Given Safely via the SC Route

Dexamethasone
Hydrocortisone
Solu-Medrol
Haloperidol
Hyoscine butylbromide (scopolamine)
Hyoscine hydrobromide
Octreotide
Morphine
Hydromorphone
Methotrimeprazine
Metoclopramide
Midazolam
Lorazepam
Prochlorperazine

Concerns about chemical compatibility and stability of such mixtures are justified. Most of the published data on compatibility speaks to drugs that can be mixed with morphine (see Table 2). In every instance, the infusion should be observed for precipitation or discoloration. A one-to-one dose-conversion ratio is used initially when converting from oral to sublingual, buccal, rectal or subcutaneous, with the exception of morphine and hydromorphone, for which the conversion from oral to subcutaneous is 3:1 and 4:1, respectively.

Table 2. Medications That Have Been Safely Mixed with Morphine

Haloperidol
Lorazepam
Midazolam
Dexamethasone
Hydrocortisone
Metoclopramide
Hyoscine butylbromide (scopolamine)
Methotrimeprazine
Octreotide
Methylprednisone

In order for the home plan of care to be effectively implemented and maintained, it is strongly recommended that a home hospice program be involved. Hospice is the gold standard for providing comprehensive "whole person" palliative care in the home setting. Hospice uses an interdisciplinary team to address the physical, psychological, spiritual, and social components that a dying patient and family experience. The members of the interdisciplinary team share the mutual goal of improving the quality of life of the patient and family. In fact, expert symptom management in the home care setting, as demonstrated in the present case, is routine for a skilled home hospice team.

For the present patient, home-based management strategies included treatment of his nausea and vomiting with metoclopramide 10 mg every 6 hours SC for its antinausea effects of dopamine blockade and prokinetic action, and lorazepam 0.5mg, scheduled every 6 hours and every 1 to 2 hours as needed, sublingually or SC, was initiated as both an antiemetic and anxiolytic. Corticosteroids were initiated as an anti-inflammatory to relieve dyspnea associated with tumor metastasis and lymphangitic carcinomatosis. Dexamethasone 20 mg SC once daily was chosen because it has low mineralocorticoid activity, which aides in minimizing fluid retention, and its long half-life of 36 to 54 hours, which permits once-daily dosing. Additionally, it served as an adjuvant antiemetic. As the patient was opioid naïve, short-acting morphine 2.5 to 5.0 mg sublingually or SC every hour as needed for management of his dyspnea was available.

The oxygen was continued at 3 liters per nasal cannula, as he felt this aided in relieving his breathlessness. A fan, blowing directly on the patient's face was initiated (it is thought that this assists in relieving dyspnea by cooling the trigeminal nerve). Oral candidiasis was treated with an elixir of fluconazole. Aspiration precautions were instituted, and Thick-it™ was added to thicken the texture of food. In addition to the above measures, the home hospice nurse taught the patient's wife the nonpharmacologic strategies of guided imagery and massage and reassured her that there was expertise available 24 hours a day to ensure her husband's comfort.

As the patient neared the end of his life, medications were titrated to maintain effective symptom control. He eventually needed a metoclopramide SC continuous infusion at 5 mg/hr mixed with a morphine SC continuous infusion at 2 mg/hr. He died at home peacefully 3 weeks later, free of nausea, vomiting, and dyspnea, with his wife at his bedside. His family reflected that his time at home had been meaningful to the patient and family and that he had enjoyed a good quality of life with adequate symptom control.

Clinical Pearls

1. Most symptoms in patients with advanced chronic illness can be managed at home through a multimodal, team-based approached.

2. Clinicians must be knowledgeable of and comfortable with alternative routes of drug administration (sublingual, buccal, rectal, subcutaneous).

3. Clinicians should know medications that can be mixed and are thought to be compatible (see Table 2).

4. Home hospice services are the gold standard for the delivery of palliative care in the home. The expertise of the interdisciplinary team in addressing the physical, emotional, and spiritual needs of patients and families is well recognized, althoughhospice remains significantly underused.

5. Knowing the palliative effects of dexamethasone can be very helpful. While it is generally used as an anti-inflammatory, it has antiemetic, appetite-stimulating, mood-elevating, and fatigue-reducing effects. In the palliative setting, its long half-life allows for once-daily dosing, the absence of mineralocorticoid effect minimizes salt and water retention, and the risks of immunosuppression are less relevant.

REFERENCES

1. Fainsinger R, Miller M, Bruera E, et al. Symptom control during the last week of life on a palliative care unit. J Palliat Care 1991;7:5–11.
2. Mannix KA. Palliation of nausea and vomiting. In Doyle D, Hanks GWC, MacDonald N (eds). Oxford Textbook of Palliative Medicine. Oxford: Oxford University Press; 1993: pp 489–499.
3. Roberts CJC, Keir S, Hanks G. The principles of drug use in palliative medicine. In Doyle D, Hanks GWC, MacDonald N (eds). Oxford Textbook of Palliative Medicine. Oxford: Oxford University Press; 1993: pp 223–236.
4. Twycross R, Regnard C. Dysphagia, dyspepsia, and hiccup. In Doyle D, Hanks GWC, MacDonald N (eds). Oxford Textbook of Palliative Medicine. Oxford: Oxford University Press; 1993: pp 499–512.
5. Twycross R, Lichter I. The terminal phase. In Doyle D, Hanks GWC, MacDonald N (eds). Oxford Textbook of Palliative Medicine. Oxford: Oxford University Press; 1993: vol pp 977–992.
6. Chandler SW, Trissel LA, Weinstein SM. Combined administration of opioids with selected drugs to manage pain and other cancer symptoms: initial safety screening for compatibility. J Pain Symptom Manage 1996;12:168–171.
7. Baines MJ. Nausea, vomiting and intestinal obstruction. BMJ 1997;315:1148–1150.
8. Ahmedzai S. Palliation of respiratory symptoms. In Doyle D, Hanks GWC, MacDonald N (eds). Oxford Textbook of Palliative Medicine, 2nd ed. Oxford: Oxford University Press; 1998: pp 583–616.
9. Bruera E, Ripamonti C. Dyspnea in patients with advanced cancer. In Berger AM, Weissman DE (eds). Principles and Practice of Supportive Oncology. Philadelphia: Lippincott-Raven Publishers; 1998: pp 295–308.
10. Pasero C, Portenoy RK, McCaffery M. Opioid analgesics. In McCaffery M, Pasero C (eds). Pain: Clinical Manual, 2nd ed. St. Louis: Mosby; 1999: pp 161–299.

Jennifer Rhodes-Kropf, MD
Barbara Paris, MD

PATIENT 39

A 78-year-old woman intubated for COPD and lung cancer whose family states that she had never wanted to be on a ventilator

A 78-year-old woman with stage IIIb lung cancer and a long history of COPD experiences a respiratory arrest and is intubated. She has been cared for by the same primary medical doctor for 10 years and also has an oncologist whom she has seen for 4 months. She is fully cognitively intact, but her functional status has declined over the last few months. She is homebound but needs assistance with all of the activities of daily living. The patient does not have a living will or durable power of attorney for health care.

Physical Examination: Blood pressure 80/50, pulse 100, temperature 39° C, respirations 18. General: thin, pale, eyes closed. Cardiac: tachycardic, no murmurs. Chest: decreased breath sounds and dullness to percussion throughout the right lung field. Neurologic: responsive only to painful stimuli. Extremities: cool, doppler pulse 1+ bilaterally, 1+ edema bilaterally.

Laboratory Findings: Hct 32%, WBC 12000/μl with elevated neutrophils, sodium 140 meq/l, bicarbonate 35 meq/l, BUN 40 mg/dl, creatinine 1.5 mg/dl, with normal potassium, chloride, magnesium, and phosphate. ABGs (FIO_2 60%, rate 12/min, pressure support 8 cm H_2O, tidal volume 600 ml): pH 7.40, PCO_2 50 mm Hg. EKG: multifocal atrial tachycardia. Chest radiograph: pleural effusion involving the entire right lung, bilateral hilar adenopathy, and a 2 cm × 2 cm nodule in the left upper lobe.

Hospital Course: Over the next 24 hours, the patient's condition deteriorates with increasing hypoxia and evidence of biventricular failure. Her blood pressure of 85/55 is dependent on dopamine. She continues to be febrile on broad-spectrum antibiotics. The family states that the patient had never wanted to be on a ventilator.

Question: What reasons might this patient have had not to complete advance care planning?

Diagnosis: Terminal pulmonary disease with a very low chance of survival.

Discussion: Advance care planning refers to a person's wishes for resuscitation and choice of a health care proxy. A survey of a random sample of 800 outpatients found that only 11% of patients had ever discussed resuscitation with a physician, 67% had thought about the issue, and 44% had discussed it with someone other than a physician. The data are similar for patients who require hospitalization. So why are there so few conversations on advance care planning?

Limited time is one reason cited by physicians for their lack of advance care planning discussions. It is appropriate and preferable to discuss advance care planning in the outpatient setting. These discussions are effective, even in 5-minute intervals, integrated into regular visits. The conversations can transpire over a few visits and lead to a good understanding by the physician of the patient's wishes, values, and beliefs. Patients can be encouraged to discuss the topic with their proxy and other family members. These discussions form the basis for the clinician and patient to review preferences for care and confront major treatment decisions when serious illness, disability, or other significant changes in health status occur.

Because discussions on advance care planning are infrequent in the outpatient setting, most patients who enter the hospital do not have advance directives. The problem often persists during admission. Patient discussions on this topic are limited by the belief of physicians that the patient is unlikely to die during the hospital stay and, therefore, a discussion about advance directives is irrelevant. However, it is extremely difficult to discuss resuscitation with a patient who is acutely ill, and even more difficult when a patient becomes mentally incapacitated and the burden of making decisions suddenly falls to a surrogate. Unfortunately, this is the case in the vast majority of end-of-life discussions. The level of stress on families who must decide on withdrawal of life-sustaining treatments is tremendous. Physicians are wise to plan ahead, even if it is felt that the patient's death is not imminent. The more the doctor and family know about a patient's wishes, the less stress there will be when a patient is acutely ill and decisions regarding treatment must be made.

Physician discomfort with end-of-life issues contributes to the paucity of clinical conversations about dying, death, and grief. The discomfort is present for various reasons. Reticence reflects a taboo in American culture. The physician does not know the patient well and wonders whether it is his or her role to broach the subject. There is a lack of training in residency programs. The physician is fearful of his or her own mortality. One way to help ease this discomfort is to plan ahead what needs to be said to a particular patient and in what way. If the physician appears at ease and open to discuss advance care planning, the patient is more likely to feel at ease.

Some physicians worry that a conversation on advance care planning will be distressing their patients. A study of hospitalized patients found that patients are comfortable with and welcome the opportunity to have these discussions. Patients are able to set limits on the subjects they wish to avoid. Sometimes there are cultural, religious, or personal reasons why patients want to avoid advance care planning. It is important to ask patients about these issues, to listen to and acknowledge their concerns, and to answer questions and correct misconceptions they may have.

Physicians and patients are sometimes concerned that a DNR order leads to less attentiveness in patient care. DNR does not mean "do not treat." When goals of care shift to an emphasis on comfort and quality of life, patients can continue to get close monitoring and frequent therapeutic adjustments as required to achieve these therapeutic goals. Physicians can reassure patients that they will not be abandoned—that they will be their companion throughout all aspects of care. It is also noteworthy that DNR orders vary by diagnosis. In one study, the percentage of patients with DNR orders ranged from a high of 98% on an oncology service to a low of 43% on cardiology. Patients of all diagnoses deserve discussion about advance care planning.

The present patient has terminal pulmonary disease and is intubated despite having expressed to her family that she did not want ventilation. The primary medical doctor had missed an important opportunity of prospectively addressing issues in advance of a crisis. The physician had a close relationship with her, but had put off discussion of this issue because he had not thought her decline was imminent. The ICU attending and primary care doctors met with the family. The physicians and family felt that there was no hope for meaningful recovery and decided to withdraw life-sustaining treatment. Palliative measures were continued for fever, pain, and dyspnea. The patient expired without signs of distress.

Clinical Pearls

1. Effective discussions on advance care planning can occur with brief integrated discussions during regular visits.

2. Most patients welcome the opportunity to discuss end-of-life issues with their physician.

3. Encourage patients to share their feelings regarding resuscitation with their proxy.

4. It is extremely important to talk about advance care planning before patients are acutely ill.

5. Physicians and patients should understand that DNR does not mean "do not treat."

REFERENCES

1. Bedell SE, Delbanco TL: Choices about cardiopulmonary resuscitation in the hospital. N Engl J Med 1984;310(17):1089–1093.
2. Maksoud A, Jahnigen DW, Skibinski CI: Do not resuscitate orders and the cost of death. Arch Intern Med 1993; 153(10):1249–1253.
3. Paris BE, Carrion VG, Meditch JS Jr, et al: Roadblocks to do-not-resuscitate orders: a study in policy implementation. Arch Intern Med 1993;153(14):1689–1695.
4. SUPPORT Principal Investigators: A controlled trial to improve care for seriously ill hospitalized patients: the study to understand prognoses and preferences for outcomes and risks of treatments (SUPPORT). JAMA 1996;274:1591–1598.
5. Ebell MH, Smith MA, Seifert G, Polsinelli K: The do-not-resuscitate order: outpatient experience and decision-making preferences. J Fam Pract 1990;31(6):630–636.
6. Carney MT, Morrison RS: Advance directives: when, why, and how to start talking. Geriatrics 1997;52(4):65–73.
7. Elliason AH, Parker JM, Shorr AF, et al: Impediments to writing do-not-resuscitate orders. Arch Intern Med 1999; 159(18):2213–2218.

Alan Carver, MD

PATIENT 40

A 56-year-old man in need of palliative care in anticipation of end-of-life distress

A 56-year-old man with a 4-year history of amyotrophic lateral sclerosis (ALS) has experienced worsening dyspnea, poor secretion control, dysphonia, and coughing in the past 2 months. Upon arriving for a home visit, the patient's neurologist finds him in mild to moderate respiratory distress. The patient also complains of diffuse muscle pain and cramping. His wife sits near him, holding his hand. She breaks down in tears when he tells the neurologist how guilty he feels about the emotional and financial burdens he is placing on her and their two adult children.

During the home visit, the neurologist reviews invasive and noninvasive options for mechanical ventilatory assistance, and the man declines. The patient informs his neurologist that he has thought a great deal about his disease and prognosis, and that he does not want to "prolong the inevitable." The man requests that everything possible be done to help make him comfortable and to ease the burden he has placed on his wife and two adult children in recent months. He is notably dyspneic and frequently coughs when speaking.

Physical Examination: Blood pressure 100/65, pulse 110, temperature 37.0°, respirations 26. Oxygen saturation 90%. General: thin, ill-appearing in moderate distress, dyspneic in conversation. Cardiac: tachycardic, no murmurs. Chest: no crackles or rhonchi, decreased breath sounds bilaterally. Abdomen: soft, nontender, no masses, bowel sounds present. Neurologic: Mental status: awake, slight lethargy when not verbally stimulated; oriented to person, place, time; unable to perform serial 7's or serial 3's; registration intact; recalls 1/3 objects in 5 minutes; naming and repetition intact, follows 2- but not 3-step commands. Cranial nerves: no deficits. Motor: moderate spasticity with diffuse atrophy and 1/5 strength in all muscle groups, prominent fasiculations noted in all four extremities. Sensory: no deficits to multi modality testing. DTRS: 3+ throughout with ankle clonus bilaterally.

Question: What strategies should be employed to ensure that this patient's physical and psychological needs are met now and in the future?

Discussion: The World Health Organization (WHO) defines palliative care as "the active total care of patients whose disease is not responsive to curative therapy." Because ALS is a progressive and incurable disorder, patients with this condition benefit from the time of first diagnosis from caregivers with expertise in the principles and precepts of palliative medicine. Palliative care is especially important considering that distressing symptoms of dyspnea (seen in 88% of patients), dysphagia (88%), pain (76%), weight loss (68%), and dysarthria (60%) are common in patients with ALS at or near the end of life.

Delaying considerations of palliative care until patients are near the end of life is a common error in managing patients with progressive illnesses. One expert in palliative care has stated that "the crucial issue in symptom control at the end of life is preparedness. It is a wholly inadequate response to the onset of a distressing symptom if control has to wait on a doctor's order or the pharmacist's acquisition of the medication required." Advances in the evaluation and treatment of pain, dyspnea, and other symptoms at the end of life have engendered scientifically based guidelines that define comprehensive approaches to patient assessment and management. The Quality Standards Subcommittee of the American Academy of Neurology has published an especially valuable clinical practice guideline for palliative care of patients with ALS. Recent guidelines also focus on the management of pain, dyspnea, and other more general end-of-life challenges.

A successful palliative strategy depends on a comprehensive **pain assessment.** The cornerstone of this strategy is a trusting relationship between the physician and patient that accepts the patient's complaints as real and deserving of a detailed and thoughtful evaluation. Regular use of one of the widely available, scientifically validated pain measurement scales is critical when making a pain assessment. Asking the patient to rate his or her pain on a scale of 0 to 10 (0 = no pain, 10 = the worse pain imaginable) allows quantification of symptoms and an evaluation of the response to treatment. The WHO three-step analgesic ladder provides a useful framework for selecting analgesic drugs. The ladder recommends that clinicians match pain severity with choice of drug, thereby ensuring that patients with mild, moderate, and severe pain are managed appropriately.

Morphine remains the drug of first choice in managing severe pain. Established guidelines recommend that opioid-naïve patients with moderate to severe pain should be treated with 5–10 mg of i.v. or s.c. morphine, titrated according to anal-gesic efficacy and side effects. Opioid-tolerant patients whose pain has escalated should receive an initial bolus at a dose adjusted for the dose of medication that they are currently taking. Many patients receiving substantial doses of opioids may require 10–15 mg of i.v. or s.c. morphine and titrated to response.

The fundamental concept that underlies this approach is individualization of pharmacotherapy. The correct dosage is the amount of medication that provides maximal pain relief with minimal side effects. As there is no ceiling effect for opioid drugs, patients should be titrated upward until satisfactory pain relief is achieved or dose-limiting side effects occur. For patients who are sedated but obtaining adequate analgesia, psychostimulants may reverse sedation and improve cognitive function. Depressed patients with a short life expectancy may benefit from a psychostimulant as a quick-acting adjuvant antidepressant.

No more frightening sensation exists than intense air hunger. Treatment of **dyspnea** depends on the underlying cause. Some patients may benefit from antibiotics, diuretics, or supplemental oxygen depending on clinical circumstances. In the absence of specific therapy, palliative interventions can alleviate dyspnea at the end of life. These interventions include the use of bronchodilators, benzodiazepines, corticosteroids, and i.v. or nebulized morphine. Low-dose i.v. morphine is the palliative treatment of choice, with the goal of striking a balance between the patient's level of comfort and the risk of oversedation. Opioid-naïve patients should be given 1–2 mg of i.v. morphine, titrated to maximal efficacy or dose-limiting side effects.

Respiratory depression is a concern in treating patients with advanced ALS who require an opioid drug for the relief of pain and/or dyspnea. It is important to remember that tolerance develops to all opioid side effects except constipation. Treatment of a patient's dyspnea requires not only knowledge of how to manage side effects (including the use of stool softeners, laxatives, stimulants, and antiemetics), but also the maintenance of comfort by prescribing equianalgesic dosages of alternative opioids when it is necessary to change drug regimens.

Balancing symptom control while maintaining full consciousness is sometimes difficult to achieve for patients with far-advanced disease or who are imminently dying. A family meeting may be essential to clarify concerns, ensure a trusting bond with the healthcare team, and establish the goals of care.

Some family members may voice concerns that opioids or other palliative drugs may **hasten death.**

At present, no evidence exists that opioid medications accelerate the time to death. Some data suggest that opioids may actually prolong life by decreasing the work of breathing, pain, dyspnea, and generalized stress. In a study of dying patients who received morphine as compared to those who receive saline during withdrawal of ventilatory support, patients treated with morphine lived longer, suggesting that morphine may have protected these patients from the acute stressors of critical illness.

Drugs used to control intractable symptoms should be titrated according to the needs of the patient and in concert with the established goals of care. Doses of sedatives and analgesics should not be titrated upward in the absence of clear indications for their use. High doses that may depress respiratory drive are morally, ethically, and legally acceptable if the intent is to relieve symptoms. Continuous infusions rather than bolus injections are preferable to prevent acute rebound or breakthrough pain, dyspnea, or agitation. Patients recognize a caregiver's offer for sedation at the end of life as an empathic acknowledgment of the severity of their suffering. A promise of nonabandonment even when sedation is required can be a great comfort to dying patients and their families and friends.

The present patient was reassured that the neurologist's commitment to providing care would not stop with the patient's refusal of life-sustaining interventions. The physician outlined the palliative interventions that were available and promised that the patient would not suffer at the end of life. The family pastor was invited to discuss with the patient and his wife how he had cared for his family and how it was acceptable for the family to now care for him.

Home hospice implemented the neurologist's palliative care plan with medications to relieve his dyspnea and muscle pain. One month later, he died at home, having enjoyed a relatively comfortable period under hospice care with his family.

Clinical Pearls

1. Nothing has a greater impact on improving the quality of life for patients with advanced ALS than the implementation of currently available, scientifically validated guidelines, symptom assessment tools, and practice parameters for effective palliative care.

2. Opioids do not hasten death or the progression of disease. However, the routine use of morphine for dying patients in the absence of a target symptom should be avoided.

3. When a troublesome single side effect occurs while using opioids for pain or dyspnea, physicians can usually treat the symptoms attached to the side effects rather than discontinue opioid therapy. If multiple side effects occur, the opioid should be replaced with an alternative agent.

4. Ongoing open communication among the physician, patient, and family is essential at all stages of illness and critically important in advanced illness in order to clarify concerns, alleviate patient fears, and establish the goals of care.

REFERENCES

1. Cancer Pain Relief and Palliative Care: Report of a WHO Expert Committee. Geneva, World Health Organization, 1990 (WHO Technical Report Series, no. 804).
2. Wilson WC, Smedira NG, Fink C, et al: Ordering and administration of sedatives and analgesics during the withholding and withdrawal of life support from critically ill patients. JAMA 1992;267:949–953.
3. Oliver D: The quality of care and symptom control—the effects on the terminal phase of ALS/MND. J Neurol Sci 1996;139(suppl): 134–136.
4. Ingham JM, Portenoy RK: The measurement of pain and other symptoms. In Doyle D, Hanks GWC, MacDonald N (eds): Oxford Textbook of Palliative Medicine, 2nd ed. New York, Oxford University Press, 1998, pp 203–219.
5. Quality Standards Subcommittee, American Academy of Neurology: Practice parameter: The care of the patient with amyotrophic lateral sclerosis (an evidence-based review). Neurology 1999;52:1311–1323.
6. Sykes N: End of life care in ALS. In Oliver D, Borasio GD, Walsh D (eds): Palliative Care in Amyotrophic Lateral Sclerosis. Oxford, Oxford University Press, 2000, p 164.

Thomas Prendergast, MD

PATIENT 41

A 73-year-old woman with multiorgan failure
and a contentious, divided family

A 73-year-old woman gradually develops diffuse upper abdominal discomfort, nausea, and vomiting of bilious material over 24 hours. Her primary care physician admits her to a local hospital for diagnostic evaluation. The patient has a history of autoimmune hepatitis for which she was treated for six months 2 years ago with corticosteroids.

Physical Examination: Blood pressure 98/62, pulse 108 and regular, SpO_2 92% on room air, temperature 37.9°. General: awake, interactive and appropriate, but appears acutely ill. Chest: normal. Cardiac: normal. Abdomen: slightly obese, soft, mild diffuse tenderness without any masses. Stool: negative for occult blood.

Laboratory Findings: Hct 35%, WBC 14,800/μl with 32% band forms. Electrolytes, renal indices, and liver function tests: normal. Urine: no leukocytes or bacteria. Abdominal CT scan: normal. Abdominal ultrasound: normal. Chest radiograph: The primary physician reads it as normal, but a radiologist later interprets it as showing a subtle right-lower-lobe infiltrate.

Hospital Course: The patient is treated with intravenous piperacillin and tazobactam for an ill-defined abdominal disorder. Over the first 24 hours, her abdominal discomfort improves, but she becomes dyspneic and hypoxemic. A repeat chest radiograph shows diffuse pulmonary infiltrates consistent with acute respiratory distress syndrome (ARDS). On her third hospital day, she is intubated and transferred to the ICU of a teaching hospital for continued care.

On arrival to the teaching hospital, the patient is sedated on a midazolam infusion. She does not respond to voice or gentle shaking. Over the next 4 days, she develops renal dysfunction, severe hypoalbuminemia, progressive hypoxemia, and hypotension requiring fluid boluses and vasopressors. All cultures remain negative.

The patient is a retired college professor who lives alone. Her husband of 47 years died of lung cancer 5 months ago. The patient has an advance directive instructing that she would not want prolonged aggressive treatment if there were "no reasonable prospect of regaining my ability to think and act for myself." There is no documentation in the record of any discussion at the community hospital regarding intubation or the patient's wishes in the event of prolonged intensive care.

She has four adult children who describe her as dynamic, independent, and very caring. They openly express their desire for her to recover. The patient's eldest son points out that the patient agreed to intubation after the referring physicians told her that she would be intubated for "no longer than a few days." There appears to be some resentment by youngest daughter toward her older brother's handling of his role as proxy decision-maker.

The ICU team approaches the children about continuing therapy. The discussion does not go well. The children are critical of the community hospital for what they perceive as a failure to diagnose a respiratory problem. They are frustrated by their mother's decline in the absence of a specific diagnosis. They want to know the patient's prognosis with greater precision than you believe is possible. Their interactions are consistent with an apparent history of internecine sibling squabbles. Your discussion with them ends when the youngest daughter storms out after accusing her brother of giving up on their mother.

Question: What do you do next?

Diagnosis: An incompetent, elderly woman with systemic inflammatory response syndrome leading to ARDS, shock, and multiorgan dysfunction syndrome.

Discussion: Considerable skill is needed in managing critically ill patients whose family members have a history of internal dissension and who disagree among themselves regarding appropriate levels of care. For healthcare providers to succeed in these difficult situations, it is crucial to understand three principles of communication in the ICU:

First, **communicating with a family** is as much the intensivist's job as managing a patient's multiorgan failure. One should take appropriate advantage of local resources to facilitate specific problems—nursing staff, chaplain services, social work, and psychiatry may all provide invaluable help—but the focus of treatment decisions remains with the attending physician who is responsible for medical treatment.

Second, **complicated communications** with families are not rare. Critically ill patients have complex medical problems that arise unexpectedly, present diagnostic challenges, and demand ongoing management decisions despite uncertain outcomes, which are usually difficult to predict. Disagreements and misunderstandings between physicians and families about the medical facts or their interpretation are common. The goal of communications in the ICU is to identify and diffuse those disagreements before they harden into conflict that makes it impossible to reach reasonable decisions.

Third, a skilled intensivist recognizes that **resolution of disagreement** requires the participation of the parties involved. Unilateral decision-making is almost never the proper response to disagreement. Many physicians are tempted to declare a course of treatment futile. The practical import of labeling a direction of care "futile" is to avoid the difficult, time-consuming, and unpredictable process of working through a decision with the participation and understanding of the family. Similarly, if families do not believe that their concerns are being addressed, they may be unable or unwilling to consider difficult decisions involving limitations of life support.

Several facts in this case are not in dispute. First, the patient is gravely ill. She has been hospitalized only 4 days, but her progressive respiratory deterioration, continued vasopressor dependency, hypoalbuminemia, and renal dysfunction all point to a high mortality. Up to 10% of patients with systemic inflammatory response syndrome and multiorgan dysfunction syndrome have no clear cause of their disorder; the prognosis is worse in those without as compared to those with a documented

site of infection. Also not in dispute is the fact that the patient has an advance directive that sets some limits on her acceptance of ICU care but is vague regarding her wishes in the current circumstances. The document appoints a proxy decision-maker but does not tell how to weigh a small but real chance of survival against her desire not to have her treatment unnecessarily prolonged. Questions regarding the boundaries of care must be raised with the patient's legal surrogate.

Another fact not in dispute is the observation that a family dialogue regarding boundaries of care is both appropriate and a common occurrence in the ICU. Multiple studies from the United States and Canada confirm that approximately 75% of critically ill patients who die have some form of life-sustaining therapy withheld or withdrawn following a discussion with the family.

Multiple surveys confirm that families want **clear and accurate information** delivered to them in language that they can understand. They also want their physicians to be **optimistic.** In the ICU, however, when decisions regarding continued care depend so clearly on accurate information, naïve optimism and hope for cure must be replaced with a considered hope that, whatever the outcome, the person will be free of physical distress and treated in a dignified manner, consistent with his or her wishes. This is a modern, responsible approach to the old dictum that one should never take away a patient's or family's hope.

Physicians tend to view continuing or withdrawing life support as a decision made on a rational, probabilistic weighing of the medical facts. Families experience the same circumstances not as an event but as a process with cognitive, affective, and interpersonal aspects. They need information to understand the illness; they need a trusting relationship with medical care providers to be able to accept the implications of that information and to find meaning therein; and they need to make a decision that protects and preserves relationships within the family so that they can live with themselves and each other in the days, months, and years ahead.

Skilled, experienced intensivists recognize the importance of this process by their willingness to orchestrate a "good death" that values the ethics of care as well as the social, cultural, and aesthetic values of families. Physician behavior affects family decision-making. Frequent, timely communication with clinicians who make themselves available builds trust with the family. In contrast, failure to address significant changes in status or impending death creates suspicion. A skilled communicator encourages consensus by respecting different opinions while maintaining focus on what the patient would want in the current situation. This focus on the patient's wishes helps to avoid placing the burden of decision-making on one person, who may be made to feel responsible for the patient's death.

Families need and deserve accurate information delivered compassionately and in a timely fashion. This information must not come at the expense of sensitivity to the emotional and interpersonal aspects of their decisions. For example, **denial** is the inability to recognize facts because of psychological consequences such as grief or guilt. To misconstrue denial as a failure to understand the facts of the case may lead to cognitive interventions (e.g., painfully detailed discussions of the physiology of sepsis) that confuse families and lead to bilateral frustration. To attempt to overwhelm denial with information is analogous to the habit of speaking progressively louder to a patient who does not understand English.

Recognizing the emotional pain within family conversations that confront decisions of limiting treatment reveals the possibility of clinically effective strategies. Open-ended listening, respectful silence, and nondefensive or neutral responses that reflect and validate family members' emotions allow families to gradually come to terms with the most difficult decision of their lives.

Physicians and nurses are not required ethically or legally to provide medically inappropriate care. However, the definition of medically inappropriate is not made theoretically but is determined through conversations and negotiations over time with patients and their families. With the present patient, her condition did not improve. The physician met informally with individual members of the family over the next several days. They needed time to struggle with two realizations: that their mother was dying, and that to honor the person that she was, they needed to respect her wishes not to have disease-directed treatment prolonged. On the sixth ICU day, the four children and their spouses met with the attending physician and agreed to withdraw ventilatory support. Afterwards, they thanked the intensivist for allowing them time to work through the decision as a family. They also agreed to an autopsy on the grounds that their mother would have wanted to contribute to expanded medical knowledge in any way that she could.

Clinical Pearls

1. Disagreement over prognosis and therapy is common in the treatment of critically ill patients. Conflict is a maladaptive response to that disagreement. Effective physician communication can reduce conflict.

2. Futility is a strategy to resolve disagreement through the power to impose a unilateral decision. It is rarely effective and even more rarely appropriate. The frequency of invoking the notion of futility reflects the lack of training and discomfort physicians have with negotiating complex, end-of-life care decisions.

3. Physicians and families often approach decisions to limit life-support differently. Physicians should adapt their information-based communication to acknowledge and facilitate the family's process of coming to a decision, which includes informational, emotional and interpersonal elements.

4. Families want honest, accurate information while they want physicians to be optimistic. The skilled intensivist can provide accurate information about prognosis while supporting hope for a good death consistent with the patient's wishes.

REFERENCES

1. Hickey M: What are the needs of families of critically ill patients?: a review of the literature since 1976. Heart & Lung 1990;19:401–415.
2. Tilden VP, Tolle SW, Garland MJ, et al: Decisions about life-sustaining treatment: impact of physicians' behaviors on the family. Arch Intern Med 1995;155:633–638.
3. Swigart V, Lidz C, Butterworth V, et al: Letting go: family willingness to forgo life support. Heart & Lung 1996;25:483–494.
4. Prendergast TJ: Resolving conflicts surrounding end-of-life care. New Horiz 1997;5:62–71.
5. Jastremski CA, Harvey M: Making changes to improve the intensive care unit experience for patients and their families. New Horiz 1998;6:99–109.
6. Cook DJ, Giacomini M, Johnson N, et al: Life support in the intensive care unit: a qualitative investigation of technological purposes: Canadian Critical Care Trials Group. CMAJ 1999;161:1109–1113.
7. Kutner JS, Steiner JF, Corbett KK, et al: Information needs in terminal illness. Soc Sci Med 1999;48:1341–1352.
8. Goold SD, Williams BC, Arnold RM: Handling conflict in end-of-life care. JAMA 2000;283:3199–3200.

Cynda Hylton Rushton, DNSc, RN

PATIENT 42

A 26-month-old child with severe developmental abnormalities, hydrocephalus, and recurrent ventricular shunt infections

A 26-month-old, mentally retarded boy presents with fever, vomiting, and lethargy complicated by failure of his long-term intravenous access. He was born at 24 weeks' gestation and developed multiple medical problems related to his premature birth. These problems included grade III intraventricular hemorrhage, shunted hydrocephalus, subglottic stenosis with tracheostomy dependence, brochopulmonary dysplasia, cerebral palsy (spastic diplegia), and dysfunctional swallow necessitating a gastrostomy tube for nutrition and fluids. After birth, he had an extended stay in the neonatal ICU until he could be discharged home. He subsequently required frequent hospitalizations for multiple shunt malfunctions and infections, in addition to episodes of sepsis and intravenous access failure. During one of these hospitalizations, he suffered cardiopulmonary arrest that resulted in further deterioration in his neurologic condition.

During previous admissions, the patient's parents have requested that their son receive all available life-sustaining treatments, even though his physicians at times recommended a more conservative approach. Despite their son's diminished awareness and poor functional ability, they see value in his life.

The patient is now admitted with the diagnoses of a shunt infection and obstruction. After numerous conversations with the physicians, the patient's parents agree to a do-not-resuscitate (DNR) order. They refuse to accept, however, any other limitations to his care. The physicians offer hospice care, but the parents do not want to "give up." The health care team, most of whom are familiar with this child and the parents, believes that they would be subjecting the patient to burdensome and inappropriate care if they aggressively treated him again with aggressive life-sustaining treatments.

Question: How should the health care team respond to the parents' request for aggressive, life-sustaining care?

Diagnosis: Hydrocephalus with a shunt infection in a patient for whom aggressive care would seem to present more burden than benefit.

Discussion: Nothing seems so tragic as the death of a child. Whether death comes quickly after a sudden accident or expected after a long-term illness, parents and caregivers struggle to accept the reality of a dying child. This acceptance is made all the more challenging when parents face decisions regarding the withholding or withdrawing of life-sustaining care.

Although the intention of clinicians is to minimize pain and suffering, these decisions force parents to acknowledge that death is imminent, and therefore, they are a source of distress. To reach some level of acceptance, parents must consider their deep-seated beliefs about life, death, and disability against the backdrop of the protective love a parent holds for a child. Conflicts arise between a parent's desire to protect their child from pain and suffering and a universal parental instinct to safeguard their child's life. Resolution of such intrinsic conflicts requires parents to realize that at some point the goals of preserving life and alleviating distress are often mutually exclusive. Clarifying the goals of care assists in choosing treatment alternatives that maximize benefit and minimize harm.

The possible medical goals for the present patient include: 1) aggressive life-prolonging care to stabilize the patient's condition, in preparation for another shunt revision and placement of intravenous access; 2) maintenance of the current level of support and provision of palliative care without surgical interventions; and 3) "comfort care," foregoing any life-sustaining treatments and allowing the natural history of the underlying disease to unfold.

Supportive goals include: 1) allowing the child's parents sufficient time to accept the reality of their son's death; 2) assisting the parents to reframe their options, allowing them to be faithful to their vision of being "good parents" while acknowledging that their son's life is coming to an end; 3) creating opportunities for memory making and life closure, such as scrapbooks or hand prints; and 4) developing a plan and offering the family the opportunity to care for their son at home with the support of home care hospice providers.

In considering choices among the available goals for a patient, caregivers should weigh the outcomes attached to each goal and the likelihood that each outcome could be achieved. For the present patient, the following questions bring to focus the relationship between goals and outcomes.

Is it surgically feasible to revise the shunt and re-establish intravenous access? The physicians believed that it was possible to revise the shunt, treat the infection, and re-establish venous access but voiced concern that aggressive intervention became more difficult for the child to endure with each shunt infection.

How likely is it that the proposed treatment will reduce symptoms and improve the quality of the child's life? With treatment of the hydrocephalus and infection, the present patient would most likely survive but would experience a further decline in his functional capacity.

If life-sustaining treatment were not escalated and palliative interventions were initiated, what would become the goals of therapy? If further surgical interventions were not pursued, the goal for the child's care would focus on symptom treatment, comfort care, selection of a site for care (home or hospital), and strategies for managing morbidities that may arise. Care would extend to support for the pateint's family through his death and during their initial period of bereavement.

What degree of risk, intrusiveness, or discomfort is associated with the treatment of the shunt obstruction? Surgical interventions will include short-term burdens that may be tolerable, especially from the parent's perspective, if they will restore the patient to his previous functional level. The health care team reports that the child tolerates each of his hospitalizations and shunt revisions less well. He has required more pain medications and sedative control with each revision to prevent intractable crying, grimacing, stiffening, and related signs of distress.

What is the patient's capacity to experience pain and to appreciate and enjoy life? Opinions are changing regarding the impact of pain on infants and young children. In the past, infants might not receive sedation or analgesia for some painful procedures because of a conception they would not remember pain or suffer consequences from painful experiences. Recently, the ill effects of untreated pain on infants and children have been more fully recognized. Despite the present patient's young age and developmental disabilities, it must be assumed that another shunt revision would be a painful experience. Caregivers often use parents as the most reliable proxy to assess the ability of their young children to experience pain and suffering. The patient's parents recognized the pain attached to the shunt revisions that their son had undergone but believed it acceptable if a favorable outcome could occur.

What is the level of certainty about the prognosis and outcomes? Decisions regarding the treatment of children with life-threatening conditions often occur under conditions of uncertainty. It may be difficult to discern when a patient has become terminal from when a degree of recovery remains a reasonable hope. Moreover, it is frequently difficult to predict with accuracy a child's trajectory of disease. This uncertainty may stimulate caregivers and parents to pursue extensive diagnostic testing and innovative therapies in hopes of clarifying a child's prognosis. The greater the uncertainty of the prognosis, the more likely parents will accept burdens of treatments in hopes of benefiting their children.

Will the proposed treatment alter the natural course of the disease? Revising the present patient's shunt will not improve the baseline cognitive impairment, although it may prevent further acute deterioration.

Will life-sustaining treatments only prolong the dying process? The caregivers believed that treatment of the shunt obstruction would merely delay the patient's inevitable death, which appeared likely in the coming weeks or months. The patient's parents held that every moment of their son's life was precious, and he had not yet begun to die.

Inevitably, many disagreements in the appropriateness of different health care options derive from values held regarding the nature of a "meaningful" life and the competing goals that comprise caring for a patient. The health care team did not believe that aggressive interventions were in the patient's best interest because of the patient's short life expectancy and his poor baseline quality of life. Although the parents remained convinced that every day of their son's life was precious, they began to recognize the full range of goals available for caring for their

son. They slowly grew more open to the perspective that palliative care was not "giving up," that it could be an affirmation of life and their love for their child in granting him relief from pain and suffering. Although they valued his life and wished to delay his death, they learned to value other ways of expressing their paternal love and care.

In resolving the present dilemma, a meeting of the Ethics Committee was convened to provide a forum for the caregivers and parents to express their viewpoints. One of the primary values expressed by the patient's parents was their wish to care for him at home for as long as possible. They eventually conceded during the meeting that they knew their son would not get better and that he was dying. This acceptance allowed caregivers to assist the parents to redirect their concerns from life prolongation to comfort, symptom relief, and preparation for their son's death. The patient's primary pediatrician and the parents agreed on a plan for handling potential situations in which medical intervention might be considered. The parents feared that they would be alone when their child began to die. The physicians and hospice team offered their support and immediate assistance whenever it was needed.

Shunt revision was not performed. Antibiotics were discontinued. The child was discharged home with hospice care. Antiseizure medications were administered and subcutaneous opioids were titrated to comfort. The patient died 36 hours after discharge at home in his mother's arms, with a hospice nurse in attendance.

Clinical Pearls

1. By discussing the need for decision-making regarding palliative care, physicians often present parents with their first opportunity to recognize that their child is near death.

2. Pediatric care centers on the family unit and acknowledges the important role of parents in knowing their children's needs and advocating for their interests. At times, however, parents require assistance in recognizing the treatment goals that will promote their children's best interests.

3. Because the course of illness in children often remains uncertain and unpredictable, palliative care should be integrated early into treatment plans for all children who have life-threatening conditions.

REFERENCES
1. Shelton T, Jeppson E, Johnson B: Family-Centered Care for Children With Special Health Care Needs. Bethesda, Association for the Care of Children's Health, 1987.
2. Rushton CH, Glover J: Involving parents in decisions to forgo life-sustaining treatment for critically ill infants and children. AACN Clin Issues Crit Care Nurs 1990;1:206–214.
3. Fleishman AR, Nolan K, Dubler N, et al: Caring for gravely ill children. Pediatrics 1994;94:433–439.
4. American Academy of Pediatrics Committee on Bioethics and Committee on Hospital Care. Palliative care for children. Pediatrics 2000;106:351–357.
5. Woods NS, Marlow N, Costelow K, et al: Neurologic and developmental disability after extremely preterm birth. N Engl J Med 2000;343:378–384.

Kelly A. Wood, MD, MHS
Derek C. Angus, MD, MPH

PATIENT 43

A 73-year-old man with a subdural hematoma and poor prognosis
based on an ICU scoring system

A 73-year-old man with a history of hypertension and chronic obstructive lung disease requiring home oxygen therapy is found collapsed at home. He is intubated and placed on mechanical ventilation in the emergency department. A subdural hematoma is evacuated operatively and he is admitted to the ICU. The patient retired 8 years ago and has been living at home by himself.

Postoperatively, the patient remains unresponsive and continues to require mechanical ventilation. He suffers a brief episode of hypotension that responds to fluid resuscitation alone. Subsequently, his creatinine increases from 0.8 to 2.8 mg/dl. He is persistently febrile (39.2°) during the first 3 days of ICU care, with an initial WBC count of 20,000/μl and heart rate in the 110 to 120 range. On the third ICU day, he is noted to have a right middle lobe infiltrate on his chest radiograph and his PaO_2 is 78 mm Hg with a concentration of 60% inspired oxygen.

The ICU scoring system in use defines the patient's prognosis as poor. The incorporation of this scoring system into the patient's clinical assessment persuades the ICU team to encourage the family to consent to withdrawal of life support. The family wishes to discuss the patient's prognosis with the ICU team and to learn more about the ICU scoring system.

Question: What role should ICU scoring systems play in the decisions of withdrawing life-supportive care?

Diagnosis: Critically ill patient with a poor prognosis estimated by a scoring system that should serve only as an adjunct to decision-making.

Discussion: Most patients who die in ICUs in the United States do so during the withholding and withdrawing of life support. As demonstrated by the present patient, ICU scoring systems appeal to physicians because they offer a potential for assisting in the difficult decision to withdraw life-supportive care. The Acute Physiology and Chronic Health Evaluation (APACHE) system published in 1981 was the first major severity scoring system. Subsequently, the Mortality Prediction Model II (MPM), the Simplified Acute Physiology Score II (SAPS), and APACHE III have been developed.

ICU scoring systems were developed by analyzing clinical data from large, heterogeneous populations of critically ill patients. APACHE II is an updated version of the APACHE system that used data from 13 U.S. hospitals in a logistic regression equation to give a mortality probability. The APACHE III system was developed in 1991 using data from 40 hospitals. APACHE III includes an increased list of physiologic variables, an enlarged diagnostic list, and coefficients for the time and source of admission.

SAPS II and MPM II models were developed from a large data set collected in 139 ICUs from 12 countries. SAPS II uses logistic regression to choose both the variables included in the model and the ranges and weights for those variables. SAPS II is a general model and does not require a single diagnosis to obtain the probability of hospital mortality. MPM II uses similar methodology extended to include probabilities at the time of ICU admission and at 24, 48, and 72 hours after admission.

ICU scoring systems have proven valuable in comparing groups of patients in randomized trials and for quality assurance. Some clinicians have proposed the use of ICU scoring systems for prognostic purposes to reduce physician uncertainty during clinical decision-making. Because these systems are based on large databases, it has been suggested that they may provide more accurate predictions of patient outcomes than physician judgment.

Use of these systems for prognostication, however, is a subject of debate. APACHE, for example, is designed to classify groups of patients rather than individuals. Group classification was selected for APACHE because previous systems designed to predict survival for individual patients required extensive data collection and, at that time, physicians were reluctant to accept estimated probabilities as the basis of limiting or stopping therapy.

Since the inception of the APACHE scoring system, there has been a dramatic increase in withholding or withdrawing life support.

Because many patients die in the ICU during the withholding or withdrawing of life support, an objective means of identifying patients for whom aggressive medical care is futile would be a valuable aid in decision-making. The use of scoring systems for identifying patients with poor prognoses, however, is controversial for the following reasons:

1. Prognostic scoring systems are generally based on first day score.
2. There is the potential to apply a prognostic scoring system inappropriately to a group of patients with a diagnosis not included in the original database.
3. There can be significant variability not only between different data collectors, but also between scoring systems themselves.
4. Ethical issues exist in the application of scoring systems to individual patients.

Most prognostic scoring systems are based on data collected from the initial day(s) of intensive care. The prediction of a patient's clinical outcome, however, is dynamic and changes relative to responses to therapy or unforeseen complications. Systems based on a static analysis of admission data from groups of patients therefore provide limited value for decisions to withhold or withdraw therapy from patients in the ICU. Moreover, some scoring systems are subject to lead-time bias, which depends on whether data collected before ICU admission is included in the analysis. Thus, the application of a mortality prediction based on first-day scores to patients on day 4 of their ICU stay, as exemplified by the present patient, may not provide accurate information.

The selection process used to classify diagnoses in the original database strongly influences scoring systems. In the APACHE III system, for instance, patients are classified by the one nonoperative or operative diagnosis that is considered to have precipitated admission to the ICU. The selection of a single diagnosis as the cause for admission is highly subjective and can be difficult to ascertain, particularly for the trauma patient who may have multiple injuries, including neurologic disorders, as demonstrated by the present patient. One study prospectively evaluated residents and nurses as severity-score data collectors. Although the study demonstrated only a minimal effect of interobserver variability between resident and nurse data collection on predicted mortality rates in large patient groups, significant variability occurred in predicting outcomes for individual patients.

Important ethical issues surround any discussion of withdrawal of life supportive care. As stated by Watts and Knaus, "Prognostic systems will never be able to predict outcome with 100% specificity, and high severity scores therefore never will be indicative of absolute irreversibility of disease or impossibility of survival." Consequently, scoring systems have inherent inaccuracies that create ethical concerns if they are used to identify patients with high severity scores for whom restorative care is predicted to be "futile." The inaccuracies of scoring systems are less problematic when low scores are used to predict survival for patients who later die in the ICU.

While predicting survival in the ICU is uncertain and often difficult based on the clinical picture, one cannot unilaterally rely on ICU scoring systems. Alternatively, there are no data that support the accuracy of physician judgment alone as compared with predicted mortality from severity scoring systems. Instead, data indicate that the best survival estimates combine an objective prognosis with a physician's clinical estimate. Thus, as demonstrated by the present patient, scoring systems can provide helpful guides in conjunction with clinical judgment and patient and family input.

The family of the present patient was influenced by the ICU team's recommendations for withdrawal of life-supportive care. While waiting for out-of-town relatives to arrive, however, the family observes the patient purposefully moving his left hand. Despite the poor prognosis predicted by the scoring system, they decided to continue full support. One month later, the patient underwent a tracheotomy and required treatment for pneumonia as well as a hospital-acquired urinary tract infection. The patient's condition stabilized, and he subsequently opened his eyes and followed a few simple commands. The family was pleased with his limited progress and gratified that they did not withdraw life-sustaining care.

Clinical Pearls

1. Clinicians should use ICU scoring systems cautiously when considering withdrawal of life-supportive care for individual patients. Severity scores provide only supportive information that should be combined with the physician's clinical assessment and input from the patient and family.

2. Considerable differences exist between ICU scoring systems in predicting mortality.

3. ICU scoring systems were developed from heterogeneous populations of critically ill patients. They cannot be customized to improve their accuracy in prognosticating for individual target populations.

4. Large errors in mortality predictions can occur when inadequately trained personnel collect data for ICU scoring systems.

REFERENCES

1. Knaus WA, Zimmerman JE, Wagner DP, et al: APACHE—acute physiology and chronic health evaluation: a physiologically based classification system. Crit Care Med 1981;9:591–597.
2. Chang RWS: Individual outcome prediction models for intensive care units. Lancet 1989;2(8655):143–146.
3. Holt AW, Bury LK, Bersten AD, et al: Prospective evaluation of residents and nurses as severity score data collectors. Crit Care Med 1992;20:1688–1691.
4. Knaus WA, Watts CM: The case for using objective scoring systems to predict intensive care unit outcome. Crit Care Clin 1994;10:73–89.
5. Knaus WA, Harrell FE, Lynn J, et al: The SUPPORT prognostic model: objective estimates of survival for seriously ill hospitalized adults. Ann Intern Med 1995;122:191–203.
6. Clermont G, Angus DC: Severity scoring systems in the modern intensive care unit. Ann Acad Med Singapore 1998;27:397–403.
7. Prendergast TJ, Claessens MT, Luce JM: A national survey for critically ill patients. Am J Respir Crit Care Med 1998;158:1163–1167.

Stephen W. Crawford, MD

PATIENT 44

A 68-year-old women with respiratory failure who requests in writing to "end it now"

A 68-year-old Australian-born widow with severe emphysema is admitted to the ICU with acute respiratory failure. She undergoes endotracheal intubation for respiratory failure. During the last several years, she has had two hospitalizations requiring mechanical ventilation. During both previous admissions, she required a temporary tracheotomy to wean from the ventilator.

The physicians who managed the patient during her previous hospitalizations considered her an "extraordinarily difficult patient" and refused to assume her care after hospital discharge. The patient lives alone and takes pride in her fierce independence. She has repeatedly dismissed offers of assistance from her children. She is short-tempered, argumentative, and extremely demanding. She demands perfection from all around her. During the last 3 years, she has fired all but one home health worker sent to provide assistance.

The patient's present physician recognizes her as a frightened woman who fears losing control. He views her belligerence as an attempt to cope with uncertainty. The physician has developed a good rapport with the patient and has offered his forthright opinion that she needs to "stop being so mean." The patient has gained trust that her physician will remain involved with her care regardless of her attitudes and behavior. She also trusts that he will tell her when her behavior becomes inappropriate. They have developed a mutual respect.

Several days into the present hospitalization, the patient begins to improve. Her physician anticipates successful extubation within the next several days. The patient appears alert, recognizes her physician, and knows the date and her location. She writes profuse messages to caregivers on a notepad throughout the day. Her physician is surprised when she begins writing messages stating that she wants her care to stop. She requests removal of her endotracheal tube so that she can be allowed to die. These requests are repeated multiple times during the day. Despite the apparent urgency with which she write these messages, however, she makes no effort to remove any tubes, interfere with her care, or harm herself.

Question: What is the proper response to the patient's request?

Diagnosis: Respiratory failure due to severe emphysema.

Discussion: Conventional teachings in ethics in Western society hold that autonomy is a preeminent principle governing healthcare decision-making. All legally competent adults—those clinically assessed to have decision-making capacity—have the right to refuse unwanted medical interventions. In addition, patients are assumed to be competent until proven otherwise.

Specific circumstances of individual patients, however, often complicate attempts to adhere to the principle of autonomy. Consider first the issue of **capacity.** Physicians need to determine when a patient is speaking in a clear and reasoned mind. Although a patient may be alert and oriented, further assessment is needed to ensure that decisions are rational, reflect reasoning on the part of the patient, and are durable over an appropriate period of time.

The issue of **durability** of decision-making also must be considered. Persons who make end-of-life decisions during periods of stable health occasionally alter those decisions when faced with a critical illness and the possibility of death. This is exemplified by patients who make "last-minute" requests for life-supportive interventions despite previously expressed wishes to withhold "aggressive" medical care. But it is also true that patients who have wanted "everything done" may eventually relent in the face of inexorable progression of symptoms and disease.

It is certainly understandable for patients' decisions to shift over time in response to changes in their condition, particularly in response to increased disease burden and an accompanying diminished sense of physical well-being. Although some physicians assume that patient decisions made while facing the possibility of death are more "true" to their convictions, others voice concerns that the stress of critical illness and situational depression can diminish patients' decision-making capacity and the validity of their end-of-life decisions. Clearly, assessments of this nature can be complex and must consider patients' previously stated preferences, long-held values, and the current clinical situation. Although a clear and durable request of a competent patient to refuse treatment must be honored, **timing** is a critical issue. This is especially true when the request is for termination of life-sustaining treatment.

Because withdrawal of life-sustaining care from a critically ill patient usually results in death, the irreversible nature of this decision mandates that it be approached in a cautious and deliberate manner. It should be first recognized that the withdrawal of life-support is not a medical emergency.

While responding urgently to any physical distress the patient may have as well as to any emotional sense of hopelessness or despair, time should be taken to analyze all aspects of the request. This includes a careful assessment of treatable confusion or depression, meticulous reassessment of the patient's capacity to make decisions, and an examination of any inconsistencies with previously stated beliefs. These deliberations provide sufficient time to allow identification of any issues that may be clouding a patient's decision-making capacity and driving the patient to make a decision that they might later wish to rescind were they to survive.

The present patient was by all measures "competent," considering that she was alert and oriented to person, place, and time. Her request to "end it now" was persistent, consistently stated, and emphatic. Moreover, she had experience with respiratory failure and mechanical ventilation, and she did not appear suicidal.

The patient's physician, however, noted that the patient did not attempt to communicate her reasons for requesting the withdrawal of life support. The physician knew the present patient well enough to recognize her inclination to act rashly and impulsively in times of depression and stress. He feared that feelings of loss of control could compel her to make "foolish" decisions. Despite the patient's clear sensorium, he was concerned that the severity of her illness had clouded her decision-making capacity. Consequently, he did not discontinue ventilator support. He communicated empathy with her circumstances and conveyed that he recognized that she was upset and depressed. He reassured her of his expectations that she would survive the hospitalization and would soon no longer require ventilatory support. With this reassurance, she stopped writing her requests.

The patient was successfully extubated and transferred a few days later from the ICU. While sitting next to her bed, her physician said, "We need to talk about the notes you were writing in the ICU." "What notes?" she asked. When told about the requests to end her life-supportive care and "end it now," she exclaimed, "I said what?" She had no memory of the events and could not understand nor explain why she would have made such requests. She reaffirmed that she did not want to die. She said that she would especially want to live considering that she had been on her way to recovery when she wrote the notes. The patient and her physician reflected how honoring her repeated and urgent requests to end her life would not have been consistent with her wishes after her recovery.

In this instance, the physician felt fortunate that he had a preexisting relationship with the patient and knew her propensity for depression, anger, and rash action. Being aware of her nature made his refusal to honor her request to "end it all" not especially difficult. He considered, however, how he could make a mistake in honoring such requests for other patients with whom he did not have a prior relationship or insight into their life values and goals. This experience reconfirmed his interests in maintaining extreme vigilance in evaluating the consistency and appropriateness of all patient requests for termination of life-supportive care.

Clinical Pearls

1. Withdrawal of life-support is not an emergency procedure. Care, caution, and vigilance must be exercised before implementing this often irreversible decision.

2. Delaying withdrawal of life-support is appropriate until all questions about the mental state of the patient are clarified.

3. Patients cannot be assumed to be "competent" to make durable, consistent decisions regarding life-support merely because they are oriented to person, place, and time.

4. Someone knowledgeable of the patient's emotional responses and attitudes should be consulted before proceeding with an unexpected request to withdraw life support.

REFERENCES

1. Jonsen AR, Siegler M, Winslade WJ (eds): Clinical Ethics: A Practical Approach to Ethical Decisions in Clinical Medicine. New York, MacMillan Co., 1992.
2. Wenger NS, Oye RK, Bellamy PE, et al: Prior capacity of patients lacking decision making ability early in hospitalization: implications for advance directive administration: The SUPPORT Investigators. J Gen Intern Med 1994;9:539–543.
3. Roach MJ, Connors AF, Dawson NV, et al: Depressed mood and survival in seriously ill hospitalized adults: The SUPPORT Investigators. Arch Intern Med 1998;158:397–404.
4. Covinsky KE, Fuller JD, Yaffe K, et al: Communication and decision-making in seriously ill patients: findings of the SUPPORT project: the Study to Understand Prognoses and Preferences for Outcomes and Risks of Treatments. J Am Geriatr Soc 2000;48:S187–193.

Carla Alexander, MD

PATIENT 45

A 36-year-old African-American mother with terminal AIDS

A 36-year-old African-American mother of four with a previous history of drug addiction is seen at home by her palliative care nurse with recurrent complications of HIV/AIDS. She acquired HIV infection from her husband, who died 3 years ago.

She first presented with advanced, stage C3 HIV/AIDS with an episode of cryptococcal meningitis. Her CD4 lymphocyte count was 24 cells/ml at that time. After a hospitalization for treatment of meningitis, she began therapy with HAART (highly active antiretroviral therapy) that included three drugs. She soon developed a diffuse erythematous macular rash and painful numb sensations from her feet to thighs that required discontinuation of HAART. Her rash resolved, but the peripheral neuropathy required therapy with gabapentin 100 mg tid and oxycodone 5–10 mg every 3 hours, which resolved her symptoms over 4 weeks. The patient limited her use of oxycodone because of her fear of falling back into her previous drug addiction.

She resumed HAART with a decrease in her HIV RNA load from 650,000 copies/ml to 60,000 copies/ml, but she again stopped her medications because of watery diarrhea. After her diarrhea resolved, the patient refused to resume HAART therapy. The clinic staff convinced her to continue her prophylactic medications against opportunistic infections.

The patient did not return to the clinic for 3 months and presented with severe oral candidiasis. She had lost 35 lbs, and her feet had numbness and burning when she walked. She refused hospitalization because she wanted to remain home with her children. Her nurse practitioner requested assistance from a palliative care nurse, who suggested itraconazole oral suspension 200 mg/day and oxycodone 5–10 mg on a regular basis with a double dose at bedtime. She offers to visit the patient in her home.

The palliative care nurse and a spiritual care provider visited the patient's row home the next day. The first floor windows were boarded up. They found the patient after climbing a dark staircase. Although it was midafternoon, there were multiple partially clad children present and two older African-American women sitting by the window in a room where the patient was lying on a bed without sheets. The room was otherwise empty.

The patient improved and was able to drink four cans of nutritional supplement per day. Pain was controlled with long-acting oxycodone 20 mg bid, but the oral white patches and symptoms remain unchanged. She weighed 96 pounds, and the infectious disease specialist recommended daily intravenous fluconazole for her presumed *Candida* esophagitis because of its resistance to oral therapy. Although her mouth improved, she developed hiccups unresponsive to household remedies, chlorpromazine, or metoclopramide. Endoscopy revealed white patches throughout and intravenous amphotericin was prescribed. Over the next 2 weeks, her hiccups and a "sticking" sensation in her throat resolved.

Despite weekly suppressive amphotericin therapy, her symptoms have recurred. The patient tells the palliative care nurse that she refuses further treatment. She tells her sisters that she is dying and does not want to go back to the hospital or clinic. After much encouragement, the patient finally agrees to a hospice referral on the condition that she can remain at home. The palliative care nurse observes that the patient appears withdrawn and asks about her concerns. She expresses worry about who will care for her children if she dies. She also says that she is the "entertainer" in the family and does not feel up to making jokes.

Question: What special circumstances and beliefs may influence the care decisions of inner city dwellers with AIDS?

Diagnosis: Terminal HIV/AIDS in a patient who requires symptom management, spiritual and emotional support.

Discussion: Managing a patient with HIV/AIDS in the inner city entails the difficulties inherent in an environment of endemic poverty and a high prevalence of illicit drug use. Within the African-American culture, hospice care may be suspected of being second-class care. Attempts to control pain may be perceived as misguided or even ill-intended efforts to encourage previously addicted patients to relapse. These suspicions can best be countered by developing a trusting relationship, ongoing demonstration of concern, and home care visits by nurses who recognize the importance of their patients' emotional and spiritual needs.

Morbidity in advanced HIV disease is related to control of opportunistic infections, which occur more frequently as the immune system declines. Prophylactic therapies should be continued for anyone with a CD4 cell count $< 75/\mu l$. Sulfamethoxazole-trimethoprim prevents *Pneumocystis carinii* pneumonia (PCP) with the added benefit of preventing toxoplasmosis. PCP also can be prevented with dapsone 100 mg/day, aerosolized pentamidine 300 mg/month, or atovaquone suspension 750 mg bid in patients allergic to sulfa drugs. Cryptococcal suppression is required life-long. It is reasonable to discontinue preventive therapies when patients become bed-ridden and no longer pursue active antiviral treatment. Preventive treatments can always be re-instituted for symptom control if needed later.

Despite the existence of effective care for patients with HIV/AIDS, a myriad of reasons lead some people to not seek, refuse, or discontinue treatment. Young African-American women who lose a spouse to HIV/AIDS may not seek HIV testing or treatment for themselves because of a belief that such care is experimental. Also, some fear that treatment will enroll them into experimental programs that will exploit their illness, as occurred in the infamous Tuskegee incident. In the Tuskegee experiment, poor African-Americans were unknowingly denied treatment for syphilis so that researchers could observe the natural history of the disease. Because of their reluctance to seek care, many inner-city African-Americans present with opportunistic infections related to HIV/AIDS that have become rare in other patient populations since the advent of HAART.

Drug-related side effects and complicated medication regimens also hinder use of HIV/AIDS medications among disadvantaged patient populations. Moreover, inner city residents may not have access to adequate housing, refrigerators for storing medications, or phones to receive reminders from treatment clinics. All of these hurdles result in a higher likelihood that disadvantaged patients with HIV/AIDS will reach the end of life without ever having received consistent treatment for their underlying disease.

Oral candidiasis reflects the degree to which the AIDS virus has been controlled. Candidiasis becomes increasingly difficult to control as HIV/AIDS progresses. Overgrowth with *Candida* may occur despite use of cryptococcal prophylaxis with fluconazole, resulting in the need for combination antifungal therapy for patients with established candidiasis. Patients with advanced oral and esophageal candidiasis often have poor absorption of oral drugs and require an intravenous route of therapy. Chewable and liquid medications should be discontinued in these patients because the high sugar content in these preparations can stimulate fungal growth.

Peripheral neuropathy can occur in any stage of HIV/AIDS. The sensation of burning, tingling, or numbness (without bowel or bladder involvement) affects the feet first, although hands can also be affected. The clinical examination reveals hyperesthesia, decreased vibratory sensation, and decreased or absent ankle jerks. Peripheral neuropathy that occurs as a consequence of HIV disease itself may respond to treatment of the HIV infection with antiviral agents and symptomatic interventions.

Symptomatic interventions include avoidance of tight footwear, minimizing walking, and intermittent application of ice on the feet. As with any neuropathic pain, appropriate pharmaceuticals include NSAIDs, antidepressants, anticonvulsants, and opioids. In order to avoid rapidly dropping drug levels that might "trigger" the urge to use street drugs in previously drug-abusing patients, a long-acting opioid can be selected to initiate therapy. Patients receiving steroids for other reasons have noted a relief of symptoms. In communities where drug use is prevalent, multiple approaches are needed to convince people to use opioids for the legitimate purpose of pain relief.

Disadvantaged, inner city women with HIV/AIDS often reject traditional hospice care until the last days of life because they are young with dependent children and desire to live as long as possible. They may associate hospice care with "giving up." Acceptance of such care can be promoted by tapping into patients' religious and spiritual heritage. Hospice workers can have a member of the patient's church, preferably a leader of the congregation, accompany them to the home to convey the message that they are interested in more than just the patient's physical problems. Family members can learn from the church about community resources available to assist with care.

The most important efforts to gain patient's trust center on the willingness of caregivers to remain present and accompany the patient through the course of the disease, even after curative options no longer exist.

The present patient quickly came to value the visits by the palliative care nurse. After gaining trust, she accepted recommended treatment of her candidiasis to resolve her hiccups. The patient learned from the caregivers that treatment for her infections was required to alleviate her symptoms. She also learned the importance of receiving preventive therapy for infections—even in the late stages of disease when HAART has been forgone—to promote comfort and an improved quality of life.

Hearing the patient tell the palliative care nurse that she worried about who was going to care for her children and that she no longer felt up to making jokes, her sister turned and said, "We all are going to watch over your babies. And we still haven't stopped laughing from all of your jokes. What makes you think that just because you're dying we can't laugh with our memories?" The patient smiled. She died peacefully with her children and sisters at her bedside 3 weeks later.

Clinical Pearls

1. Despite the common clinical adage that admonishes clinicians to define a unifying diagnosis for signs and symptoms of disease, patients with AIDS often have more than one etiology for their problems.

2. After the discontinuation of HAART, continuing prophylactic agents can prevent opportunistic infections and symptoms that cause suffering. Prophylactic drugs can be held when the patient has < 2 weeks' prognosis.

3. Previously addicted patients typically fear pain medications, even when prescribed for bonafide indications. Their concerns must be acknowledged by clinicians, who can help patients distinguish between abuse and legitimate use of these medications. Careful adjustment and monitoring of opioids is required to ensure patients get the symptom relief they deserve.

4. Management of fungal infections near the end of life in patients with HIV/AIDS may require combination therapy and parenteral routes of administration.

5. Invasive diagnostic procedures may be appropriate to determine optimal management for symptoms caused by infectious agents, even near the end of life.

REFERENCES

1. Alexander CS. Palliative and End of Life Care. In A Guide to the Clinical Care of Women with HIV 2001 Edition. Ed. Anderson, Jr. HIV/AIDS Bureau, HRSA, US Dept HHS, Rockville, MD, 2000.
2. Arribas JR, Hernandez-Albujar S, Gonzalez-Garcia JJ et al. Impact of protease inhibitor therapy on HIV-related oropharyngeal candidiasis. AIDS 2000;14:979–985.
3. Bartlett JG and Gallant JE. Medical Management of HIV Infection, 2001–2002 Edition. Johns Hopkins University, Division of Infectious Disease, Baltimore, 2001.
4. Bruckenthal P. Managing non-malignant pain; Challenges for physicians. Conference Coverage 20th Annual Meeting of the American Pain Society. http://www.medscape.com/viewarticle/416591
5. Haddad NE, Powderly WG. The changing face of mycoses in patients with HIV/AIDS. AIDS Read 2000;11(7):365–378.
6. Portenoy R. Opioid therapy for chronic non-malignant pain: A review of the critical issues. J Pain Sx Mgmnt 1996;11:202–217.
7. Selwyn PA, Arnold R. From fate to tragedy: The changing meanings of life, death, and AIDS. Ann Int Med 1998:129(11);899–902.
8. UPHS/IDSA Guidelines for the prevention of opportunistic infections in persons infected with human immunodeficiency virus. MMWR 1999;48:RR–10.

Natalie Moryl, MD
Richard Payne, MD

PATIENT 46

A 46-year-old African-American man with widely metastatic cancer who "will fight for his life till the end"

A 46-year-old African-American man with a chordoma primary to his pelvis with wide metastases presents with chills and lethargy. His tumor has grown massively over the last months, producing severe body deformity with 85° of kyphosis, paraplegia and bilateral paraparesis, urinary and bowel incontinence, and chronic pain in both lower extremities and his lower back. The pelvic tumor drains foul-smelling purulent material through cutaneous fistulae. The patient is divorced and a former actor who lives alone. He states that he "is concentrating on fighting for my life." He is totally dependent for personal hygiene and other care. The patient has always asked that "everything be done" for him, including CPR.

Physical Examination: Blood pressure 90/60, pulse 124, temperature 38°. General: diaper in place; body deformity that forces him to lean forward, with his torso touching his thighs. Abdomen: pelvic tumor 3.5 by 2 feet in size draining foul-smelling necrotic material mixed with fresh blood. Neurologic: lethargic, paraplegia and bilateral paraparesis.

Laboratory Findings: Pelvic CT performed 1 year earlier: huge soft tissue mass with almost complete bony destruction of the entire pelvis and sacrum.

Hospital Course: The patient was hospitalized and treated with intravenous antibiotics, opioids, and red cell transfusions. During the next 3 days, his condition continued to deteriorate, and he became obtunded. The patient's mother, who was the designated health care proxy, and his sisters expressed their wishes for the patient not to be resuscitated.

Question: How does one discuss forgoing life-sustaining interventions with African-American patients?

Diagnosis: Terminally ill man with extensive metastatic disease who cannot be intubated because of body deformity.

Discussion: Increased public awareness of racial and ethnic health care disparities has brought new understanding of the barriers to end-of-life communication with minority patients. Some of these barriers derive from the lower access to medical care faced by African-Americans and other minority groups. Minority patients are less likely to undergo heart surgery, hemodialysis, or organ transplantation. They also have decreased access to cancer screening, curative cancer treatment, and even pain management. Consequently, cancer-related mortality rates in black men are 50% higher than rates for white male Americans.

Racial disparities also exist in end-of-life care. Even though African-American patients prefer more aggressive use of life-prolonging interventions than the general public, they are less likely to receive "high-tech" critical care during serious illnesses and at the end of life. To resolve disparities in end-of-life care, it is important for clinicians to examine their cultural sensitivity and the potential influence of their racial biases and preconceptions on their medical decision-making. Culturally sensitive dialogue should be targeted to the needs of the particular patient and family to respect inter- and intracultural differences. The discussion will benefit from the physician's acknowledgment of current and past injustices in the health care system, rather than ignoring or denying them or somehow defending "the system."

Cultural barriers, both real and perceived, complicate communication with patients and families about end-of-life issues. Many African-American patients request **aggressive care** at the end of life because they believe signing advanced directives increases the likelihood of receiving inferior care. They also may associate the completion of a living will with loss of hope, "giving up," and decreased expectations for quality medical care. These patient perceptions appear to be shared by African-American physicians, who are five times more likely to request aggressive treatments and tube feedings when they themselves become gravely ill compared with other physicians. African-American physicians are also more likely than other physicians to state a preference for aggressive care if they develop an illness that results in a persistent vegetative state.

These patients also may question the "humanitarian" motives of hospice workers, who are often white. Caregivers should explain, therefore, that palliative care goals are not an alternative to curative treatment, but rather a part of appropriate medical care for a particular stage of illness.

African-American patients and families are also more likely than other ethnic groups to **deny death** when faced with a serious illness. This denial must be understood in the context of the high infant mortality, homicide, and accidental death rates within their ethnic group and the lower access to specialized medical care they experience. Also, some of their religious traditions consider death to be a "welcomed friend" after prolonged suffering of chronic illness. African-American patients may be more accepting of death as compared with other ethnic groups in these circumstances.

Faith-based traditions, family-centered decision-making, and cultural values are important in the African-American community. Although caregivers must always respect patient autonomy, it is critical to involve the family in discussing end-of-life care. One can conceptualize a "family-centered" style of medical decision-making and autonomy as being particularly important even when there are disagreements within the family.

The present patient's family states that the patient had discussed his attitudes toward life and illness with them. They confirm that his life-long need "to fight for everything he had" was consistent with his personality, shaped by his African-American heritage. He had become determined to fight for his life and preserve it as long as possible at any cost, even beyond the point where his family thought his quality of life was unacceptably poor. The patient had considered earlier discussions of a do-not-resuscitate (DNR) order and supportive symptomatic care as "giving up" hope. The physician assured the family that their interests in developing appropriate goals of care were not an effort to deny care.

The physicians continued their close communication with the patient's family throughout the hospitalization. As the patient's condition deteriorated and he became more unresponsive, his mother asked that a DNR order be written and that her son would receive comfort care only. She stated, with her large family in agreement, that he had suffered enough. Medications were carefully adjusted to ensure physical comfort, and meticulous nursing care was continued. The patient died a few days later surrounded by the family.

Clinical Pearls

1. Honest, culturally sensitive discussion about end-of-life care responsive to the particular patient and his or her ethnic background is the cornerstone of successful communication with minority patients.

2. Clinicians' awareness of the patient's sociocultural history and sensitivity to documented health system inequalities in access and quality of services are essential when discussing the end-of-life issues with African-Americans.

3. Palliative care goals must never be positioned as an alternative to curative treatment, but rather as an integral part of appropriate medical care for a particular stage of illness.

4. A patient's family, clergy and other community can be important contributors to end-of-life discussion and in developing achievable goals of care. Close ongoing communication with family throughout the illness is paramount in achieving positive outcomes in the context of progressive, incurable disease.

REFERENCES

1. Yergan J, Flood AB, LoGerfo JP, Diehr P: Relationship between patient race and the intensity of hospital services. Med Care 1987;25:592–603.
2. Neubauer BJ, Hamilton CL: Racial differences in attitudes toward hospice care. Hosp J 1990;6:37–48.
3. Caralis PV, Davis B, Writght K, Marcial E: The influence of ethnicity and race on attitudes toward advanced directives, life-prolonging treatments, and euthanasia. J Clin Ethics 1993;4:155–165.
4. McKinley ED, Garrett JM, Evans AT, Danis M: Differences in end-of-life decision making among black and white ambulatory cancer patients. J Gen Intern Med 1998;11:651–656.
5. Sondik EJ: Cancer and minorities: learning from the differences in prevalence, survival, and mortality. Cancer 1998;83:1757–1764.
6. Mebane EW, Oman RF, Kroonen LT, Goldstein MK: The influence of physician race, age, and gender on physician attitudes towards advance care directives and preferences for end-of-life decision-making. J Am Geriatr Soc 1999;47:579–591.
7. Crawley L: Death and difference: the value of narratives in cross-cultural work. Center for Literature, Medicine and the Health Professional News 2000;12:p 5,6.

Sheryl B. Movsas, DO
Russell K. Portenoy, MD

PATIENT 47

A 33-year-old man with active substance abuse and metastatic colon cancer who requires analgesia for pain control

A 33-year-old man presents to the emergency department with severe and rapidly progressive back pain. He has a 9-month history of metastatic colon cancer, stage 3BT3N2, and has previously undergone surgical resection, chemotherapy, and radiation therapy. He also is an active substance abuser, which includes intravenous heroin and cocaine during the past month. His sister reports that he has been estranged from the family and has been intermittently destitute since cancer diagnosis. On several occasions, he has refused recommended therapies and he did not complete his course of radiation. He was hospitalized twice during the past 4 months and both times left against medical advice. His nutrition has been poor and weight loss has accelerated during the past month. His sister reports that his mood has been anxious and depressed.

Physical Examination: Blood pressure 130/80, pulse 90, temperature 37.2°. General: awake, alert, anxious. Abdomen: palpable masses, hepatomegaly, functioning colostomy. Neurologic: mild paraparesis at a T6 sensory level. Patellar and Achilles reflexes: absent. Extremities: 2+ edema of the bilateral lower extremities.

Laboratory Findings: Hct 23.7%, BUN 29 mg/dl, creatinine 1.1 mg/dl, calcium 8.2 mg/dl, alkaline phosphatase 530 IU/L, albumin 2.3 g/dl. MRI of the thoracic spine: epidural metastases at T3 and T4 causing moderate spinal cord compression; multiple metastatic lesions in the thoracic and lumbar spine; large prevertebral lymph nodes present.

Hospital Course: In the emergency department, intravenous access is obtained and the patient is given morphine 10 mg i.v., which is repeated three times before his arrival on the oncology unit, with some reported benefit. After the results of the MRI are known, spinal radiation therapy is strongly recommended, but the patient refuses. He states that pain medicine is all that he will accept. Told that a corticosteroid could help the pain, he accepts treatment with dexamethasone. He is given another i.v. bolus injection of morphine 10 mg, and his history is obtained in more detail. As part of a detailed history, he states that his only drugs of abuse recently have been cocaine and heroin, and he readily provides a urine sample.

Question: What pharmacologic agents should be prescribed to maximize pain control in this patient with recent polysubstance abuse?

Diagnosis: Far advanced colon cancer in a patient with active addiction and other physical and psychosocial comorbidities, who now has severe pain due to spinal metastases and epidural spinal cord compression.

Discussion: The prevalence of substance abuse among patients with progressive medical illnesses has been estimated to be 3% to 25%, depending on the underlying diagnosis and site of care. The treatment of pain in patients with a substance abuse history who are at the end of life presents a unique challenge. Treatment is aided by categorizing patients with a history of abuse and chronic pain into three groups:

1) actively abusing patients (distinguishing subgroups based on the drugs of abuse);
2) those in drug-free recovery (distinguishing subgroups based on the duration of recovery and the use of peer-support groups); and
3) those in opioid-based recovery, usually methadone maintenance (distinguishing subgroups based on the stability of treatment and the incidence of relapses).

Patients with terminal conditions and active drug abuse commonly have the additional problems of destitution, malnutrition, lack of social support, and psychiatric problems. These difficulties complicate care and often hinder the development of a therapeutic alliance and a mutually trustful relationship with healthcare providers. For such patients, pain management is usually the most pressing need, but only one of several components of aggressive palliative care. Successful treatment of pain can encourage a patient to accept other modalities of care, such as radiation therapy, to prevent complications related to an underlying cancer. Palliative radiation for cancer patients may also provide more effective analgesia than drug therapy alone.

Often, however, patients who actively abuse drugs only accept drug therapy for pain management. Such patients require urgent inpatient treatment with establishment of an effective medication regimen. Pain management is complicated by mood disorders that hinder pain assessments, mistrust of medical professionals, and opioid addiction. Selecting and adjusting doses of opioids is often compromised by uncertainties related to the quantity and types of illicit drugs patients have recently used.

A team approach facilitates assessment and palliative care for patients actively abusing drugs. Palliative teams benefit from the expertise of palliative care physicians, nurses, social workers, consultants in psychiatry or psychology, and addiction medicine specialists. Communication with the primary medical team — in the instance of the present patient, the oncologists — is essential.

The success of opioid therapy depends on individualization of the dose. The goal is to obtain a favorable balance between efficacy and side effects through gradual dose escalation. Well-grounded concerns exist, however, that opioid titration may lead to aberrant drug-related behaviors, such as purposeful requests for overmedication, manipulation of the staff for specific drugs or routes of drug administration, acquisition of drugs from outside the hospital, and other **drug-seeking behaviors.** Caregivers should recognize this potential for abuse, implement strategies to reduce the likelihood of these behaviors, and promptly identify inappropriate drug-seeking activities when they occur.

Concern regarding drug-seeking behaviors, however, never justifies the undertreatment of pain. Indeed, it is an irony that undertreatment itself can lead to aberrant drug-related behaviors, which is termed "pseudoaddiction." The patient with addictive disease who has unrelieved pain and engages in an aberrant drug-related behavior may be demonstrating the impact of both the addictive disorder and the iatrogenic pseudoaddiction associated with undertreatment.

In the inpatient setting, severe pain should be managed with an opioid. Therapy is usually initiated with an estimated maintenance dose of oral long-acting opioid (such as controlled-release or sustained-release morphine or oxycodone) or methadone. Alternatives include transdermal fentanyl or continuous i.v. or s.c. infusions of opioids, such as morphine or hydromorphone. Maintenance doses are complemented by "rescue" doses of a short-acting opioid. Some patients benefit from devices that allow the i.v. or s.c. delivery of patient-controlled analgesia (PCA). As a general rule, repeated doses of short-acting opioids should not constitute the primary pain management regimen, because this approach undertreats most patients with chronic pain and increases the risk of addiction relapse. It may also promote aberrant drug-related behaviors.

Selection of a specific regimen depends on the patient's ability to exercise self-control. Transdermal regimens and PCA are subject to abuse when used for extremely distressed patients who have poor self-control. Such patients may be more appropriately managed with long-acting oral drugs complemented by rescue doses delivered by a nurse upon request. Nonpharmacologic interventions, such as patient education and cognitive therapies that include relaxation techniques and music therapy, provide adjunctive benefits.

Management strategies for patients who are actively abusing drugs include a private room close to the nursing station to allow patient monitoring. Visitations should be restricted to family and friends known to be drug-free. Additional interventions include searching packages brought to the hospital by patient visitors for illicit drugs, enacting a written contract outlining expectations for patient behavior, and requiring periodic urine drug screens to detect drugs not included in the patient's therapeutic regimen.

It is important for healthcare providers to institute these interventions without punitive attitude. Caregivers should explain that these safeguards are intended to allow aggressive pain management with the patient's best interests in mind. Patients should be informed that aggressive interventions to manage pain can only occur in the absence of ongoing drug abuse. Open discussions about management guidelines allow optimal treatment for the disease and the most sensitive and compassionate palliative care possible.

The present patient agreed to accept periodic urine drug screens and not to visit with friends out of his hospital room, which was near the nursing station. He understood the purpose of these arrangements, which were intended to ensure that illicit drugs were not being used, thereby allowing intensive efforts to control his pain. In the presence of his sister, the patient was told that evidence of

drug abuse would require tighter restrictions and could jeopardize the use of opioid therapy for pain management.

The patient was initially treated with a long-acting oral morphine formulation at a dose of 60 mg twice daily. He experienced periods of breakthrough pain. The nursing staff upon request administered i.v. morphine, 15 mg every 2 hours. His anxiety was treated with clonazepam.

During the first day, he requested morphine every 2 to 3 hours. On the second day, the dose of the long-acting opioid was doubled. He reported a greater degree of comfort for several hours, after which he experienced a flare in pain. At this point, the team felt comfortable proceeding with a PCA device. He was switched to a continuous i.v. infusion of morphine at 5 mg/hr by PCA with self-administered i.v. rescue boluses of 5 mg of morphine every 15 minutes as needed. The nursing staff monitored him every hour and observed that he administered boluses until he became mildly sedated and pain-free. His basal infusion rate was adjusted after 6 hours based on the number of rescue boluses he used. Several hours later, his use of rescue boluses declined. There were no aberrant drug-related behaviors associated with this therapy. He continued to refuse radiation therapy and remained in the hospital for another 3 weeks before his death.

Clinical Pearls

1. In patients with serious illness and a substance abuse disorder, the use of an opioid is usually appropriate if pain is moderate or severe.

2. Patients must undergo a careful assessment of their drug abuse history in an effort to judge the risk of aberrant drug-related behavior during pain treatment.

3. Accepted guidelines for opioid therapy still apply for the patient with a substance use disorder, particularly the need to individualize the dose to obtain a favorable balance between analgesia and side effects. Undertreatment can complicate the management of drug addiction by promoting aberrant behaviors that reflect the desperation of uncontrolled pain.

4. Long-acting opioid preparations with short-acting rescue doses can reduce the likelihood of aberrant drug-related behaviors. Concurrent non-drug approaches may be valuable adjunctive therapies.

5. It is essential to develop a structured management plan based on the risk of aberrant drug-related behavior. Interventions include placing the patient in a private room close to the nursing station to allow monitoring, inspecting packages brought by visitors, and performing periodic urine drug screens.

REFERENCES

1. Passik SD, Portenoy RK, Ricketts, PL: Substance abuse issues in cancer patients: p 1. Prevalance and diagnosis. Oncology 1998;12:517–521.
2. Passik SD, Portenoy RK, Ricketts, PL: Substance abuse issues in cancer patients: p 2. Evaluation and treatment. Oncology 1998;12:729–734.
3. Passik SD, Portenoy RK: Substance abuse issues in palliative care. In Berger A, Portenoy RK, Weissman DE (eds): Principles and Practice of Supportive Oncology. Philadelphia, Lippincott-Raven Publishers, 1998, pp 513–529.
4. Passik SD, Portenoy RK: Substance abuse disorders. In Holland JC (ed): Psycho-Oncology. New York, Oxford University Press, 1998, pp 576–586.

Horace M. DeLisser, MD
Jacquelyn R. Evans, MD
Rashmin C. Savani, MD

PATIENT 48

A 500-g preterm infant born to parents who must make decisions about life-supportive care

A 24-year-old gravida 1 para 0 woman presents in preterm labor after 23 5/7 weeks of gestation. She had been in good health until she developed abdominal cramping. Her membranes are intact and ultrasound examination reveals an appropriately grown fetus with an estimated weight of 530 g. There is no evidence of fetal compromise. Betamethasone is administered to the patient to accelerate fetal lung maturity and ampicillin is started for presumed amnionitis. Tocolysis is attempted with ritodrine infusion.

After 2 days on magnesium sulfate with relatively good tocolysis, spontaneous rupture of the membranes occurs, and preterm labor is now unable to be stopped. Labor and subsequent delivery by caesarian section are performed without complications. A vigorous infant weighing 530 g is born with Apgar scores of 7 at 1 minute and 8 at 5 minutes. The infant develops increased work of breathing with retractions and tachypnea soon after birth, requiring intubation and manual bag ventilation. Usual neonatal resuscitation includes insertion of central arterial and venous catheters and administration of surfactant.

The infant is managed with fluids, antibiotics, and ventilatory support. For the first 7 days, the infant remains relatively stable on low ventilatory settings with modest oxygen requirements. The infant develops a patent ductus arteriosus that is treated successfully with indomethacin. On day of life 8, the infant shows evidence of increased work of breathing with worsening arterial blood gases. A chest radiograph shows generalized haziness. Blood cultures are obtained and antibiotics are started for possible nosocomial infection.

Over the next 2 days, the infant's respiratory status rapidly deteriorates, requiring increasing ventilatory support. By day 10 of life, the infant develops pulmonary interstitial emphysema with an inability to oxygenate or ventilate. The infant also demonstrates hypotension requiring a dopamine infusion. The health care team believes that the lungs are not recoverable and that the infant will not survive.

Question: How do you counsel parents as to the potential viability for their preterm child and to the withdrawal of care from an nonviable neonate?

Diagnosis: Nonbeneficial therapy at the margins of viability.

Discussion: Advances in neonatal intensive care over the last 20 years have extended the boundaries of infant viability to increasingly younger gestational ages. Technological improvements, however, have outpaced ethical discussions, and the outcomes for the tiniest of infants delivered after extremely short gestations remain highly uncertain. No national consensus has emerged for the care of infants born at the threshold of viability.

In general, intact survival with good functional outcomes for infants < 600 g and < 24 weeks' gestation is poor, and the burden of intensive care for such infants is great. The outcome for an individual infant, however, is difficult to determine. The American Academy of Pediatrics has set guidelines where the standard is to weigh the benefits and burdens of treatment from the infant's (and not the parents') perspective. The uncertainty between provision of comfort care versus aggressive life-sustaining interventions lies in the balance between the possibility of prolonged suffering ending in a poor outcome versus the possibility of intact survival.

Some experts suggest that medical interventions at the limits of viability be judged in one of four operational modes:

1. Unreasonable—unacceptable interventions because the outcome is certain to be extremely poor
2. Mandatory—necessary interventions because the anticipated outcome based on national and local statistics is expected to be reasonable and outweighs the burdens placed on the infant
3. Optional—interventions of uncertain value because the outcome is uncertain ("gray zone") and parental influence on decision-making is of central importance
4. Investigational—a "therapeutic trial" of active intervention for infants born in the gray zone, with discontinuance of that intervention if the response is poor

To fully inform couples who are about to become parents of a premature infant at the edge of viability, it is important to have **accurate outcomes** data regarding such births from national and local sources. These data promote informed decisions by both the healthcare team and parents. Certain caveats exist when reviewing published data on mortality and morbidity at the limits of viability. For instance, centers with good survival and aggressive approaches are more likely to publish their results. Furthermore, institutional philosophies regarding the provision of life-sustaining care for infants at the edge of viability strongly influence survival. Lastly, population differences and the use of different denominators may grossly affect the published data and make it difficult to compare one center to another. Currently, babies born at > 25 weeks and > 600 g birth weight have a > 50% chance of survival to discharge. Importantly, fetal compromise and multiple gestations have dramatically negative effects on survival.

It must be stressed that despite careful efforts at dating the pregnancy, gestational age estimates can be off by as much as 2 weeks. Furthermore, birth weight varies widely for babies of the same gestational age. As a result, the parents must be informed that a definite decision to start or forgo initial resuscitative treatments can usually be made only after the neonatologist assesses the newborn and determines whether the infant's initial condition is consistent with the prenatal estimates of gestational age and maturity.

Although little data exist that are stratified by small birth weight or gestational age groups, certain neonatal morbidities appear to adversely affect short- and medium-term neurodevelopmental outcome. These include severe brain injury, bronchopulmonary dysplasia, nosocomial infection, retinopathy of prematurity, and necrotizing enterocolitis. It is unclear, however, whether these early morbidities serve as adequate predictors of very late outcome or the quality of life.

Healthcare providers, parents, society, and patients themselves are interested parties in the decision regarding the provision of aggressive life-sustaining care for infants with borderline viability. One investigation has studied the assessment of **quality of life** in parent-child cohorts of extremely low birth weight infants who survived to adolescence (ages 13 and 14 yrs). While one-quarter of the extremely low birth weight infants had measurable neurosensory defects as teenagers, only 12% reported complex limitation of cognition, self-care, sensation, and pain. Indeed, 73% of affected teens (versus 71% of control teens) rated themselves in a high functional state and 34% reported perfect health. It is noteworthy that healthcare professionals (both physicians and nurses) rated hypothetical situations of disability much worse than either parents or the children who had been born at the limits of viability.

Therefore, families who are about to experience the birth of an infant at the limits of viability should be counseled in a manner consistent with full disclosure of national and local outcomes data and on the potential options for active interventions or comfort care in the delivery room. The influence of the healthcare team and society is maximal for the areas where more certainty exists about medical outcome. Parental wishes assume greater importance when the outcome is uncertain and the infant falls in the "gray zone."

Taken in context with current outcome data, "unreasonable" would constitute all infants <23 weeks and 500 g birth weight and "mandatory" all infants ≥ 25 weeks and 600 g. A "gray zone" exists regarding the utility of aggressive care for infants 23 to 24 % weeks and 500 to 600 g for whom parental wishes assume greatest influence. It is critical to emphasize the process of continued and ongoing evaluation of the infant who has been offered treatment. The parents should be advised that should severe complications occur, further discussions of the appropriateness of continued provision of care would become necessary.

Clinicians need to consider the **withdrawal of life-sustaining care** when borderline infants fail to improve with aggressive treatment. Unlike the adult for whom notions of autonomy hold sway, the "best interest of the child" guides the decision-making for infants and children. This approach requires that we forgo treatment if the anticipated burdens of life-sustaining care exceed the expected benefits. Inherent in this standard is the recognition that it may not always be in a child's best interest to receive medical intervention. While widely accepted, determining when the best interest of an infant is no longer served by continued treatment can be difficult.

There is, however, consensus, as reflected in the work of the President's Commission on Ethical Problems in Medicine, that aggressive treatments are not required in certain circumstances. These circumstances include situations where (1) the infant is irreversibly comatose, (2) treatment would merely prolong dying or otherwise be futile in terms of promoting the survival of the infant, or (3) treatment itself would be inhumane. More recently, the Royal College of Paediatrics and Child Health has defined five circumstances in which the withdrawal of treatment is ethically appropriate. These circumstances include (1) brain death; (2) permanent vegetative state; (3) prolonged survival with unreasonable suffering; (4) further treatment would only delay death without alleviating suffering; and, (5) when the child is older, both the child and family believe that continued treatment is unbearable, despite what they are told by healthcare providers.

Neonatal intensive care necessarily must never be an end to itself. It is a means to be used only when the patient is expected to derive lasting benefit and when there is a reasonable chance that the infant will survive with an acceptable level of long-term morbidity and disability. Despite this concept, a number of studies have reported that it is not uncommon for neonatologists to continue to provide failing treatments well beyond the time when they have become convinced that the burdens of treatment exceed the benefits. Reasons for this include concern over further distressing the parents provision of time for the parents to accept the reality of their infant's dying, a perceived need to give the parents the sense that "everything" was done, fear of being sued, and and the belief that respect for autonomy requires continuance of care if demanded by the parents. We emphasize once more that the best interests of the child should prevail.

If treatment is initiated for an infant in the "gray zone", care should be guided by patient-centered goals involving continued clinical assessment and defined time-limited trials of treatment. Once the treatments have failed to attain their desired therapeutic goal(s), they should not be continued. The availability of life-sustaining technology should not drive care. Furthermore, while parental input assumes increased influence, there is no obligation to "do whatever the parents want." The best interests of the child, particularly in terms of preventing suffering, remain paramount.

It must be emphasized that while a decision may be made to forgo life-sustaining interventions, at no point do we withhold or withdraw caring, comfort, or compassion. As life-prolonging therapies are limited, the staff must be careful to guard against also withholding or withdrawing their emotional support of the parents and family. To provide warmth, the infant should be wrapped in a blanket and the head covered with a hat. As much as possible, it is important that the infant be held by the parents (if they desire to do so) and/or staff. Monitoring of the patient need only involve intermittent evaluation of the heart rate. For newborns in whom life-prolonging therapies are being withheld or withdrawn, all infusions should be stopped, except for those required to treat pain or provide sedation. Morphine, at appropriate dosage, may be administered as needed based on clinical signs of discomfort. Spiritual/pastoral care (baptisms, blessings, and other rituals) should be offered and mementos provided.

We have found that the transition to comfort care is aided by physicians who work closely with parents from the outset of their infant's care. Ongoing communication is required to report the response to therapeutic trials and to acknowledge the tragedy of their situation, their disappointment, and grief. Parents rightfully come to trust that physicians are working with them to come to a decision about what is in the infant's best interest.

After discussing with the parents their child's inability to survive, the family conferred and asked for the withdrawal of life-supportive care. The infant was held by his mother and died without any appearance of distress minutes after the withdrawal of ventilatory support.

Clinical Pearls

1. Antenatal counseling for parents of preterm infants should center on a full disclosure of national and local data on outcomes.

2. A clear presentation of the definitions of the mandatory, unreasonable, and "gray zones" for determining the appropriateness of life-sustaining care is a necessary component of decision-making.

3. Therapeutic trials of life-prolonging care can be presented as options for infants who are in the gray zone.

4. In all decisions, it is paramount that clinicians work with parents to develop treatment plans that are in the best interest of the child.

5. Neonatal intensive care is a means to be used when the patient is expected to derive lasting benefit with a reasonable chance of survival with acceptable long-term burden.

REFERENCES

1. President's Commission for the Study of Ethical Problems in Medicine and Biomedical Behavioral Research: Making Health Care Decisions: The Ethical Legal Implications of Informed Consent in the Patient-Practitioner Relationships. Washington, DC, Government Printing Office, 1983.
2. Allen MC, Donohue PK, Dusman AE: The limit of viability-neonatal outcome of infants born at 22 to 25 weeks' gestation. N Engl J Med 1993;329:1597–1601.
3. Lantos JD, Tyson JE, Allen A, et al: Withholding and withdrawing life sustaining treatment in neonatal intensive care: issues for the 1990s. Arch Dis Child 1994;71:F218-F223.
4. American Academy of Pediatrics Committee on Bioethics, 1992 to 1994: Guidelines on forgoing life-sustaining medical treatment. Pediatrics 1994;93:532–536.
5. American Academy of Pediatrics Committee on Fetus and Newborn 1994 to 1995, American College of Obstetricians and Gynecologists Committee on Obstetric Practice 1994 to 1995: Perinatal care at the threshold of viability. Pediatrics 1995;96:974–976.
6. Tyson JE, Younes N, Verter J, Wright LL: Viability, morbidity, and resource use among newborns of 501- to 800-g birth weight. JAMA 1996;276:1645–1651.
7. Royal College of Paediatrics and Child Health: When life saving treatment should be withdrawn in children. BMJ 1997;315:834.
8. Paris JJ, DeLisser HM, Savani RC: Ending innovative therapy for infants at the margins of viability: case of twins H. J Perinatol 2000;4:251–256.
9. Saigal S: Perception of health status and quality of life of extremely low-birth weight survivors: the consumer, the provider, and the child. Clin Perinatol 2000;27:403–419.
10. Jobe AH: Predictors of outcomes in preterm infants: which ones and when? J Pediatr 2001;138:153–156.
11. Leuthner SR: Decisions regarding resuscitation of the extremely premature infant and models of best interest. J Perinatol 2001;21:193–198.

Karin T. Kirchhoff, PhD, RN

PATIENT 49

A 54-year-old man with intractable heart failure who transitions to palliative care in the ICU

A 54-year-old man with a long-history of intractable heart failure is admitted to the emergency department with severe shortness of breath. He has a history of multiple myocardial infarctions and has undergone two coronary artery bypass procedures. The patient was in his usual state of health until this morning, when he became dyspneic, orthopneic, and restless. His wife accompanies him and provides the patient's living will, which requests no aggressive life-sustaining care if his condition is terminal.

Physical Examination: Blood pressure 100/45, pulse 120, temperature 36.4°. General: thin, pale, confused, markedly dyspneic, and disoriented. HEENT: distended head and neck veins, raised jugular veins. Chest: crackles heard over both lungs. Abdomen: distended, liver enlarged. Extremities: moderate edema.

Laboratory Findings: Hct 27%, creatinine 3 mg/dl, BUN 50 mg/dl, Arterial blood gases (100% oxygen by facemask): PaO_2 80 mm Hg, $PaCO_2$ 55 mm Hg, pH 7.20. Radiography: diffuse pulmonary edema.

Hospital Course: The patient is transferred to the ICU, where a tight-fitting facemask is placed to initiate noninvasive positive pressure ventilation. An echocardiogram demonstrates a 15% left ventricular ejection fraction. Over the next 3 days, his condition worsens with unremitting dyspnea and progressive renal failure despite aggressive medical therapy with red cell transfusions, diuretics, intropic drugs, intermittent doses of morphine, and left ventricular unloading therapy. His previous cardiac catheterization is reviewed, and he is not considered a candidate for invasive procedures. A repeat echocardiogram demonstrates worsening ventricular function, and the ICU team determines that no additional therapy is available. A continuous infusion of morphine with intermittent doses of the sedative lorazepam are ordered to provide relief from his intense dyspnea.

Question: What palliative care interventions should the nurses consider for the patient and family in the ICU?

Diagnosis: Terminal heart failure and a need for palliative care for the patient and family.

Discussion: Nurses in a critical care setting need to be alert for circumstances in which palliative care is the best treatment option. Once palliative care is initiated, they also should recognize the need for patients and families to express to each other their thoughts and feelings. For example, before nurses begin palliative treatment with sedatives to assist patients with intractable dyspnea, they should ask family members and the patient whether they wish to talk about important issues before sedatives interfere with communication. Some sedated patients may be able to hear and understand conversation from their family but become unable to respond. Unfortunately, many families have reported that they did not know that the use of paralytics and sedatives in the ICU precluded later goodbyes. Because nurses usually are the ones administering these drugs, they need to be mindful of the unintended effects on closure at the end of life.

Nurses caring for patients at the end-of-life have clinical responsibilities—and therapeutic opportunities—to provide family support in critical clinical situations. When physicians complete discussions with families about a patient's poor prognosis and the potential need for life-supportive care or withdrawal of life-supportive interventions, families look to the nurse for support when the physician leaves the room. Nurses can acknowledge the difficulty of hearing a poor prognosis and making decisions that might limit aggressive life-prolonging care for a loved one. Nurses can also validate the emotional stress that arises from such decisions, expressing how difficult it is to follow a patient's advance directives to limit therapeutic interventions when family members wish to have their loved one with them longer. Nurses can reassure the family that they are acting in accord with their loved one's wishes and that in doing so, they are being both respectful and loving.

When patients are expected to die within a few hours after decisions are made to limit therapeutic interventions, it is often best for care to continue in the ICU because of the value of maintaining existing supportive relationships with the staff and, conversely, because of the potential for disruption in transferring the patient care and family support to unfamiliar providers. In these instances, critical care nurses are key to facilitating the transition from life-extending critical care to comprehensive and intensive palliative care, which includes family support as the patient dies. When patients are expected to linger for days, it is preferable to transfer them to a less clinically aggressive setting, perhaps a room that will be larger and allow more private space for the family to gather, conduct any religious or cultural rituals, and say their goodbyes. In such situations, critical care nurses can ease the transition of care to the new clinical team by communicating the personal details they have learned about the family to new caregivers.

In anticipation of death, the nurse can ask the family what, if any, arrangements have been made ahead of time. Often families have not selected a funeral home despite the presence of long-term serious disease. Nurses can provide family members with information and resources and can direct them to others who care assist with their planning. The nurse can prepare family members for changes to expect as the patient dies: cooling of the skin, cyanosis of extremities and lips, somnolence, and patterns of breathing. As these changes occur, the nurse can again explain that the patient is not experiencing any discomfort. Often, explanations of this nature can diminish the anxiety family members feel as they witness these progressive signs of imminent death.

Family members become concerned as to whether the patient will be comfortable if life-supportive treatments are withheld. Questions emerge regarding hunger and thirst and what comfort measures are available. Nurses can explain that as death approaches, the need for food and drink lessens and the body's ability to handle them is weakened. Nurses should be prepared to call for a palliative care consult to assess the patient and suggest additional comfort measures. Some aspects of palliative care can be managed by the ICU staff nurse, such as communication and preparation for the time of death. Additional expertise of the palliative care team may be necessary for management of symptoms not responsive to usual drugs and treatments.

Families also worry whether they will be able to communicate with the patient and whether children will be able to talk to a dying patient. Nurses can explain that patient's hearing may be present for a long time and should encourage families to hold a patient's hand and express their thoughts and love. Nurses can lower a bed and drop bed rails and suggest to spouses that they may lie in bed with the patient if they wish. It is vital that nurses provide privacy for family members who are saying their final goodbyes, yet remain available when needed. Special signs can be hung on a patient's door to alert unit staff that a patient is dying and receiving palliative care and that privacy of family interaction has assumed high priority.

The nurse should ask family members about the patient's spiritual interests and whether a pastor or other religious counselor should be called to visit the patient. Families often forget to attend to their own spiritual needs when they are focusing on the immediate events associated with a dying loved one. Nurses can facilitate family prayer when a spiritual counselor arrives to the unit. As family members gather away from the patient, the nurse can encourage them to come close, say their goodbyes, and touch the patient as they would normally. The physical changes in the patient may cause the family to withdraw. If so, nurses can make it safe for family members to move closer to the patient and encourage a more natural expression of love and concern.

The nurse caring for the present patient recognized that the order for lorazepam and continuous morphine represented the initial efforts for palliative "comfort" care. Before she begins the morphine infusion to relieve his dyspnea, she asked both the patient and his wife whether there was a need for a two-way conversation. She gently explained that after the sedative was administered, the patient may be able to hear but may have difficulty responding. She asked whether the children have been called and told about their father's serious condition. She helped the wife make phone contact with her children. She also made a call to the family pastor who arrived within the hour.

Through the afternoon, the family remained by the bedside talking with the patient, praying, and holding hands. The physician adjusted the patient's sedation to provide maximal relief of dyspnea. The patient died peacefully several hours later in the ICU, surrounded by his family.

Clinical Pearls

1. Communication with the family and patient to provide information and ascertain their wishes and desires is an important activity for critical care nurses as they coordinate care at the bedside.

2. Nurses have a key role of facilitating goodbyes between patient and family at end-of-life.

3. Palliative care can be initiated in the ICU by the staff with additional help from the palliative care team.

4. Assisting the family to express love and affection is helpful.

5. Nurses should ask whether patients and families have unfulfilled spiritual needs as patients approach the end of life and assist in meeting those needs.

REFERENCES

1. Jett LG: Comfort at the end of life: palliative care policy. J Nurs Adm 1995;25:55–60.
2. Jenkins C, Bruera E: Assessment and management of medically ill patients who refuse life-prolonging treatments: two case reports and proposed guidelines: Capital Health Authority Regional Palliative Care Program. J Palliative Care 1998;14:18–24.
3. Henkelman WJ, Dallinis PM: A protocol for palliative care measures: p2. Nurs Manag 1998;29:36c,36f-36g.
4. Henkelman WJ, Dalinis PM: A protocol for palliative care measures: p1. Nurs Manag 1998;29:40–42,45–6.
5. Levetown M: Palliative care in the intensive care unit. New Horizons 1998;6:383–397.
6. Zerzan J, Stearns S, Hanson L: Access to palliative care and hospice in nursing homes. JAMA 2000;284:2489–2494.
7. Kirchhoff KT, Spuhler V, et al: Intensive care nurses' experiences with end-of-life care. Am J Crit Care 2000;9:36–42.
8. Billings JA: Recent advances: palliative care. BMJ 2000;321:555–558.
9. Rushton CH, Sabatier KH: The Nursing Leadership Consortium on End-of-Life Care: the response of the nursing profession to the need for improvement in palliative care. Nurs Outlook 2001;49:58–60.

David J. Gattas, MB, BS
William J. Sibbald, MD

PATIENT 50

A 78-year-old man who is unconscious and ventilator-dependent after a stroke with a family that requests transfer of care

A 78-year-old man arrives at the ICU from a referring hospital after 6 weeks of care following an ischemic stroke that left him unconscious. The family requested the transfer because of their disappointment with the care the patient had received.

The patient was admitted 6 weeks ago to the referring hospital after sudden loss of consciousness. A head CT and MRI scan both demonstrated extensive areas of brain infarction involving the left parietal hemisphere along with most of the midbrain and pons. A separate, smaller area of infarction existed in the right hemisphere.

During that admission, the patient never regained consciousness and demonstrated abnormal flexor posturing of the left arm to deep pain. Some spontaneous eye opening and chewing motions were observed. The patient was ventilator dependent and had experienced several episodes of ventilator-associated pneumonia. A tracheotomy and percutaneous feeding tube were placed 10 days before transfer.

Because of the critical care physicians' rotating schedule at the referring hospital, the patient's family interacted with four different physicians during their father's 6-week hospitalization. From the family's perspective, all four physicians expressed different values and beliefs regarding the appropriateness of withdrawing life support. The family voiced frustration that the nurses and physicians seemed to provide different versions of how life support would be withdrawn if consent were given to "let their father go." The referring hospital had no explicit policy governing the withdrawal of life support. It also had not created educational opportunities for staff in end-of-life care or the withdrawal of life support.

Conflict developed between the physicians and the family during the last 2 weeks of the patient's hospital stay. A few days before transfer, the patient's wife and adult child became resistive to discussions about withdrawing or even limiting aggressive life-supportive care. They stated their belief that the patient's wishes would be for them to "fight for him to survive against all odds until the end." They began to discuss extended care, suggesting the patient might eventually regain consciousness and return home. They threatened to discuss the situation with their lawyers whenever approached about withdrawing life-supportive care. The resulting stalemate was resolved by transferring the patient to the current tertiary-care teaching hospital for a second opinion.

The patient has a history of non-insulin-dependent diabetes mellitus. He has experienced a gradual decline in gait and short-term memory over the last 2 to 3 years. He had lived, however, independently at home with his wife. On arrival at the ICU, the patient is unconscious. Examination confirms the previously documented neurologic findings. He remains ventilator dependent.

Question: What measures might have avoided the conflict between the family and physicians? How can clinicians work with the family to make sound decisions now?

Diagnosis: Massive stroke affecting a patient who has no apparent chance for meaningful recovery and needs coordinated end-of-life care.

Discussion: The health of communities is the shared responsibility of the many organisations and interests that the communities comprise. Healthcare providers, hospitals, patients, and patients' families represent only a few of these community interests. To satisfy the needs of these diverse stakeholders with varying perspectives, open communication must occur through a political process. *Politics* represent the negotiating process by which society decides who gets what, when, and how. The political process leads to the creation of *policy*. A hospital board, for instance, creates *policy* in representing its community by selecting a course of action from among alternatives that guides and determines its present and future decisions in light of given conditions.

In contrast, *guidelines* are those directions or principles that present the current rules contained within policy. As systematically developed statements, guidelines assist practitioners and patients in decisions about appropriate healthcare delivery for specific clinical circumstances. Guidelines make explicit recommendations, often on behalf of health organisations, with a stated intention of influencing what clinicians do.

Two observations highlight the importance of creating both policy and associated guidelines to direct care in the ICU for patients who are at the end of life. First, most patients who die in ICUs do so after decisions are made to limit treatment. Because the withdrawal of life-supportive care occurs so commonly, it has become increasingly important that it be done well. Success in withdrawing life-supportive care requires proactive involvement of medical leadership to ensure that medical staff have the requisite skills and interests to discuss end-of-life care with patients and their families in an effective and meaningful way.

Second, observational studies demonstrate variations in how physicians withdraw life-supportive care. Practices in end-of-life care vary between countries, between hospitals in the same region, and even between physicians in the same hospital. Differences exist between community and teaching hospitals in the use of family meetings before the withdrawal of life-supportive care and specific steps used to discontinue life-sustaining interventions. Prescribed doses of morphine and sedative drugs vary by 10-fold between physicians during the withholding or withdrawal of life-supportive care.

Hospital policies can decrease practice variation, improve end-of-life care, and avoid conflicts between healthcare providers and their patients. Policies provide a framework for discussing difficult topics, such as the withdrawal of life-supportive care, and facilitate decision-making at difficult times for both families and caregivers. Policies also provide guidance for the negotiation and management of any conflicts that might arise.

Most policies originate with efforts by physician leaders who work in the units to which the policies apply. Formulation of an effective policy requires discussion and debate among members of the multidisciplinary critical care team responsible for a patient care. Proposed policies should be informed by a critical review of the profession's local governing bodies, as well as by relevant literature. Practices should advance the ethical principles of patient autonomy, beneficence, and nonmalfeasance.

Policy developers should also consider statements from agencies and professional organisations charged with oversight and accountability for the institutions and healthcare professionals involved. Policy development is aided by reviewing authoritative summaries of legal issues related to withholding and withdrawing life support.

A policy about withdrawal of life-sustaining interventions should include a preamble that establishes linkage with the hospital's value set. For example, a policy might begin with a statement such as the following: "This hospital requires that its care processes include the respect of life and human dignity by providing care to patients that is medically and ethically appropriate. Care should address issues of patients and families as they define them, in order to relieve as much discomfort and distress as possible. Care also includes help for patients and surrogate decision-makers who face decisions about life-supportive interventions proposed by their physicians."

Policies related to the withdrawal of life-supportive care should contain several elements. The policy should explicitly emphasize the necessary concern caregivers should direct toward patient comfort and the prevention of suffering during treatment withdrawal. Concern for the family should also be included as an important policy directive.

Policies that pertain to the withdrawal of life support should also discuss the critical importance of involving patients' families in discussions about treatment withdrawal, unless the patient has expressly requested otherwise. Policies can guide caregivers toward approaches that promote meaningful and cooperative discussions of difficult and painful topics among patients, their families, and the ICU team. When conflicts are anticipated, policies should suggest approaches for negotiation and conflict resolution to serve the patient's best interests. Policies should remind clinicians that open and unhurried communication is the fundamental approach to avoiding and resolving conflict.

Because caregivers must individualise care to meet patient needs, policies should not mandate any particular medication or dosing regime. Rather, they should focus on important principles for withdrawing life support. The general policy is designed to support the development of a guideline that provides more explicit recommendations for care derived from consensus among the critical care team. The guidelines should describe best clinical practices for managing patient suffering and distress in a manner that respects the patient's wishes and concerns.

Well constructed guidelines cannot alter caregiver behavior unless a well-conceived process for their implementation is put into place. Clinician "champions" who promote the best clinical practices contained within the guideline can foster the implementation process. End-of-life care is a competency that can be taught and learned.

Von Gunten and colleagues have identified competencies necessary for good end-of-life care, including skills in communication, decision-making, and building relationships. They have proposed a seven-step approach for physicians for structuring communication regarding care at the end of life. In step one, physicians prepare for these discussions by confirming medical facts and establishing an appropriate environment. Subsequent steps include establishing what the patient (and family) knows through open-ended questions; determining how information is to be handled at the beginning of the patient-physician relationships; delivering the information in a sensitive but straightforward manner; responding to emotions of the patients, parents, and families; establishing goals for care and treatment priorities when possible; and establishing an overall plan. Families also need to know treatment discussions in the ICU will be accompanied by pastoral care as necessary and will include a

"doctor-in-charge," family conference rooms, and a lenient visitation policy.

Finally, a formal approach may be considered to create a "guide" to the process of withdrawing life support, a process that ideally should involve all ICU stakeholders. In this proactive approach, a guideline can be created and documented that clearly articulates the unit's approach to the alleviation of suffering and distress in these circumstances. The primary intent of administering medication during the withdrawal of life support is to relieve suffering and distress, not to hasten death; the proprietary of such action is based on the nature of the physician's intentions, not on the consequences of the actions themselves. Medication administered to alleviate suffering or distress during the withdrawal of life support should be titrated against symptoms and signs of these problems. A guideline should indicate the need for advance discussion by the multidisciplinary team members who will be involved in the patient's bedside care during this process, with the results of such discussion documented.

The present patient was evaluated by the critical care team, with initial ventilator adjustments to relieve his work of breathing. The senior physician met with the family and listened patiently to their experiences at the other hospital. The physician communicated her impressions regarding the patient's grim prognosis and reviewed the available care options, which included maintaining patient comfort and considering withdrawal of life-supporting interventions. The family asked how the ventilator would be withdrawn and what their family member would experience. The physician was able to refer to not only her personal experience with end-of-life care but also described the unit's guidelines and safeguards for palliative and end-of-life care. The next day, the family agreed to withdraw life-supportive care. Morphine was titrated to maintain patient comfort. The patient died soon after removal of the ventilator, with the family and physician in attendance.

Clinical Pearls

1. Withdrawal and withholding of treatment in hospitals should occur in harmony with the values of surrounding society. The process must be an open one guided by prospectively identified policy.

2. Hospitals should have policies and procedures (guidelines) for the withdrawal and withholding of treatment. These policies should define the principles and practices through which it may be carried out. They should be taught to all members of the multidisciplinary team in an active learning approach.

3. Open communication and time are the fundamental approaches used to present and resolve conflict. Involvement of the legal system signifies failure of communication and hospital policy to prevent or resolve conflict.

REFERENCES

1. Field MJ, Lohr KN (eds): Clinical Practice Guidelines: Directions for a New Program. Washington, Institute of Medicine, National Academy Press, 1990.
2. Tunis SR, Hayward RSA, Wilson MC, et al: Internists' attitudes about clinical practice guidelines. Ann Intern Med 1994;120:956–963.
3. Prendergast TJ, Luce JM: Increasing incidence of withholding and withdrawal of life support from the critically ill. Am J Respir Crit Care Med 1997;155:15–20.
4. Prendergast TJ, Claessens MT, Luce JM: A national survey of end-of-life care for critically ill patients. Am J Respir Crit Care Med 1998;158:1163–1167.
5. Hall RI, Rocker GM: End-of-life care in the ICU: treatments provided when life support was or was not withdrawn. Chest 2000;118:1424–1430.
6. Keenan SP, Busche KD, Chen LM, et al: A retrospective review of a large cohort of patients undergoing the process of withholding or withdrawal of life support. Crit Care Med 1997;25:1324–1331.
7. Asch DA, Christakis NA: Why do physicians prefer to withdraw some forms of life support over others?: intrinsic attributes of life-sustaining treatments are associated with physicians' preferences. Med Care 1996;34:103–111.
8. Luce JM, Alpers A: Legal aspects of withholding and withdrawing life support from critically ill patients in the United States and providing palliative care to them. Am J Respir Crit Care Med 2000;162:2029–2032.
9. Meisel A, Snyder L, Quill T: Seven legal barriers to end-of-life care: myths, realities, and grains of truth. JAMA 2000;284:2495–2501.
10. von Gunten CF, Ferris FD, Emanuel LL: The patient-physician relationship: ensuring competency in end-of-life care: communication and relational skills. JAMA 2001;284:3051–3057.
11. Abbott KH, Sago JG, Breen CM, et al: Families looking back: one year after discussion of withdrawal or withholding of life-sustaining support. Crit Care Med 2001;29:197–201.

Christina M. Puchalski, MD

PATIENT 51

A 52-year-old woman with metastatic cancer who asks, "How does a Jewish person die?"

A 52-year-old woman with terminal ovarian cancer who is being cared for by home hospice asks her physician one day, "How does a Jewish person die?" During the last 7 years since her original diagnosis, the patient experienced multiple tumor recurrences that required several surgeries and many courses of chemotherapy. After her husband's sudden death 2 years ago, she became depressed. She improved after joining Jewish Healing Services, a spiritual support group.

Two months ago, she was diagnosed with recurrent metastases to her liver and spleen. During another course of chemotherapy, she required hospitalization for a bowel obstruction and sepsis. After extensive discussions between the patient, her family, and oncologist, the patient entered home hospice care. She has received effective pain management, and there has been no recurrence of her previous depression. However, until this time, she has avoided talking about death and remains uncertain about whether she should request further chemotherapy.

Question: How might this patient's spiritual beliefs assist her in coping with her terminal illness?

Diagnosis: Terminal ovarian cancer in a patient who needs spiritual support at the end of life.

Discussion: Spirituality represents a vitally important factor in maintaining good health for many persons. No single definition of spirituality suffices to encompass the many forms and range of spiritual experience and expression. We express spirituality in our search for ultimate meaning through various pursuits, such as a belief in God and participation in religion, through family, or through active expression of naturalism, rationalism, humanism, and the arts. Spirituality in its multiple forms influences how patients and their healthcare providers perceive and experience health and illness. Peoples' spiritual orientation also influences how they interact with one another.

Spirituality plays a critical role in our patients' lives. Illness and the prospect of dying can call into question the very meaning and purpose of a person's life. By eroding a sense of life's purpose, a serious illness can generate profound suffering. All people seek meaning and purpose in their lives. Victor Frankl wrote, "Man is not destroyed by suffering; he is destroyed by suffering without meaning." The search for meaning becomes intensified when we face death. To address spiritual suffering, caregivers need to engage patients on a spiritual level.

Spirituality helps people find hope in the midst of despair. A relationship with God or a felt connection with any sense of the transcendent can add meaning and purpose to life's joys and sufferings. Spirituality is concerned with transcendental or existential aspects of one's life and, at a deeper level, "with the person as human being."

Religious and spiritual beliefs may affect patients' decisions about treatment and care. For some people, religious doctrine can strongly influence—or flatly determine—decisions regarding whether or not to withdraw life-supportive care or to accept blood transfusions or feeding tubes.

People who are faced with their own mortality may survey their life and re-prioritize what is important to them. It is not uncommon for people with potentially life-limiting illnesses to quit jobs, start new projects, question relationships, or travel to places that give them new-found meaning. As professional caregivers, we can best serve our patients by creatively modifying standard treatment plans to accommodate their wishes and personal priorities.

The present patient expressed a need to travel to the mountains in Washington several times after being diagnosed with cancer. Being in nature helped her feel grounded and, she said, helped her "touch a sense of the divine." This was as important to her and her well-being as her medical therapy. Chemotherapy schedules were modified to accommodate her travel needs.

It is important for physicians, nurses, other healthcare providers and family to recognize and respond to a seriously ill person's spiritual needs. Multiple resources are available to assist patients in these needs.

Pastoral care providers are trained in spiritual care and counseling. Chaplains may be clergy or lay people who are trained to be spiritual care providers familiar with assisting patients to explore issues of meaning, reconcile suffering, and draw strength from one's values and beliefs. Chaplains work with people of all faiths as well as with those with no faith. Clergy are typically trained to provide religious care within the traditions, customs, and rituals of their specific denominations. Chaplains and clergy for individual patients should be recognized as valuable members of the interdisciplinary healthcare team. As with other members of the team, chaplains and clergy can contribute their insights as well as their unique services to care and support for the patient and family.

Religion and religious beliefs can play an important role in how patients understand their illness. In a study, structured interviews were conducted with a sample of 40 community-dwelling adults aged 65–74 in Durham County, North Carolina. These older adults were asked about God's role in health and illness; many (60%) of respondents saw health and illness as being partly attributable to God and, to some extent, seventy-seven percent saw health and blessings as gifts from God. Prayer, in this study, appeared to complement medical care rather than compete with it. Symptoms never discussed with a physician were less likely to be prayed about than those that had been discussed with a physician. Meditation has been found to be a useful adjunct to conventional medical therapy for chronic conditions such as headaches, anxiety, depression, premenstrual syndrome, AIDS, and cancer.

In addition to assisting in the innate quest for meaning and purpose, spiritual and religious belief and experience can foster hope in the midst of despair. Hope can change during a course of an illness; early on, the person may hope for a cure. Later, when a cure becomes unlikely, the person may hope for time to finish important projects or goals, make peace with loved ones or God, and have a peaceful death. These efforts can result in a healing, which can be manifested as a restoration of one's relationships or sense of self. While cures are not always possible, the possibility of healing, the restoration of wholeness, remains to the very end of life.

Spirituality can also offer patients a sense of control in the face of serious illnesses. Some people can gain a sense of control by turning worries or a situation over to a higher power or God. Religious and spiritual beliefs can help patients to let go of their need for control and to accept a higher wisdom.

The present patient's physician discussed "how Jewish patients die" from his perspective and asked the patient to welcome her rabbi into her home. After the rabbi visited, the patient appeared more content and comfortable with thoughts of "letting go." Her family reported that she sought comfort through prayer and meditation, both of which seemed to relieve her anxiety and stress. Over the next few months, the patient spent time talking with her family and friends, sharing stories, crying, laughing, and, as she put it, "living while I am dying." The day before she died, she was surrounded by her loved ones who sang with her, shared more stories, and frequently hugged and kissed her. Her physicians visited her, as did the rabbi. At her funeral, the rabbi remarked that during her last week, she appeared at those times to be so full of life.

Clinical Pearls

1. Illness and the prospect of dying can call into question the meaning and purpose of a person's life, generating profound suffering. Spirituality can help restore hope and purpose.

2. Patients with life-limiting illness may re-prioritize their lives to address new goals, travel, or personal relationships. Clinicians should attempt to modify treatment plans to accommodate patient's wishes and new-found personal priorities.

3. Physicians can call on pastoral care providers associated with the hospital or on local clergy to minister and support their patients with spiritual needs.

REFERENCES

1. Frankl V: Man's Search for Meaning. New York, Simon & Schuster, 1984, p 135.
2. Conrad NL: Spiritual support for the dying. Nurs Clin North Am 1985;20:415–426.
3. O'Connor P: The role of spiritual care in hospice Am J Hospice Care 1988;5:31–37.
4. Bearon LB, Koenig HG: Religious cognitions and use of prayer in health and illness. Gerontologist 1990;30:249–253.
5. Doka KJ, Morgan JD (eds): Death and Spirituality. Amityville, NY, Baywood Publishing Comp., 1993, p 11.
6. Benson H: Timeless Healing: The Power and Biology of Belief. New York, Simon and Schuster, 1996.
7. Interfaith Committee, Department of Chaplaincy Services and Pastoral Education, University of Virginia Health System: Religious Beliefs and Practices Affecting Health Care [pamphlet]. Charlottesville, VA, Chaplaincy Services and Pastoral Education, 1997.
8. Puchalski CM, Romer AL: Taking a spiritual history allows clinicians to understand patients more fully. J Pallia Med 2000;3:129–37.
9. Post SG, Puchalski CM, Larson DB: Physicians and patient spirituality: professional boundaries, competency, and ethics. Ann Intern Med 2000;132:578–583.
10. Puchalski CM: Spirituality and end-of-life care: a time for listening and caring. J Palliat Med 2002 (in press).
11. Puchalski CM: Spirituality and end of life care. In: Berger AM, Portenoy R, Weissman D (eds): Principles and Practice of Palliative Care and Supportive Oncology. Philadelphia, Lippincott Williams & Wilkins (in press).

Linda Emanuel, MD, PhD

PATIENT 52

A 74-year-old man with acute respiratory failure who has not had prior discussions with his family about life-supportive care

A 74-year-old man presents to his physician's office with a 2-day history of cough and fever. He has a history of adult-onset diabetes managed with insulin and mild congestive heart failure treated with an angiotensin-converting enzyme inhibitor. He has remained active, working part-time. Last year, the patient and his wife designated each other as health care proxy. No specific wishes were discussed except that both wanted to avoid "being a vegetable on a machine."

Physical Examination: Blood pressure 105/75, pulse 110; temperature 103°; respiratory rate 22. Neck: jugular venous distension. Cardiac: normal heart sounds. Chest: bibasilar crackles, dullness at both lung bases. Extremities: moderate pitting edema.

Laboratory Findings: Hct, normal, WBC 22,000/μl with left shift. Glucose 290 mg/dl. Electrolytes and renal indices: normal. Sputum: polymorphonucleocytes with gram-positive cocci suggestive of *Staphylococcus aureus*. Chest radiograph: bilateral infiltrates.

Hospital Course: Despite appropriate therapy for bacterial pneumonia and congestive heart failure, the patient declines rapidly. He becomes confused and severely dyspneic. When asked about life support, the patient mumbles his response but seems to indicate that he is refusing intubation. His wife supports her husband's apparent decision, explaining his long-term fear of "being stuck on a machine." The nurse protests this interpretation of the patient's advance wishes. The nurse asserts that he need not become "stuck" on the ventilator because life-supportive care could be withdrawn if the patient fails to improve after an initial trial of mechanical ventilation.

Question: How can the health care team assist the patient and his wife in making a wise decision whether to accept intubation and mechanical ventilation?

Diagnosis: Respiratory failure, secondary to pneumonia and exacerbation of congestive heart failure, in a patient with a good chance of surviving with aggressive medical treatment.

Discussion: Many people who complete advance directives limit their planning to the designation of a health care proxy. Comprehensive advance directives, however, can anticipate future health care situations and structure discussions with health care proxies of hypothetical decisions about which treatment options would be acceptable or unacceptable. Although many people find discussion of such future eventualities difficult, the omission of these considerations may leave a proxy in the stressful situation of making life-and-death decisions with little or no guidance.

The best way to avoid this dilemma may be the use of user-friendly **worksheets** when making advance care plans that present important, clinically relevant scenarios and key decisions. To help patients become comfortable with planning their end-of-life care, such worksheets can be provided as a part of routine office visits. In selecting a worksheet, clinicians should determine whether it has been designed and tested for its ability to cover the most pertinent issues, to be understood correctly by all parties, and to elicit answers that reflect the patients' wishes in a sensible and reliable fashion. Validated worksheets exist for general use and for people with particular diseases or disease groups. They employ patient scenarios and most of them use goals for care as well as specific intervention choices. Without this level of specificity regarding conditions, treatments and goals, a patient's general values and wishes may be hard to translate into actual clinical decisions.

A step-wise approach to advance-care planning that employs worksheets can make good use of the physician's time during an office visit and allow the patient and family to take ownership of their future care. Physicians can orient patients to the worksheet and let them pencil in their choices on their own time. Patients can read through the scenarios and consider goals for care before focusing on specific examples of life-sustaining interventions. Physicians should schedule a follow-up visit to review the patient's worksheet. At that time, the patients' preferences can be clarified and discussed. The physician can respond to any question and further explore any apparent inconsistencies or clinical misconceptions. The physican can also discuss any wishes expressed that caregivers at the bedside could not morally support. Sessions of this nature can be timed for patient convenience with another reason for a visit, and the discussion of advance-care planning can be billed as counseling.

When the physician, patient, and family become comfortable with all aspects of the advance directive, a signed copy should be entered into the patient's contact information within the medical record. Copies should be provided to the patient and proxy. The advance-care planning document should be reexamined every 3 to 5 years and at the time of any serious illness or significant functional change.

As occurred with the present patient, omission of advance-care planning leaves proxies with little to guide their decisions. Physicians can assist decision-making by leading proxies through an examination of the issues. For instance, the wife of the present patient only knew that, were he in a persistent vegetative state, her husband would not want long-term mechanical ventilation. Empiric research indicates that when people are presented with a range of scenarios and decisions about life-sustaining interventions, a previously expressed wish to avoid life support for vegetative states does not imply that the person would decline short-term life-sustaining care for acute and potentially reversible conditions.

Caregivers can ask proxies whether they recall previous comments by their ill family member indicating what decision he or she might have made. Often, a proxy may remember such comments and gain a greater insight into the relative desirability of life-supportive care in light of the likelihood of meaningful recovery and anticipated disabilities. Worksheets are available to estimate these personal thresholds and extrapolate estimates to real-life decisions. After working through these discussions, proxies may gain greater confidence of being able to act in accordance with the wishes of a seriously ill and incapacitated patient.

With the present patient, the wife could not recall any prior comments about the desirability of life-supportive care in different clinical circumstances. Consequently, there were no specific statements, written or verbal, to help her make an informed substituted judgment. In such circumstances, proxies may be better able to make an emphathic substituted judgement, based on their knowledge of the patient as a person, or a best-interests judgment.

An **empathic substituted judgment** takes into account anything that the proxy thinks the patient would have considered, such as the feelings and wishes of children. Unfortunately, extensive research has demonstrated that substituted judgments are often quite inaccurate. When faced with hypothetical life and death situations, individuals and their chosen proxies often make different choices. A **best-interests judgment** follows what appears to be in the patient's "best interests." Best-interests judgments are subjective by nature and may appear similar to substituted judgment because it is hard to imagine what is in the patient's best interests in the absence of considering what the patient would have wanted.

Despite having thought she and her husband had attended to their advance-care planning, the patient's wife was left to fall back on substituted judgment. The healthcare team first suggested that she consider what the appropriate goals were for her husband's care. They also explained that the in emergency decision-making, standard principles are to err on the side of intervening to preserve life and are employed when no knowledge exists of patients' wishes.

Upon reflection, the patient's wife felt that if her husband could decide, he would probably pursue a cure as long as he could feel sure that life support would be withdrawn if recovery seemed unlikely. She opted for aggressive intervention, including intubation. Unfortunately, the patient continued to decline despite ventilatory support and died several days later. In addition to their sadness, the patient's wife and family expressed a sense of confidence in the choice they had made and comfort from the guidance and support they received from the healthcare team.

Clinical Pearls

1. Physicians should use the opportunity of routine patient encounters to broach the topic of advance-care planning, with designation of a proxy and completion of written statements regarding the desirability of various life-sustaining interventions.

2. In the absence of prior considerations of care, the decisions of a proxy often fails to promote the care patients would have selected for themselves. Substituted judgment and best-interests judgment are burdensome for proxy decision-makers, highly subjective, and often inaccurate.

3. Validated worksheets can assist the completion of written statements about preferences for care in potentially life-limiting situations.

4. In using worksheets, advise patients and their families to first consider and decide on the goals of care for each scenario before addressing the specific life-sustaining treatment that they would choose.

5. Patients and families should consider the patient's thresholds for accepting or declining intervention on the basis of the burden of the treatment, the likelihood of survival, and the nature of any anticipated disability. Thresholds for decision-making generally emerge once a range of scenarios, goals, and interventions have been considered.

REFERENCES

1. Pearlman R, Starks H, Cain K, et al: Your Life Your Choices, Planning for Future Medical Decisions: How to Prepare a Personalized Living Will. Seattle, WA, Patient Decision Support, 1992.
2. Emanuel LL: Advance directives: what have we learned so far? J Clin Ethics 1993;4(1):8–16. Available at: www.medicaldirective.org.
3. University of Toronto Joint Centre for Bioethics: The Joint Centre for Bioethics Cancer Living Will Form. Available at: http://www.utoronto.ca/jcb/canchap5.htm; accessed October 22, 1998.
4. Emanuel LL, von Gunten CF, Ferris FD: EPEC Series: Advance Care Planning. Arch Fam Med 2000:9:1181–1187.

Thomas G. Heffron, MD
Todd Pillen, PA-C/SA

PATIENT 53

A 4-year-old boy with fulminant hepatitis whose "terminal" course is altered by liver transplantation

A 4-year-old boy presents to the emergency department with a 1-week history of nausea and vomiting. His mother states that he has alternated between being irritable and lethargic over the last 2 days and that his personality and activity levels have changed remarkably. She brings him in today because she noted his eyes to be slightly yellow.

Physical Examination: Blood pressure 80/50; pulse 125, temperature 37.2°, pulse 120, weight 22.5 kg. General: well-nourished, irritable, jaundiced, arousable to voice but confused. HEENT: icteric sclera with PERRL. Chest: clear to auscultation. Cardiac: tachycardia without murmur. Abdomen: soft and nontender without ascites, organomegaly, or venous distention. Extremities: full range of motion, capillary refill of < 2 sec; no asterixis, cyanosis, or edema.

Laboratory Findings: Hct 33% with normal indices, WBC 7,600/μl with normal differential, platelets 150,000/μl. BUN 55 mg/d, creatinine 1.2 mg/dl, total bilirubin 14 mg/dl, AST 5,500 IU, ALT 6,900 IU. Prothrobin time 32 sec, factor V 13 (normal 50–150), factor VII 12 (normal 50–150). Serologic and microbiologic studies including bacterial and viral cultures, HIV, hepatitis A,B, and C, EBV, and CMV: negative.

Hospital Course: The patient is admitted to the pediatric ICU, where he receives fresh frozen plasma and volume resusciation with i.v. saline via a large-bore catheter in the left femoral vein. Vitamin K is administered. Blood levels of factors V and VII show no improvement. His prothrombin time worsens to 35 sec despite transfusion of blood products and vitamin K. He becomes progressively more somnolent.

Question: What type of liver transplant should be offered to this child given the survival rate and potential risks to a living donor?

Diagnosis: Fulminant hepatic failure (FHF).

Discussion: All treatments for fulminant liver failure prior to the era of liver transplantation almost always ended in death. With the development of liver transplantation during the 1970s and 1980s, survival was dependent on the condition of the recipient patient at the time of referral as well as the ability to transplant at an optimal time with a viable, high-quality organ. A child with signs of multiple organ failure directly related to the acute liver disease, especially hepatic encephalopathy, may have a 40% to 50% chance of surviving a liver transplant compared to a 70% to 80% survival in children with chronic, "early end-stage" liver disease.

Children with FHF often present with symptoms similar to a mild case of gastroenteritis. Even after the child becomes jaundiced, he or she may act only slightly irritable. However, the child may progress to coma and brain death over a period as short as a few hours secondary to brain edema or toxic metabolic waste products. In the present patient, the exceedingly low factor V and VII levels, worsening prothrombin time refractory to treatment with vitamin K and fresh frozen plasma, high bilirubin, and negative testing for hepatitis A, B, and C almost surely indicates FHF as the cause of acute liver decompensation.

This child's only chance for survival is emergent liver transplantation. He was emergently placed on the liver transplant list at the highest status. This means that this child has the first chance to receive a donor liver from a brain-dead person in the region whose family is willing to provide organs to persons on the national waiting list. The donor would need to have a body weight between one-half the present patient's body weight (11 kg) to twice his weight (44 kg) in order to provide a whole cadaveric liver. The patient could receive a partial liver (a piece of liver such as a left lateral segment) from a donor up to 20 times the patient's weight. Because most cadaveric donors are adults, the ability to transplant a partial liver greatly increases the donor pool available for the present patient and the likelihood of finding a suitable match before his metabolic encephalopathy becomes irreversible and brain death occurs.

Unfortunately, cadaveric organ donation remains the standard in liver transplantation, and a chronic shortage of suitable donors limits the availability of this life-saving surgery. Between 40% to 50% of transplant candidates die on the waiting list as a result of donor shortages. In response to this growing shortage of cadaveric organs, **living liver donation** was introduced as a therapeutic option in 1989. Technical advances in liver surgery allowed children with chronic end-stage liver disease to receive a partial liver from a living donor. In addition to increasing the donor pool for seriously ill patients, living liver transplantation allows the procedure to be performed in an elective rather than emergent basis (although the seriousness of illness in the recipient dictates an emergent procedure in approximately two thirds of instances).

Usually, a parent, relative, or emotionally related person serves as the living donor for patients in need of transplantation. Living donors can donate up to 60% of their liver and still maintain adequate hepatic function. For the present patient, it was estimated that a left lateral segment of liver approximating 15 to 30% of the total liver volume from an adult living donor would be needed. Unlike kidney or heart transplantation, the donated liver only needs to be matched to the recipient by size. With the use of current immunosuppression and plasmapheresis, matching of blood types and HLA tissue types does not alter expected graft and patient survival and is unnecessary.

Considering the severity of the present patient's FHP, an emergent transplantation was needed to avoid death from brain swelling. Both the mother and older sister wished to donate. The sister was disqualified because of a previously unrecognized viral illness. The mother's CT scan revealed an inappropriately sized left lateral segment. The father was too large on screening examination. Fortunately, the child's church mobilized 30 possible donors between 20 to 30 years of age who were willing to donate. A 28-year-old married man with two small children had an appropriately sized left lateral segment for donation. An angiogram confirmed satisfactory arterial diameter and architecture for donation. He subsequently provided the portion of liver that saved this child's life.

The call for a donor, the entirety of the donor evaluations, and the transplantation procedure itself were all performed within 36 hours of the patient's hospital admission, thereby halting the typically rapid deterioration to death that occurs with fulminant liver failure. Both the patient and the living donor are alive and well 8 months after transplantation.

Clinical Pearls

1. Fulminant hepatic failure represents a life-threatening condition that requires emergent consideration of liver transplantation.

2. Advances in surgical techniques offer the opportunity of living donor transplantation, which greatly increases the donor pool and likelihood of providing a transplanted liver before death occurs.

3. Because of the effectiveness of modern immunosuppression, possible organs for donation must be matched only by size. Mismatched blood and tissue types do not alter organ or patient survival.

REFERENCES

1. Broelsch CE, Whitington PF, Emond JC, et al: Living Related Liver Transplantation: patient Selection and Procedures. Chicago, American Surgical Association, Dec 1990.
2. Rogiers X, Emond JC, et al: The concept of reduced size liver transplantation, including a living related liver transplantation. In: Abouna GM (ed): Recent Advances and Current Practice in Organ Transplantation. Amsterdam, Kluwer Academic Publishers, 1991.
3. Stevens LH, Piper JB, Heffron TG, et al: The role of reduced-size liver transplantation in pediatric liver disease: rationale and results. In: Rodes J, Arroya V (eds): Therapy in Liver Disease. Barcelona, Edi Doyma, 1991.
4. Dhawan A, Langnas AN, Vanderhoof JA, et al: Outcome of liver transplantation for fulminant liver failure in children: 10 year experience. Hepatology 1995, 22(4, pt 2):08A #407.
5. Heffron TG, Matamoros A Jr, Langnas AN, et al: Preoperative evaluation of hepatic segmental volume in living related donor (LRD): clinical application. Presented at the Southwestern Surgical Congress Annual Meeting, April 28, 1996.

Anthony L. Back, MD

PATIENT 54

A 58-year old woman with ovarian cancer who requests physician-assisted suicide

A 58-year-old woman with metastatic ovarian cancer comes to the clinic for a routine followup and casually mentions that she has been thinking about hastening her death. She was diagnosed with ovarian cancer 2 years ago and underwent debulking surgery and chemotherapy with paclitaxel and cisplatin. Aside from side effects related to cycles of chemotherapy, she was free of cancer-related symptoms for 11 months. Unfortunately, her disease recently relapsed with recurrent ascites and positive ascitic fluid cytology for ovarian cancer. The patient was subsequently treated with second-line chemotherapy comprised of carboplatin and paclitaxel. Although her ascites initially improved, her disease soon progressed. Most recently, she has been receiving liposomal doxorubicin as a third-line treatment.

Her chemotherapy has been complicated by two admissions for fever and neutropenia, a laparotomy for bowel obstruction that proved secondary to adhesions, and fatigue. She has actively participated in her cancer care, extensively researched her condition on the internet, and sought other medical opinions. She lives alone and remains independent in activities of daily living.

Her physical exam shows a pale, chronically-ill-appearing woman with alopecia and an intense smile. She has a venous access port in the left chest wall. Significant findings include mild ascites, 1+ lower extremity edema, and moderate sensory neuropathy.

Near the end of the visit, she mentions that she has been thinking "about what would happen at the end." After a pause, she asks the physician if he would "consider helping her hasten her death."

Question: How should her physician respond?

Diagnosis: Patient interest in physician-assisted suicide that has not been assessed.

Discussion: Physicians who receive requests for physician-assisted suicide (PAS) have a complex task. A physician must clarify the patient's request and explore the reasons underlying the request as well as related concerns. A competent and compassionate response does not mean that a physician must share a patient's views on the moral acceptability of PAS. Moreover, a caring and therapeutically effective response to a patient's inquiry also need not resolve the moral and social debate over legalizing PAS. This discussion will lay out some practical steps to ensure that the patient receives the best possible care, but it does not attempt to resolve the ethical debate surrounding PAS.

The terms *physician-assisted suicide* and *euthanasia* are not always used by patients and physicians to mean the same thing. In the medical literature, PAS refers to the prescription by a physician of lethal medications with the intention of causing or hastening death. Euthanasia refers to situations in which a physician causes death, for example, by injecting a medication intended to cause death. These practices are morally controversial; euthanasia is illegal in all states, and in all except Oregon, PAS is illegal as well. Among PAS advocacy groups, the term *hastening death* is preferred because it avoids negative connotations of the word *suicide*.

PAS and euthanasia are sometimes confused with withdrawing and withholding therapy. Additionally, patients, family members, and clinical staff may also confuse appropriate pain management, especially when it involves morphine or other strong opioids, with PAS or euthanasia. In the large majority of patients, however, even high doses of opioids are well tolerated and do not depress respirations or compromise vital signs. In those occasional situations in which sedating doses of opioids and other medications are required to control symptoms and the patient appears to die a hastened death, death is considered a secondary or "double effect." Aggressive pain control is ethically and clinically desirable and should not be confused with PAS.

Whether or not a physician thinks that assisting a patient with suicide is ever morally acceptable, responding to a patient's request is an important skill. On some occasions, PAS requests are a sign of patient crisis. In other situations, PAS requests are simply an individual patient's way of talking about dying. A skilled physician can approach a PAS request in ways that address suffering, strengthen the doctor-patient relationship, and often broaden options for end-of-life care.

The most common reasons for patients' requesting PAS include current physical or personal suffering, clinical depression and expressed fears of losing control, being a burden on family members or other caregivers, losing dignity, or fear of future pain. In recent studies of reasons for patients' interest in PAS, uncontrolled pain and financial concerns have been less common. Depression is of particular concern because it is under-diagnosed in terminally ill patients, is often associated with ideation about assisted suicide, and it treatable.

The U.S. Supreme Court has not recognized a federal constitutional right to PAS, but it did affirm that individual states may choose to legalize it. It also stressed the legality of withdrawing life-sustaining treatment and palliative care approaches to deal with end-of-life suffering.

A request for PAS should prompt ongoing discussion, evaluation, and active attempts to palliate distress. A seven-step protocol to address a PAS request includes:

1. Clarify the request; do not assume a patient shares your definition of PAS. It is important to distinguish between a patient's desire to forgo surgery or chemotherapy and a request for a lethal prescription.
2. Explore patient concerns underlying the PAS request.
3. Develop a care plan addressing the concerns, and explicitly affirm your commitment to care for the patient.
4. Offer to explain the dying process, and reassure the patient about having aggressive efforts at pain and symptom management, family support, and your efforts as their physician to provide maximal medical care.
5. Know the legal status of PAS where you practice.
6. Examine your own response to the request.
7. Consider consulting another physician to get a fresh perspective on the case.

In this case, the physician responded with an open-ended question, saying "Tell me more about what you're thinking." The patient described an intense interest in PAS that had developed after reading a medical textbook which indicated that death from ovarian cancer was "a drawn-out, ugly affair." She had found a formula for PAS on the internet that she wanted him to prescribe. The physician replied, "I can understand why you're interested in this. I really want to know more about your situation and why you are thinking about suicide. As we talk, I want you to know that whatever else we decide, I will do everything I can to make sure that you do not suffer or die in agony." The physician did a careful assessment of physical symptoms, psychosocial concerns, social support, and spiritual issues and concluded that a referral to a psychologist and a social worker would be helpful to address the patient's worries about being a burden.

When a physician has responded to a patient's reasons for seeking PAS, yet the request persists, the physician should address it directly. If a physician needs to decline, a clear explanation is helpful to maintain trust in the patient-physician relationship: for example, "I think I understand a great deal about why you are asking for assisted suicide. I think your concerns about what could happen when you die are very real. Giving you a lethal prescription would be deeply troubling to me, and I don't think I would be able to live with myself. But I want to say again that I will do everything in my power to ensure that you are as comfortable as possible. I intend to stick by you so that I can do everything I can to make your dying easier." Or, "I'm sad I haven't been able to help more. I think if PAS were legal, that I could see helping you with this. But I cannot accept the risk of breaking the law in this way." Or, "I'm sad I haven't been able to help more. Personally, I can sometimes imagine helping someone with PAS even though it is illegal. But for you, I am concerned that you may be depressed and that it is partially responsible for your feelings. I want to request that you work with me longer to treat any depression before you make any final decisions."

If the physician and patient live in Oregon, and both believe that sources of suffering have been identified and addressed and that assisted suicide would represent the least worst death for that patient, a state-approved procedure is available that includes suggested prescriptions. It is important for both patient and physician to work with other family members, who can sometimes experience complicated grief after involvement with a patient who dies in this way.

After meeting with a psychologist and social worker and discussing her care further with her physician, the present patient decided to pursue hospice care if her disease continued to progress despite her new chemotherapy. She gained confidence that her physician would provide sufficient palliative care to prevent the end-of-life suffering she feared.

Clinical Pearls

1. Responding to a patient's request for physician-assisted suicide involves exploration of the reasons underlying the request. Ensure that the patient has been adequately assessed, especially for depression, before discussing whether PAS is a good idea for this particular patient.

2. PAS requests may be a sign of patient crisis, but may also represent an invitation to talk about dying. Responding to a PAS request can help address suffering, strengthen the doctor-patient relationship, and sometimes broaden options for end of life care.

3. In its June 1997 decision, the U.S. Supreme Court did not recognize a federal constitutional right to PAS but did allow the possibility that individual states could craft laws making PAS legal within their jurisdictions. The Supreme Court also stressed the legality of withdrawing life-sustaining treatment and offering palliative care approaches to deal with end-of-life suffering. PAS is now only legally possible in Oregon, under a set of state-defined guidelines.

4. In some cases, alternatives to PAS include stopping eating and drinking and providing sedation for refractory symptoms in an imminently dying patient.

REFERENCES

1. Block SD, Billings JA: Patient requests to hasten death: evaluation and management in terminal care. Arch Intern Med 1994;154(18):2039–2047.
2. Back AL, Wallace JI, et al: Physician-assisted suicide and euthanasia in Washington State: patient requests and physician responses. JAMA 1996;275:919–925.
3. Foley KM: Competent care for the dying instead of physician-assisted suicide. N Engl J Med 1997;336: 54–58.
4. Chin AE, Hedberg K, et al: Legalized physician-assisted suicide in Oregon–the first year's experience [see comments]. N Engl J Med 1999;340:577–583.
5. Kohlwes RJ, Koepsell TD, et al: Physicians' responses to patients' requests for assisted suicide. Arch Intern Med 2000;161:657–663.
6. Quill TE, Byock IR: Responding to intractable terminal suffering: the role of terminal sedation and voluntary refusal of food and fluids: ACP-ASIM End-of-Life Care Consensus Panel. Ann Intern Med 2000;132:408–414.
7. Quill TE, Lee BC, et al: Palliative treatments of last resort: choosing the least harmful alternative: University of Pennsylvania Center for Bioethics Assisted Suicide Consensus Panel. Ann Intern Med 2000;132:488–493.

Joseph J. Fins, MD

PATIENT 55

A 38-year-old man with a secondary leukemia
who needs setting of goals of care

A 38-year-old man is admitted to the hospital because of cough, fatigue, easy bruisability, low-grade fever. His medical history is notable for widely metastatic testicular cancer that was successfully treated with combination chemotherapy 4 years ago. Following treatment, the patient returned to work as a high school teacher and married.

Physical Examination: Blood pressure 118/72; pulse 90, respirations 24; temperature 38.9°. General: thin, mild dyspnea, using accessory muscles of respiration. HEENT: conjunctival pallor. Nodes: none palpable. Chest: basilar: crackles bilaterally, wheezing on the right. Cardiac: normal. Abdomen: no organomegaly. Skin: fine petechiae and ecchymoses. Neurologic: alert and oriented.

Laboratory Findings: WBC 32,400/μl, Hct 22%, platelets 41,000/μl,. 92% lymphoctes with atypical forms. LDH 320 IU/L, uric acid 10.8 mg/dl. Chest radiograph: bilateral interstitial opacities. Arterial blood gas (room air): pH 7.45, pCO$_2$ 38 mm Hg, pO$_2$ 88 mm Hg.

Hospital Course: The patient is started on broad-spectrum antibiotics for pneumonia. A bone marrow biopsy reveals acute myelogenous leukemia, which is considered secondary to the previous chemotherapy. Despite the initiation of induction chemotherapy, the patient rapidly deteriorates, becoming nonresponsive and requiring mechanical ventilation for the adult respiratory distress syndrome.

When the patient's wife learns of his respiratory failure, she asks that the ventilator be withdrawn. She tells the medical student on the team that her husband had always dreaded a cancer recurrence. Given his past experiences, he was especially fearful of being on a ventilator and had asked his wife never to let this happen. Now that he has lost the ability to express his preferences, the wife feels obliged to speak for him and represent his interests.

The medical student communicates the wife's concerns to the attending physician. The attending quickly dismisses her request and states that it is "incredibly premature" to consider the withdrawal of care because the patient has just arrived in the unit. Nonetheless, the medical student continues to advocate for the preferences of the patient as communicated by his wife. The student suggests that care should be geared at pain and symptom management and the needs of the patient's wife. But after a week of advocating for palliative care, the student rotates off the ICU service and the patient remains on the ventilator. The student tells a classmate that her experiences in the MICU were causing her to reconsider a career in critical care medicine.

Question: How should the medical student reconcile her views about palliative care with her attending?

Diagnosis: Conflict over goals of care in a critically ill patient with a secondary malignancy.

Discussion: It is often during the most difficult cases that we learn the most about the sort of doctor we hope to become. So it is in this case, in which a cancer survivor develops a secondary leukemia, respiratory failure, and incapacity. The situation tests the fidelity of his wife and the professionalism of a young medical student who questions her attending's goals of care. This is not an easy position for a medical student. In asserting that palliation should guide the care of a patient who almost certainly has refractory disease, she is contesting the authority of her attending.

Studies have demonstrated that trainees can become especially disenfranchised when it comes to the provision of end-of-life care. They are in a hierarchical relationship and are often without the authority to direct the course of care. Although they are moral agents, they are often obliged to carry out a treatment plan that they did not formulate. A student or physician-in-training who advocates for a palliative approach to a patient in situations similar to that the one described in this patient have a view that is ethically appropriate and compassionate. Being frustrated in having their view incorporated, or even considered, can lead to disillusionment and "death avoidance" during the course of a trainee's subsequent medical career.

Although seeking the assistance of an ethics committee or the counsel of another attending physician might help to resolve this problematic situation, it is more productive to engage in reflective practice and to understand the roots of these conflicts. In this case, the student would be well served if she appreciated that the conflict with her attending was broader than interpersonal dynamics. A root cause analysis of that tension stems in part from a failure to set timely and reasonable goals of care in a patient who is clearly at the end of life. Here, the failure to view palliative care as a legitimate therapeutic alternative derives from the "routinized" pursuit of curative goals — in settings such as the ICU — and an often entrenched inability to reconstruct the goals of care even as the patient deteriorates. Instead of assessing the current clinical situation and asking what attainable goals might be achieved, physicians in hospital and critical care settings too often routinely pursue curative strategies, which may be ill suited to the needs of the patient and dismissive of prior preferences.

Constructive goal-setting should begin before a crisis arises in anticipation of a patient's decline. Ideally, this process should help clinicians recognize that death is near and allow for the planning of more timely and comprehensive end-of-life care strategies in conjunction with patients and their family. Clinical and narrative information are both essential to the formulation of cogent goals of care. In this case, a sanctioned process of goal-setting would have given both the patient's wife and the medical student a greater voice in helping to direct care.

A reconsideration of the goals of care should be prompted by developments in the patient's course, which herald a change in clinical status. Such prompts might include patient or surrogate knowledge about a terminal diagnosis or prognosis; articulated preferences for palliative care; a desire for death; or the completion of a do-not-resuscitate order. A reconsideration of the goals of care should also be prompted when dire prognostic or diagnostic information becomes available, when staff identifies the patient as dying, or when ICU admission or other life-sustaining therapies are being considered.

Through this process, clinicians can work collaboratively with patients and families to blend curative and palliative care strategies in a manner that incrementally evolves as the disease process progresses. Such an incremental approach to palliation attempts to track disease trajectory and appreciates that caring and curing are not dichotomous entities.

There is another advantage associated with the gentle titration of palliation into care strategies as the patient's condition deteriorates. It provides patient, family, and staff time to adjust to changing circumstances and develop expectations that may be more realistic and achievable. This process avoids precipitating tensions that might occur when care strategies are changed precipitously. Such abrupt changes in goals of care can often lead to futility disputes and complicate eventual bereavement.

More critically, by transforming the goals of care in a deliberate and incremental fashion, practitioners can be compassionate guides during a difficult journey. Constructive goal setting allows patients and families to remain hopeful, even if now they are hoping simply to die at home or have an opportunity to hug a grandchild. This is an important point, because many medical trainees view palliative care as the absence of care. They often cast treatment options in a false dichotomy of "doing everything or nothing." Such phraseology equates palliative care with nothing and can foster an uninformed choice for curative interventions that might, in fact, have marginal utility and carry significant burden.

At other times, trainees may well lament that "all that is left to do is just palliate." This too is problematic language. Viewing palliative care in this manner discounts this growing area in clinical medicine and disserves patients who might benefit from improved pain and symptom management.

It is far preferable to focus goals of care on what can be done and not simply what curative treatments will be forgone. In this way, clinicians can live up to their affirmative obligations to treat pain and relieve suffering. This is exactly what this young medical student tried to do. Students who read this vignette can emulate her idealism in the service of patients who will come to depend upon them.

The present patient continued to be unresponsive on ventilatory support for an additional week before the attending physician acquiesced to the wife's request to withdraw life-sustaining care. The medical student learned of this decision and returned to the ICU to comfort and assist the patient's wife.

Clinical Pearls

1. Constructive goal-setting and iterative review and updating of the plan of care can help prevent disputes in end-of-life care.

2. Curative and palliative care strategies should be blended in a manner that incrementally evolves as the disease process progresses.

3. Caring and curing are not dichotomous entities.

4. Palliative care should not be thought of as the absence of care but as an affirmative ethical obligation and a set of valuable clinical services.

REFERENCES

1. Solomon MZ, O'Donnell L, Jennings B, et. al: Decisions near the end of life: professional views on life-sustaining treatments. Am J Public Health 1993;83:14–23.
2. Faber-Langendon K: A multi-institutional study of care given to patients dying in the hospital: ethical and practical implications. Arch Intern Med 1996;156:2130–2136.
3. Miles SH, Koepp R, Weber EP: Advance end-of-life treatment planning: a research review. Arch Intern Med 1996;156:1062–1068.
4. Fins JJ, Miller FG, Acres CA, et al: End-of-life decision-making in the hospital: current practices and future prospects. J Pain Symptom Manag 1999;17:6–15.
5. Fins JJ, Nilson EG: An approach to educating residents about palliative care and clinical ethics. Acad Med 2000;75:662–665.
6. Fins JJ: Principles in palliative care: an overview. J Respir Care 2000;45:1320–1330.
7. Fins JJ, Solomon MZ: Communication in intensive care settings: the challenge of futility disputes. Crit Care Med 2001;29(suppl):N10–N15.

Mitchell Levy, MD

PATIENT 56

An 83-year-old woman with acute respiratory failure and a do-not-intubate status whose daughter requests noninvasive ventilation

An 83-year-old woman with a history of chronic obstructive pulmonary disease (COPD) presents with a 10-day history of cough, fever and increasing dyspnea. Two years ago, she underwent open reduction and fixation of a fractured hip. Postoperatively, the patient was extubated but required re-intubation for management of retained secretions and hypercapnea. Three days later, she was again extubated and subsequently discharged home. One year ago, she required intubation and mechanical ventilation for 3 days during a 7-day hospitalization for an acute exacerbation of COPD.

After her last hospitalization, the patient expressed to her pulmonologist and both children that she would not want to be intubated again in the event of another episode of respiratory distress. When questioned by her children 6 months later, the patient reiterated her desire to refuse intubation, saying "I just don't want to go through all that again." She made it clear that she was not depressed, was enjoying her life, but "had seen everything I wanted to see in life" and was "not afraid to die." The patient lives alone, has fully recovered from her hip surgery, and is independent with an active social life.

The patient is now admitted to the hospital and treated with azithromycin, albuterol, and prednisone. Although her cough and sputum production appear to be improving, her mental status deteriorates and she becomes lethargic, confused, and dyspneic. The daughter, clearly distraught, calls the pulmonologist and requests that her mother be treated with a "mask to help her breathe."

Question: Should noninvasive positive pressure ventilation be used for this patient? Is there an evidence-based approach to answering this question?

Diagnosis: Hypercapneic respiratory failure in a patient with COPD and do-not-intubate orders.

Discussion: The use of noninvasive positive pressure ventilation (NPPV) for patients with COPD who have requested a do-not-intubate (DNI) status is frequently encountered in clinical practice for two primary reasons. First, NPPV is now widely available and commonly applied, which has allowed clinicians to become comfortable with its routine use even in noncritical care settings. Second, multiple well-designed and conducted clinical trials have established the efficacy of NPPV in reducing mortality in acute respiratory failure for patients with chronic lung disease.

The dilemma presented by the current patient is becoming increasingly common in critical care medicine. The question faced by clinicians and families is whether patients who request DNI status should be managed routinely by NPPV with the assumption they would favor this noninvasive form of life support. This question becomes more difficult to address when patients cannot participate in medical decision-making. Traditionally, physicians have often assumed that patients who request not to be intubated base their decision on a dislike or aversion to the procedure of intubation itself, rather than a desire to forgo life-sustaining care with mechanical ventilation.

The request for a DNI order, however, may also reflect a patient's readiness for death. This request may represent recognition on the part of patients that their disease is end stage and their quality of life will not improve but, instead, will most likely worsen. For such patients, *any* intervention that serves to prolong life will not be consistent with their wishes for care. Administering NPPV to such patients might adhere to the letter of the DNI order but violate the spirit and intent of their advance directives.

Unfortunately, during care of patient with advanced, progressive illness, it is not unusual for caregivers to misunderstand the wishes of patients for life-sustaining care. In fact, a poor relationship between the level of life-sustaining therapies requested by patients and the type of such therapies they receive has been reported in the literature.

In light of recent survival data with NPPV, when clinicians ask patients and their families about the desire for intubation, a much deeper and more complex question is being posed than we have previously recognized. What do patients communicate to caregivers with the request not to be intubated—a fear or dislike of intubation itself, or a desire to let 'nature take its course" and allow the next serious event to be a terminal one? Unfortunately, many clinicians do not pursue end-of-life discussions sufficiently to answer this question. They often make assumptions on behalf of the patient or surrogate decision-makers that may not reflect the true wishes of the patient.

How can evidence-based medicine (EBM) help with end-of-life decision-making in a dilemma such as this? In order to answer that question, we must first review the fundamental principles that underlie EBM.

The core principles of EBM are threefold: EBM is based on (a) the integration of critical appraisal of the literature with (b) an appreciation of the importance of clinical experience, while taking into account (c) the preferences of individual patients. One of the common misconceptions about EBM is that it only values high-quality, randomized controlled trials data and discounts clinical experience as "anecdotal." In fact, this is not the case with EBM. In order to use EBM properly to enhance patient care, all three foundations of EBM must be brought to bear for a particular patient. For some medical decisions, patient preferences may be the dominant consideration, which is especially true for decision-making in end-of-life care. Other decisions may be based primarily on clinician judgment. Finally, other types of clinical problems may be addressed by large and methodologically sound clinical studies that provide clinicians with a high degree of confidence in the precision of the results.

Through the process of critical appraisal, EBM can help clinicians refine their skills for evaluating the research literature. By combining critical appraisal with a clear understanding of the preferences of patients, the clinician can then make an informed decision on whether interventions will not only be effective but appropriate for an individual patient. By applying clinical experience to this process, the caregiver can develop further confidence in his or her decision-making in medical dilemmas for which no clear evidence exists to guide therapeutic interventions.

The clinical application of EBM may be viewed as a five-step process:

1. Develop a focused clinical question.
2. Learn how and where to look for the answers and search the literature for published data.
3. Assess the strength of the data.
4. Evaluate clinician experience.
5. Assess the applicability to your specific patient in light of what their individual values and desires.

It is instructive to examine how a classic EBM approach may facilitate decision-making in caring for the present patient. As mentioned, the dilemma may be framed as whether or not noninvasive ventilation should be used to treat an ill and temporarily (at least) incapacitated patient with end-stage lung disease who has requested DNI status. The first step is to ask a focused clinical question; in this case, what impact on survival and quality of life will NPPV likely have in this patient? A literature search on the impact of noninvasive ventilation will reveal several randomized controlled trials that clearly demonstrate improved survival in patients with COPD who are randomized to NPPV as a first-line therapy for an episode of acute respiratory failure. Further investigation reveals a study that evaluated the impact of NPPV in COPD patients with DNI orders in their hospital chart. In that study, 50% of patients survived to hospital discharge. Therefore, critical appraisal of the literature strongly suggests that the patient in this case, if given NPPV, may survive to hospital discharge.

In regard to clinicians' experiences with NPPV, two observations can be made. Patients with COPD can avoid intubation and survive an episode of respiratory failure with the use of NPPV. If patients with severe COPD do *not* recover quickly, however, prolonged NPPV can be uncomfortable and lead to considerable distress, including breakdown of skin around the tight-fitting mask, drying of the upper airway, problems with secretions, and difficulty eating.

Combining critical appraisal with clinician experience in considering the present patient leads to an understanding that patients with COPD who have a DNI status are likely to survive to discharge, although their care may entail a fair amount of discomfort. Finally, evaluating the preferences of the patient in this case is also straightforward. This patient has made it clear that she does not identify survival and discharge from the hospital as her ultimate goal. In fact, she has made clear, to her caregivers and children, her readiness to die. For this patient, the outcome of survival with NPPV, even if comfortable or brief, is unwanted and not consistent with her stated preferences. Therefore, applying an EBM approach to this dilemma leads to a very clear conclusion: given the likelihood of survival in patients with COPD who receive NPPV, this therapy may not be desired and therefore may not be appropriate for this patient.

The physicians caring for the present patient discussed the benefits and risks of NPPV with the patient's daughter, who was her durable power of attorney for health care. They discussed her mother's goals in requesting a DNI order. The daughter understood her mother's intent and affirmed her commitment to honor her end-of-life wishes. The patient became somnolent and died 2 hours later with her daughter by her side. Her children expressed appreciation for the care their mother received.

Clinical Pearls

1. Evidence-based medicine integrates three aspects of clinical practice: critical appraisal of the literature, clinical experience, and patients' preferences.

2. By careful evaluation of each of the three fundamental principles of EBM, decision-making regarding end-of-life treatment may be facilitated.

End-of-life discussions with patients who have COPD and request a DNI status must extend beyond simple discussions about intubation. Clinicians should attempt to understand clearly their patient's desire for life-sustaining therapies of any type, including NPPV.

REFERENCES

1. Kramer N, Meyer TJ, Meharg J, et al: Randomized, prospective trial of noninvasive positive pressure ventilation in acute respiratory failure. Am J Respir Crit Care Med 1996;151:1799–1806.
2. Antonelli M, Conti G, Rocco M, et al: A comparison of noninvasive positive-pressure ventilation and conventional mechanical ventilation in patients with acute respiratory failure. N Engl J Med 1998;339:429–435.
3. Danis M, Mutran E, Garrett JM, et al: A prospective study of the impact of patient preferences on life-sustaining treatment and hospital cost. Crit Care Med 1996;24:1811–1817.
4. Cook DJ, Levy MM: Evidence-based medicine: a tool for enhancing critical care practice. Crit Care Clin 1998;14;353–358.
5. Nelson D, Short KS, Vespia J, et al: A prospective review of the outcomes of patients with "do not intubate" orders who receive non-invasive bilevel positive pressure ventilation [abstract]. Presented at the 30th International Educational and Scientific Symposium, January 2001.

Elizabeth M. Strauch, MD

PATIENT 57

A 68-year-old woman with metastatic cancer and severe pain
who cannot tolerate oral medications

A 68-year-old woman with a history of end-stage breast cancer, metastatic to bone and liver, is admitted to a home hospice service for end-of-life care. Her bone and abdominal pain are well-controlled on extended-release morphine 30 mg orally every 12 hours and ibuprofen 400 mg orally every 8 hours. She eats small amounts and has a small bowel movement every other day with the help of routine stimulant laxatives. Her intermittent nausea is controlled with PRN doses of promethazine by mouth.

Over the next several weeks, the patient declines steadily, becoming bed-bound and increasingly weak. Late one evening, her daughter calls the hospice nurse in a panic, reporting that the patient has become increasingly nauseated, is unable to swallow and retain her medications, and as a result, is experiencing bone and abdominal pain. The hospice nurse calls you for orders.

Question: How can this patient's pain and nausea be managed without using oral medications?

Diagnosis: Metastatic cancer with severe pain and an inability to swallow oral medications.

Discussion: In the treatment of symptoms at the end-of-life, the oral route for analgesic medications is preferred when possible because it is flexible, economical, and usually well tolerated. However, a large proportion of patients will require an alternate route of administration at some time during their course. Non-oral routes of drug administration are useful when a patient can no longer swallow reliably, experiences problems with gastrointestinal absorption, experiences severe nausea, or requires large doses of medications for comfort. Several alternative routes are available:

Rectal: A variety of palliative medicines can be used rectally when the oral route is no longer possible. Commercial suppositories are available for hydromorphone, morphine, indomethacin, acetaminophen, promethazine, prochlorperazine, and chlorpromazine. In addition, soluble morphine tablets and extended-release morphine preparations can be administered rectally with reliable absorption. Bioavailability is similar to oral administration of these agents. Drugs are administered starting with the patient's usual oral dose, with subsequent titration against effect. The drawbacks to this route are the relative inconvenience, embarrassment, and discomfort related to patient positioning and insertion of suppositories. This route becomes infeasible for patients with diarrhea or a nonfunctional rectum.

Sublingual or buccal: Morphine, fentanyl, and hydromorphone may be administered buccally or sublingually with good results. Hyoscyamine for secretions or cramps and lorazepam for anxiety may also be given by this route. Soluble tablets or liquid concentrates work best. The drawbacks to this route include limited volume (1–2 ml maximum) and unpleasant taste.

Transdermal: The transdermal route is an effective alternative for some patients. Fentanyl transdermal patches for pain and scopolamine patches for secretions or vestibular nausea are commercially available. Drawbacks include increased absorption in the febrile patient, adhesive failure in the presence of heavy perspiration, and a lag time that limits the effectiveness or rapid titration.

Subcutaneous: The s.c. route is often overlooked in nonhospice settings, but it can be extremely useful when other routes are impossible or undesirable or when large doses of opioids are necessary for symptom control. In using s.c. medications, it is important to make the conversion from oral to parenteral opioid doses due to increased bioavailability with the parenteral route. S.c. medications may be used as intermittent boluses, preferably through a subcutaneous port to avoid repeated injections, or via continuous infusion. Combinations of medications may be used in s.c. infusions for control of multiple symptoms. Establishing s.c. access is relatively safe, easy, and comfortable compared to i.v. access. Its drawbacks include volume limitations (usually ≤ 2 ml/hr) and site infiltration and irritation in some patients.

Intravenous: When central venous access is already in place, the i.v. route can be helpful. The duration of action is shorter than with other routes when bolus doses are used, and therefore, continuous infusion may be preferable. Establishing peripheral i.v. or central venous access in the dying patient is usually unnecessary as the subcutaneous route is very effective.

Intramuscular: I.m. injections should be avoided. They are painful, inconvenient, require a degree of muscle mass usually not present in cachectic dying patients, and result in unreliable, unpredictable absorption of medication. There is almost always a better alternative.

Epidural/intrathecal: Occasionally, patients with difficult pain syndromes may benefit from referral for more specialized routes for administration of analgesics. Clinicians, however, should exhaust less "high-tech" routes first.

Drug combinations: At the end of life, patients with terminal illness of almost any etiology may experience multiple symptoms or may have pain that requires the use of adjuvant medications in addition to opioids. Under these circumstances, combinations of medications will be necessary to provide good symptom control. An experienced compounding pharmacist can assist with custom combination suppositories. Furthermore, a number of medications are compatible in mixture for s.c. infusions. Examples include morphine, haloperidol, midazolam, glycopyrrolate, hydromorphone, scopolamine, and chlorpromazine. Although not compatible in mixtures, phenobarbital and dexamethasone are also useful via the s.c. route. Regardless of the route chosen, the medication regimen should always be tailored to the individual patient's needs for symptom control.

The present patient's initial management included rectal administration of her extended-release morphine, "ABH" (Ativan, Benadryl, and Haldol) suppositories for nausea and restlessness, sublingual morphine for breakthrough pain, and indomethacin suppositories added as an adjuvant pain medication. On follow-up, her daughter reported that the patient was not tolerating her suppositories due to painful hemorrhoids. It was also painful for her to be rolled into position for administration of rectal medications several times a day. Although her pain and nausea became controlled, she was too weak to swallow, making conversion to oral medications impossible.

At this point, an s.c. infusion was initiated, using equianalgesic doses of opioid, haloperidol for nausea, and a separate s.c. line for dexamethasone boluses as an adjuvant medication for nausea and bone pain. The patient became comfortable and was able to be managed at home until her death 2 weeks later.

Clinical Pearls

1. Avoid the intramuscular route, as it is painful, requires caregiver skill, and requires muscle mass usually unavailable in patients at end of life.

2. If i.v. access is already established, this route may be helpful, but establishing a new i.v. access should be avoided if possible in favor of less-invasive or less-traumatic routes. Bolus i.v. opioid doses tend to have a shorter duration of action than those given by other routes.

3. The rectal route is proven effective for a variety of palliative medications. Custom-compounded suppositories can facilitate medication combinations for control of multiple symptoms.

4. The sublingual route is effective for a number of palliative medications but may be limited by nausea or unpleasant taste.

5. The subcutaneous route is effective for many palliative medications, well tolerated by most patients, and can accommodate mixtures of medications for multiple symptoms. This route achieves blood opioid levels similar to i.v. dosing.

REFERENCES

1. Storey P, Hill HH, Louis RH, Tarver EE: Subcutaneous infusions for control of cancer symptoms. J Pain Symptom Manag 1990;5:33–44.
2. Warren DE: Practical use of rectal medications. J Pain Symptom Manag 1996;11:378–387.
3. Storey P, Knight C: American Academy of Hospice and Palliative Medicine Hospice/Palliative Care Training for Physicians UNIPAC Three: Assessment and Treatment of Pain in the Terminally Ill. Kendall Hunt, 1997.
4. Cherny NI, Foley KM: Non-opioid and opioid analgesic pharmacotherapy of cancer pain. Otolaryngol Clin North Am 1997;30:281–306.
5. Schonwetter R (ed): Hospice and Palliative Medicine Core Curriculum and Review Syllabus. Kendall Hunt, 1999.

Helen Sorenson, MA, RRT

PATIENT 58

A 72-year-old man with end-stage COPD and retained secretions

A 72-year-old retired truck driver with end-stage chronic obstructive pulmonary disease (COPD) is brought by his son to the emergency department because of increasing shortness of breath. The family had been providing palliative care for him at home, but they are now concerned with his progressive weakness and increased sputum production. Earlier in the day, the patient fell at home from weakness and shortness of breath. He also has a 40-pack-year smoking history, diabetes mellitus, abdominal aortic aneurysm, osteoporosis, and a compressed cervical disk. The patient was treated at home 3 to 4 weeks ago for pneumonia. He had requested a do-not-resuscitate (DNR) status 2 months earlier.

Physical Examination: Blood pressure 136/66, pulse 126, respirations 28, temperature 38.6°. General: cachectic with a loose, nonproductive, and ineffective cough. Neck: jugular venous distension. Chest: coarse rhonchi upper lobes, diminished breath sounds. Cardiac: early diastolic (S_3) gallop. Extremities: 1+ dependent edema without cyanosis.

Laboratory Findings: SpO_2 (3-L cannula O_2) 89%. ABG (40% air-entrainment mask); pH 7.36, $PaCO_2$ 54 mm Hg, PaO_2 52 mm Hg, HCO_3 30 mEq/L. Hct. 48%, WBC 12,800/μl with increased neutrophils. Blood cultures pending. Chest radiograph: right lower lobe pneumonia. Sputum Gram stain: multiple gram-negative bacteria.

Hospital Course: Despite aggressive therapy for pneumonia, the patient's condition deteriorates, with increasing dyspnea and a loud "rattling sound" when he breathes. The family insists on rescinding his previous DNR status and having him intubated and mechanically ventilated to manage his labored breathing. After 9 days of support, the patient remains critically ill, and the family discusses extubation to allow the patient to die peacefully.

Later that morning, the patient is extubated and managed with facemask oxygen. The patient's cough is weak and he has obvious difficulties with his airway secretions. Nasotracheal suctioning is attempted but not tolerated. The next morning, the patient has labored respirations with diffuse wheezes and "rattling" breathing despite aggressive bronchodilator therapy.

Question: How would you assist this patient with secretion control?

Diagnosis: Retained secretions due to pulmonary infection and end-stage COPD.

Discussion: COPD is a progressive respiratory condition most often caused by cigarette smoking and characterized by limitation of airflow. COPD is now the fourth leading cause of death in the United States and is an emerging global epidemic. The histologic features of COPD in the airway include hypertrophy and hyperplasia of submucosal glands, increased numbers of goblet cells, atrophy of columnar epithelium, and a reduced number of cilia. Even after smoking cessation, these abnormal histologic changes usually persist. Most patients with COPD have excess mucus production and chronic bronchitis, characterized by recurrent coughing and sputum expectoration. These patients are at risk for respiratory infections, such as pneumonia and acute exacerbations of bronchitis, which aggravate respiratory secretions and worsen the severity of airway obstruction.

Most patients with terminal conditions at the end of life experience retained secretions. The asthenia that occurs in patients dying with a chronic condition is associated with generalized muscle weakness that decreases their ability to generate an effective cough. Patients with end-stage COPD have particular problems with airway secretions. Excess mucus production coupled with a weak cough cause retention of airway secretions that can progress to airway obstruction and respiratory distress.

As seen with the present patient, family members who accept the terminal nature of a patient's condition may become increasingly concerned about retained secretions. This concern is heightened by the fear commonly expressed by terminal patients to family members of "choking" or "drowning" to death. Even after a patient and family acknowledge that death is anticipated and adopt a palliative approach to care, increasing fear and distress, "rattling" respirations, and labored breathing can trigger panic and result in emergency transport to the hospital in search of any intervention to relieve suffering. Poorly controlled respiratory symptoms with the "rattling" respirations of retained secretions may even encourage families to rescind a DNR status and accept intubation and mechanical ventilation.

Although intubation does provide a route for removal of secretions and a short-term solution to poor gas exchange, other less-invasive interventions can be used in the home to keep secretions under control. Before initiating therapy, however, family and caregivers should be educated about what to expect. Palliation should be described to the patient and family as active, total care of the patient whose disease is not responsive to curative treatment. The ultimate goal of palliative care is to achieve the best possible quality of life for both the patient and family. In this instance, an understanding of the cause of the excess secretions is helpful. Resolving the problem of retained secretions may not be entirely possible, but it is always possible to enlist support systems, educate, develop plans, and provide needed tools for dealing with the patient's respiratory systems. These measures can reassure the family and restore a sense of control.

Family members can be reassured that the "rattling" breathing may be more distressing to them than to their loved one. Patients who are receiving effective palliative treatment for dyspnea may not experience added suffering from the noisy breathing caused by secretions.

Antibiotics may diminish airway secretions and can be used selectively if, for instance, acute bronchitis is the suspected cause of an abrupt deterioration. Aerosolized bronchodilators may loosen secretions, stimulate cough, and activate mechanisms for mucociliary clearance. Nasotracheal suctioning can be performed at home, although patient discomfort with repeated use limits this intervention. Some patients with COPD and excessive secretions can benefit by assistance with "quad coughing," in which a caregiver squeezes the patient's chest during a coughing effort. "Huff coughing" can also promote expectoration; instead of repeated violent and ineffective coughing leading to exhaustion, the patient is taught to take a deep breath and expire in short bursts with the glottis open to transport secretions toward the upper trachea where a final cough can expel them from the airway. Inhalation of bland aerosols and airway humidification do not play a role. Although postural drainage and chest physiotherapy can be exhausting and usually ineffective in the absence of bronchiectasis, percussion vests may assist some patients with retained secretions.

As the end of life nears, oral atropine drops to the back of the throat may dry secretions and diminish rattling respirations. A semi-Fowler's position and use of a Yankaur suction wand by family members to remove secretions in the posterior pharynx may provide comfort. Management of dyspnea with opioid and sedative therapy contributes to relief from symptoms due to retained secretions. Some physicians may apply noninvasive positive pressure ventilation by facemask to palliate severe dyspnea at the end of life.

The present patient soon slipped into unconsciousness, and the family continued to note the audible rattle that accompanied his breathing. Because the physician had explained the origin of the noise and reassured them that the patient's distress was being controlled with drug therapy, they were no longer alarmed. The patient died that afternoon with the family in attendance. Although the patient did not die at home as originally planned, he received effective palliative care, as the caregivers and family developed a consensus for goals of therapy. He died with his family in attendance, which he had previously described as the most important element of a good death.

Clinical Pearls

1. Patients with end-stage COPD can be cared for at home with good symptom management when education about palliative techniques has been provided to the family and caregivers. Hospice services are available for patients with end-stage respiratory conditions.

2. Palliative care should be explained to the patient and family as total, active care of the patient when the disease no longer responds to curative measures.

3. When physicians prepare the family and caregivers about what to expect at end of life, it is much less stressful for all involved. "Rattling" breathing at the end of life usually generates more distress in the family than apparent discomfort for the patient if adequate palliative measures are initiated.

4. Palliation should not be confined to the home setting. It can and should be provided for in acute care facilities.

REFERENCES

1. American Thoracic Society: Standards for the diagnosis and care of patients with chronic obstructive pulmonary disease. Am J Respir Crit Care Med 1995;152(5 pt 2):S77–S121.
2. Wanner A, Salathe M, O'Riodan T: Mucociliary clearance in the airways. Am J Respir Crit Care Med 1996;154:1868–1902.
3. Norman D, Bradley S, Dorinsky P, Verghese A: Treating respiratory infections in the elderly: current strategies and considerations. Geriatrics 1996;52(suppl):S1–S26.
4. Conill C, Vergen E, Henriquiz I, et al: Symptom prevalence in the last week of life. J Pain Symptom Manag 1997;14:328–331.
5. Ahmedzai S. Palliation of respiratory symptoms. In Doyle D, Hanks GWC, McDonald N (eds): Oxford Textbook of Palliative Medicine, 2nd ed. Oxford, Oxford University Press, 1998.
6. Cassel CK, Foley KM: Principles for Care of Patients at the End of Life: An Emerging Consensus among the Specialties of Medicine. New York, Milbank Meml Fund, 1999.

Alexander Peralta, Jr, MD

PATIENT 59

A 66-year-old Mexican man with severe dyspnea due to pulmonary fibrosis who says, "Doctor, ayudeme, que no puedo respirar"

A hospice social worker asks a Spanish-speaking physician to make a home visit to a 66-year-old Mexican man to help translate advance directives and an out-of-hospital DNR order. The social worker wants a doctor to explain the forms to the patient. The patient's most recent pulmonologist referred him to hospice, with a diagnosis of advanced idiopathic pulmonary fibrosis, because of the patient's limited life expectancy.

As the physician enters the patient's home, it becomes clear that this stoic man is more concerned about his dyspnea and just wants to get a doctor to see him at home. When the social worker said they had a Spanish-speaking doctor, he knew this was his chance to talk to a doctor who could help him breathe.

The physician asks him when he first noticed something was wrong. "Doctor, I work in construction and I cannot work because I have no breath." About 3 years ago, he noticed that he would get short of breath at work around noontime. He would tire easily, with associated orthopnea and exertional dyspnea. He said, "I have seen many doctors and they have done many tests. The doctors say that my lungs are full of scars. I don't smoke and I don't drink, so why is this happening to my lungs?" The physician assures him he had done nothing wrong and that this scarring occurs for unknown reasons.

The patient is using oxygen by nasal cannula. He is limited to a small bedroom cooled only by an oscillating fan. He has to sit on the side of the bed most of his waking hours due to his dyspnea. His medications include furosemide, prednisone, digoxin, inhaled bronchodilators, inhaled corticosteroids, and lorazepam.

Question: What else may improve this patient's dyspnea? Are there other domains of suffering that need to be addressed?

Diagnosis: Severe dyspnea due to end-stage lung disease.

Discussion: Dyspnea, an unpleasant awareness of a shortness of breath, is the second most common symptom in end-of-life care. In its advanced form, it manifests as air hunger that may progress to suffocation and asphyxia. Dyspnea occurs in more than 70% of lung cancer patients, with one-third of them describing their dyspnea as moderate to severe. Dyspnea occurs from a mismatch between central respiratory motor activity and incoming afferent stimulation of stretch receptors from the airway, lungs, and chest wall. As changes in respiratory pressure, airflow, or movement of the lungs and chest wall become inappropriate for outgoing motor commands, dyspnea heightens.

Moderate to severe dyspnea at the end of life is best managed with opioid drugs. Patients treated with oral and inhaled morphine attenuate the normal ventilatory responses and feel less dyspneic, tolerating a greater degree of hypercapnia and hypoxemia. Opioids have been suggested to relieve dyspnea by producing cerebral sedation, vagal stimulation, vasodilatation with cardiac unloading, analgesia, and blunting of the CO_2-sensitive medullary respiratory center.

Opioid therapy is started with small oral doses that are carefully titrated. Immediate-release opioids have a short half-life of 60 to 90 minutes and reach a steady state within four to five half-lives. Drug doses can be increased, therefore, by 50% to 100% within 24 to 48 hours of starting therapy. If patients remain dyspneic after drug titration, opioids can be given by the parenteral (subcutaneous or intravenous) or nebulized route. Nebulized opioids may diminish dyspnea by acting on airway opioid receptors. The intrathecal or epidural routes for opioid administration are rarely required for dyspnea control at the end of life.

The present patient was started on both immediate-release and sustained-release morphine, with moderate improvement of his dyspnea, which he rated as "10" on a 10-point scale on admission to hospice. After titration of his morphine to 60 mg twice a day and 12 mg every 1 to 2 hours for breakthrough dyspnea, his dyspnea intensity was 5/10 on the third hospice day. Nebulized morphine at 2.5 mg via an updraft nebulizer was added, and his dyspnea and persistent cough improved to a severity of 2/10. Inhaled morphine can be started at a dose of 2.5 to 5.0 mg once or twice a day mixed with 3 ml normal saline or sterile water without preservatives. After serial dyspnea scores are assessed, inhaled morphine can be ordered every 8 hours and subsequently every 6 hours if needed. The dose of inhaled morphine can be increased by 50% to 100% if the patient remains dyspneic.

As the present patient's dyspnea and coughing improved, he became more contemplative and reflective. The staff at first thought he was withdrawn and depressed but subsequently recognized that his behavior resulted from a language barrier. The Spanish-speaking physician made weekly visits knowing full well that the patient's dyspnea would crescendo as his disease progressed. Chats during the weekly visits revealed a proud and humble man with a loving wife and caring children. His children were well educated and held good jobs.

It took a month to learn what really ached his heart. "Me quiero morir en mi casa"—"I want to die in my own home." The physician listened carefully and patiently to the man. After 30 years of working in the United States and living his dream of having a home, good food, and successful children, he wanted to return to his family's home in Mexico. "Doctor, I am not afraid of dying. I just want to feel the land of my ancestors under my feet. You have done all you can for me here, and my time is near. I did not think I would ever see my homeland again, but you have given me hope."

Racial and ethnic minorities still lag behind in access to medical care. Recent epidemiologic statistics of our diverse population prompted the President's Initiative to Eliminate Racial and Ethnic Disparities in Health and Healthy People. Its focus is to eliminate racial and ethnic disparities in cardiovascular disease, diabetes, cancer, HIV/AIDS, infant mortality, and immunization rates by the year 2010. Barriers include patients' sociocultural differences in world view, language, health-seeking processes, illness behavior, communication, and decision-making processes during clinical encounters. These differences can result in less-than-adequate adherence to therapeutic regimens and unsatisfactory interactions between patients or their families and clinicians.

The disparity between majority and minority populations is even more glaring in end-of-life care. Minority patients experience disproportionately higher rates of heart disease, hypertension, and diabetes and their subsequent complications, such as amputations, strokes, and end-stage heart, liver, and renal diseases. The National Hospice and Palliative Care Organization's 1995 hospice statistics reveal that only 3.5% of Hispanics, compared to 8.3% of African-Americans and 83.5% Caucasians, accessed hospice services. The reasons included economic, institutional, informational, and cultural factors.

The AMA Council on Medical Education Report in 1998 (5-A-98) states that "cultural competence means [acquiring] knowledge and interpersonal skills that allow providers to understand, appreciate and work with individuals from cultures other than their own. It involves an awareness and acceptance of cultural differences, self-awareness, knowledge of patient's culture and adaptation skills." Clinicians should learn to view patients in the context of ethnic and racial background, with an understanding of how this influences their conceptualization of disease and health behavior. Hispanic patients sometimes utilize traditional healing practices and seek medical care when these approaches fail. Subsequently, they present to medical providers with advanced disease and usually with a poor prognosis. To amend these shortcomings, ongoing initiatives emphasize that we all must add value to end-of-life care by remembering that our community is a rich tapestry woven of many strands and that this tapestry symbolizes the cultural diversity among people. "Somos humanos, somos fragil y somos testigos"—"We are human, we are fragile, and we are witnesses."

The hospice team, together with his family, procured medications, a nebulizer, oxygen, and special airfare with medical equipment and correspondence for the American embassy in Mexico. A week before his departure, the patient's condition deteriorated acutely with severe dyspnea and right-sided heart failure. Triamcinolone 1 mg twice daily was added to his nebulizer treatments, and methylphenidate 2.5 mg orally in the morning was added for opiate sedation. His final opioid titration was morphine 40 mg via updraft every 4 hours.

The patient made his flight to Mexico. His family stated that he was extremely happy to be home with his family. His dyspnea seemed to almost disappear according to his wife. He died peacefully in his sleep 3 days after his arrival, having overcome, with the assistance of the hospice team, language as a barrier to his physical, social, psychological, and spiritual needs at the end of life.

Clinical Pearls

1. Inhaled morphine helps in 65%–70% of patients with dyspnea. If it is not effective within 15 to 21 days, another route should be tried.

2. Inhaled morphine may be used for patients with malignant and nonmalignant advanced diseases. Morphine-induced respiratory suppression can be treated with naloxone (0.4mg/ml plus 9 cc NaCl infused slowly).

3. Methylphenidate 2.5 to 5 mg orally in the morning may be used to manage opioid-induced sedation.

4. Every clinical encounter is cross-cultural, so the physician should try to be flexible, sincere, and ethical in his or her interactions.

5. Patient- and family-centered care is the goal. There are no one-size-fits-all templates for end-of-life care. Effective care depends on a heightened sensitivity and awareness to social, cultural, psychological, and spiritual issues at the end of life.

6. Most people with chronic illness are not afraid of dying. Some may even know the time and place of their physical death. End-of-life care affords them the opportunity of a psychosocial moratorium to reflect and contemplate their spiritual transcendence.

REFERENCES

1. Bruera E, Macmillan K, Pither J, et al: Effects of morphine on the dyspnea of terminal cancer patients. J Pain Symptom Manag 1990;5:341–344.
2. MacLeod RD, King BJ: Relieving breathlessness with nebulized morphine. Palliat Med 1995;9:169–170.
3. Dugeon D, Rosenthal S: Management of dyspnea and cough in patients with cancer. Hematol-Oncol Clin North Am 1996;10:157–171.
4. Quelch PC, Faulkner DE, Yun JW: Nebulized opioids in the treatment of dyspnea. J Palliat Care 1997;13(3):48–52.
5. Tervalon M, Murray-Garcia J: Cultural humility versus cultural competence: a critical distinction in defining physician training outcomes in multicultural education. J Health Care Poor Underserved 1998;9:117–124.
6. Poole PJ, Veale AG, Black PN: The effect of sustained-release morphine on breathlessness and quality of life in severe chronic obstructive pulmonary disease. Am J Respir Crit Care Med 1998;157:1877–1880.
7. Carillo JE, Green AR, Betancourt JR: Cross-cultural primary care: a patient-based approach. Ann Intern Med 1999;130:829–834.
8. Chandler S: Nebulized opioids to treat dyspnea. J Hospice Palliative Care 1999;16(1):418–422.
9. Betancourt JR, Like RC, Gottilieb BR: Caring for diverse populations: breaking down barriers. Patient Care May 15, 2000.
10. Betancourt JR, Johnson M, Valadez A: Reducing the burden of diabetes and CVD. Patient Care May 15, 2000.
11. Peralta A: The color of disparity: advanced disease in diverse groups. CareNotes, A Physician Newsletter of Community Hospice of Texas, Winter 2000.

Graeme Rocker, MHSc, DM, FRCP, FRCPC
Monica Branigan, MD

PATIENT 60

A 78-year-old man with end-stage lung disease who requests aggressive, life-sustaining care

A 78-year-old man with advanced idiopathic pulmonary fibrosis is brought by his brother to the emergency department for management of worsening shortness of breath. The patient uses portable oxygen at home and has experienced dyspnea on minimal exertion for the last 2 years. The patient repeatedly whispers, "I don't want to die yet," and tells the staff to do "whatever they have to do" to keep him alive.

Physical Examination:　Respirations 40–50, pulse 115. General: anxious and dyspneic, on nasal prong oxygen. Chest: diffuse crackles. Cardiac: regular rhythm, distended neck veins. Extremities: digital clubbing, peripheral cyanosis, ankle edema to mid-calf.

Laboratory Findings:　ABG (O_2 5 L/min nasal cannula): pH 7.42, PCO_2 30 mm Hg, PO_2 52 mm Hg. Chest radiograph: acute right upper lobe airspace opacity, 3-cm mass adjacent to the right border of the superior mediastinum, extensive interstitial opacities compatible with idiopathic pulmonary fibrosis.

Clinical Course:　The emergency physician calls the patient's pulmonologist to inform him that a "suspicious lesion" was present on a chest radiograph 6 months earlier, but the present mass was clearly larger. The pulmonologist did not recall if he had mentioned the suspicious lesion to the patient. As the emergency physician begins discussing with the patient the possible limitations of care if his condition worsened, his brother becomes angry and shouts, "You need to do everything! I don't care what it is, but don't let my brother die!" The patient is intubated after further deterioration and transferred to the ICU.

Question:　Considering the patient's severe underlying lung disease and possible lung cancer, how can the ICU team deliver both critical care directed toward his respiratory failure and palliative care at the same time?

Diagnosis: Advanced idiopathic pulmonary fibrosis, acute pneumonia, and probable lung cancer.

Discussion: Multiple themes permeate end-of-life care in the ICU. Many patients enter the ICU in an emotionally charged atmosphere of imminent death with high expectations and inadequate information. Care providers with established relationships to the patient may no longer be involved in their care. Patients are less able to participate in ongoing decisions, and families and surrogates must take over this task. The importance of truth-telling, planning for death, and the conduct of appropriate conversation, in terms of both content and timing, becomes key to establishing a treatment plan.

To develop such a plan for the present patient, a meeting was arranged with the patient's younger brother, who was his sole-surviving close relative. It became clear that only 2 months ago, the patient was able to drive over for supper and seemed quite comfortable with a portable supply of oxygen. The visiting brother became angry when the ICU team mentioned cancer in addition to the underlying lung condition. He told the ICU team that his older brother was a fighter and had survived worse than this before. The pulmonologist arrived late for this meeting, where the atmosphere was already tense. The brother turned on him to demand why he hadn't been told about the cancer. The pulmonologist said he couldn't be sure about the diagnosis and didn't want to cause unnecessary distress, since he was likely to die anyway from his pulmonary fibrosis. The cost of thinking and acting for, rather than with, patients and families now becomes all too evident, however well intentioned.

From the position of the ICU providers and the pulmonologist, the patient's underlying condition is not reversible and is approaching the terminal stage. The likely malignancy only serves to reinforce this assessment. The ICU team finds itself in the position of wanting to provide good care to the patient without prolonging the dying process. This defines the dilemma of providing palliative care and intensive disease-specific care at the same time.

Many view these two types of care as opposite or counterintuitive: holistic versus reductionist, whole person versus organ, aiming for death versus aiming for life. What unites them is the desire to reduce suffering. Reduction of suffering is the key framework to use to make clinical decisions for the present patient. As Cassell points out though, suffering occurs in persons, not bodies or organs.

When the team next approached the brother, instead of asking "what should we do for the patient's breathing" or "how should we treat his heart," they asked instead about the patient as a person. They learned that the patient had survived the Holocaust and strongly valued his struggle to survive. He had been highly independent his whole life and never married. Until this admission, he was proud of his physical independence with his portable oxygen. In the last few weeks however, he had no stamina to clean his home, prepare his meals, or get out to visit. He had refused all assistance thus far.

Over the next few days, the younger brother came to realize that he would never visit his older sibling at his apartment again. He accepted that intensive care would not restore his brother's independence, as there would be further functional decline, even should he survive. He acknowledged that in some cases, artificially prolonging life may cause its own suffering. With these considerations and in face of his brother's continued deterioration, he agreed to a do-not-resuscitate order. This allowed for a peaceful death for the patient 2 days later when cardiac asystole occurred. The ICU providers were able to avoid traumatizing the brother by raising the prospects of withdrawal of ventilation before he was ready to consider this approach to care.

This ICU experience was difficult for both the brother and staff. Much of this difficulty could have been avoided if the patient had been asked about his preferences at an earlier opportunity. This requires truth-telling and the provision of tangible options for care, using language that recognizes the vulnerability of patients and families. More sensitive inquiries might have lead to an understanding of the family's experiences during the Holocaust. The survivor instinct can be tremendously strong. Fortunately, striving for survival does not conflict with the stance of "hoping for the best, but planning for the worst." This attitude is a hallmark of palliative care.

In planning, we can explore the patient's fear —perhaps of death, of suffocation, or becoming dependent—and develop specific strategies to mitigate these concerns. For this patient, a discussion of this nature may have avoided a final ICU admission by providing robust home-based treatment options. If the patient did prefer hospital care, an alternative course would have been to consider a therapeutic trial of intubation for a specified period of time, with clear clinical endpoints of improvement. As difficult as such discussions can be, making decisions about possible withdrawal of treatment prospectively is much less traumatic. Establishing values, wishes, and preferences can and should be done well in advance of an impending crisis. Indeed, avoiding these discussions is an abnegation of a physician's duties to patients with progressive illness and can cause unnecessary suffering when a crisis occurs.

Setting reasonable and realistic goals is the key. In working with patients with life-limiting illnesses to establish goals for care, our commitment should be to relieve suffering in both palliative and curative settings. Palliative care and intensive care can and should coexist.

The brother of the present patient called the ICU physicians a week after the patient's death. He thanked them for their efforts and for the patience, consideration, and concern they directed toward his brother's end-of-life care.

Clinical Pearls

1. Decisions regarding intensive, disease-focused care can only be made with reference to how the interventions will likely affect the whole person.

2. Relief of suffering should be a goal during critical care and in ICUs, just as much as it is in palliative care and specialized palliative care units. There may be no inconsistency between seeking to avoid premature death while preparing to die peacefully.

3. Time-limited interventions, therapeutic trials, with specific endpoints related to relieving suffering and prolonging life should be considered.

4. Unaddressed fear is a source of much suffering. Acknowledging suffering can be therapeutic.

5. Physicians caring for patients with progressive, life-limiting illness have a responsibility to discuss treatment options and end-of-life decisions prospectively, prior to a crisis.

6. Goals of care change as a patient progresses through a disease. These changes can and should be anticipated and planned for, before a crisis.

REFERENCES

1. Cassell EJ: The nature of suffering and the goals of medicine. N Engl J Med 1982;306:639–645.
2. The goals of medicine: setting new priorities. Hastings Cent Rep 1996;26(suppl):S9–S14.
3. Danis M, Federman D, Fins JJ, et al: Incorporating palliative care into critical care education: principles, challenges, and opportunities [see comments]. Crit Care Med 1999;27:2005–2013.
4. Roy D: The times and places of palliative care. J Palliat Care 2000;16(suppl):S3–S4.
5. Rocker GM, Shemie SD, Lacroix J: End-of-life issues in the ICU: a need for acute palliative care? J Palliat Care 2000;16(suppl):S5–S6.
6. Cohen-Almagor R: Language and reality at the end of life. J Law Med Ethics 2000;28:267–278.
7. Zaner RM: Power and hope in the clinical encounter: a meditation on vulnerability. Med Health Care Philos 2000;3:265–275.

James A. Tulsky, MD

PATIENT 61

A 48-year-old man with metastatic cancer who has not yet recognized the terminal nature of his disease

A 48-year-old man with colon cancer, metastatic to lung and brain, comes in with his wife for a follow-up office visit and complains of fatigue and weight loss. He was first diagnosed with cancer 3 years ago and underwent a colostomy. He did well until 8 months ago, when he developed balance problems. A head CT scan revealed a brain lesion, and he underwent excision of a solitary brain metastasis with postoperative brain irradiation. Within 3 months of his craniotomy, lung lesions were confirmed to be pulmonary metastases, and the patient underwent a course of radiation therapy to his chest. A chest radiograph performed today shows that the lung metastases have enlarged.

After treatment for his initial colon cancer, the patient suffered a deep, year-long depression. More recently, however, he has felt more positive and frequently speaks about his hope for recovery. His physicians have worried about dispelling this hope and have delayed talking with him about his prognosis or goals of care in fear of precipitating another episode of depression. The patient's physician, however, now recognizes that his terminal condition requires a discussion of his prognosis to allow planning for his affairs and end-of-life care.

Question: How can the physician initiate a discussion about goals and treatments at the end of life?

Diagnosis: Advanced terminal illness with no previous discussion of prognosis or goals.

Discussion: Patients experiencing the transition from fighting a potentially curable disease to accepting palliative goals for care face great challenges to their physical, emotional, and spiritual integrity. Some patients cope by avoiding discussion of the issues or even denying the severity of their illness.

Health care providers also struggle when caring for patients facing this transition. They may see stopping disease-modifying treatment as a failure or experience sadness at the anticipated loss of a dear patient. Or, as with this patient, they may worry about taking away the patient's hope or even precipitating serious depression. When this occurs, clinicians may deliberately avoid the topic. In an attempt to boost their patient's affect, they convey an overly optimistic prognosis, unfortunately creating unrealistic expectations.

In reality, physicians' concerns about causing emotional distress and eliminating hope generally have no foundation in fact. A patient's psychological adjustment to bad news is related more to the quality of communication about that news than to the nature of the bad news itself. In fact, most patients with advanced disease have thought about end-of-life issues and wish to discuss them with a physician, but they expect the doctor to raise the topic. Discussing the news openly allows patients to state their concerns and fears. By doing so, physicians can lessen patients' future anxiety and depression.

Furthermore, health care providers can neither steal nor instill hope. Hope is defined, constructed, and interpreted by the patient. Physicians can provide an empathic, reflective presence that will help patients draw strength from their existing resources. It is not the job of this patient's physician to "correct" his hope for recovery. Rather, the physician strives to understand the patient's perception of the illness, elucidate his coping strategies, and help him plan for the future. By "planning for the worst while hoping for the best," this patient may be able to complete his affairs, accept a palliative approach to medical therapy, and even say goodbye to loved ones while still stating that he hopes to recover.

When approaching such a patient, the first step is to avoid presuming to know the patient's agenda. For example, physicians are not very good at predicting which patients want more and which patients want less information. Instead of assuming that this patient does not want to talk about the future, one could ask, "I notice that we've never really spoken about what you can expect from your illness over time. Some patients want to know everything that is going on with their illness, the good and the bad. Other people do not want as much information and want me to speak more generally. And some would really prefer I do not discuss bad news with them but want me to discuss these issues with their family. Have you thought about this?" If the patient says he does not want to hear about his prognosis, he should then be asked to say more about this to examine his fears or concerns. If the patient suggests that he would like to be told about his disease, the doctor should "ask before telling." That is, ask the patient about his understanding of his illness before educating him about the specifics of prognosis.

It is equally important to attend to the patient's affect. Affect refers to the feelings and emotions associated with the content of the conversation. Feelings such as anger, guilt, frustration, sadness, and fear modify our ability to hear, communicate, and make decisions. For example, after hearing bad news, most patients are so overwhelmed emotionally that they are unable to comprehend very much about the details of the illness or a treatment plan. Unfortunately, conversations between doctors and patients often transpire only in the cognitive realm; emotion is frequently not acknowledged or handled directly, and physicians miss opportunities to do so.

The primary goal when responding to affect is to convey a sense of empathy. This can be done through a variety of specific responses, organized under the acronym "NURSE:"

N—*Naming* the emotion serves to acknowledge feelings and to demonstrate that this is a legitimate area for discussion. Statements such as "that seems sad for you," can serve this purpose.

U—Expressing a sense of *understanding* normalizes the patient's emotion and conveys concern. An example might be saying, "Although I've never shared your experience, I do understand that this has been a really hard time for you."

R—*Respect* reminds us to praise patients and families for what they are doing, and how they are managing with a difficult situation. Offering respect defuses defensiveness and makes people feel good about themselves and more capable of handling the future. A useful statement to this patient might be, "I am so impressed with how you have managed to keep living your life, despite the repeated surgeries and radiation treatments."

S—*Support* is essential to helping people in distress not feel alone. Simple statements such as, "I will be there with you throughout this illness," can be tremendously comforting.

E—Finally, patients will frequently make statements that deserve further *exploration*. For example, after asking about his understanding, this patient may say, "Each time I've gone through more surgery or treatments I've wondered if this is gonna be it." A simple response such as "tell me more" may help reveal the patient's fears and concerns about cancer that will be helpful in planning future treatment.

Although the present patient seems resistant to discussing his prognosis, no one has ever really probed his concerns, fears, and hopes. By asking him what he wants to know, finding out what he understands about his illness, acknowledging his emotions, and demonstrating empathy, this man is likely to begin planning for his future and to feel supported by his physician while he does so.

The physician initiated a dialogue with the patient about his understanding of his disease. The patient voiced a willingness to learn more about his prognosis. As they discussed the progression of his disease, the patient and his wife both seemed initially anxious but then began to relax as if a burden had been removed. The patient said, "Well, I expected as much. I can't say I am really surprised." Both the patient and his wife agreed to make the most of the coming months. He remained active until his last week of life and died at home with the support of home hospice care.

Clinical Pearls

1. A patient's psychological adjustment to bad news is related to the quality of communication, not to the diagnosis of serious illness and its implications.

2. Most patients with advanced disease have thought about end-of-life issues and wish to discuss them with a physician, but they expect the doctor to raise the topic.

3. Discussions of end-of-life issues are often best initiated by open-ended questions regarding the patient's understanding of the illness and prognosis prior to discussing specific clinical decisions.

4. Acknowledgment of patients' emotions, followed by an empathic response, is often the most effective way to elicit patients concerns and direct discussion toward goals of care.

REFERENCES

1. Smith RC, Hoppe RB. The patient's story: integrating the patient- and physician-centered approaches to interviewing. Ann Intern Med 1991;115:470–477.
2. Layson RT, Adelman HM, Wallach PM, et al: Discussions about the use of life-sustaining treatments: a literature review of physicians' and patients' attitudes and practices. J Clin Ethics 1994;5:195–203.
3. Butow PN, Kazemi JN, Beeney LJ, et al: When the diagnosis is cancer: patient communication experiences and preferences. Cancer 1996;77:2630–2637.
4. Lo B, Quill T, Tulsky J: Discussing palliative care with patients. Ann Intern Med 1999;130:744–749.
5. Detmar SB, Muller MJ, Wever LD, et al: The patient-physician relationship: patient-physician communication during outpatient palliative treatment visits: an observational study. JAMA 2001;285:1351–1357.
6. Tulsky JA, Arnold RM: Communication at end of life. In Berger AM, Portenoy RK, Weissman DE (eds): Principles and Practice of Palliative Care and Supportive Oncology, 2nd ed. Philadelphia, Lippincott Williams & Wilkins, 2002.

Gordon D. Rubenfeld, MD, MSc

PATIENT 62

A 52-year-old man whose family and physicians cannot agree on continuing life-supportive care

A 52-year-old patient is admitted to the ICU with a severe pneumonia that requires mechanical ventilation. After 2 days of care, he has progressed to the acute respiratory distress syndrome (ARDS) and maintains borderline oxygenation on 60% oxygen with heavy sedation. He demonstrates no evidence of other organ dysfunction.

Physical Examination: Pulse 120, respirations 28, blood pressure 110/54, temperature 37 °C. General: heavily sedated. Chest: harsh breath sounds. Cardiac: normal heart sounds. Abdomen: soft without bowel sounds. Neurologic: responds only to pain.

Hospital Course: The physician team discusses the patient's condition with the family and relates that they estimate he has a 60% chance of recovery. On the following day, the third day of hospitalization, the family approaches the physicians requesting the withdrawal of ventilator support, stating that the patient had never wanted to be "on a ventilator." They produce a signed, living will and durable power of attorney for health care. Although the physicians re-review the patient's condition and 60% likelihood of recovery, the family persists in voicing their wishes.

Question: What should the physicians do? What options are available, and what are the medical and legal issues?

Diagnosis: ARDS with reasonable likelihood of recovery.

Discussion: The right of competent adult patients to refuse any medical treatment is a cornerstone of modern western medical ethics. As long as patients are competent and the decision is informed, diabetics can refuse insulin, patients with gangrenous legs can refuse amputation, and ventilator-dependent quadraplegics can be removed from life support upon request, even if it will lead to certain death.

Situations get more complex when this right, known as *autonomy*, is extended to incompetent patients who cannot participate in informed consent. Most deaths in critical care now occur when life-sustaining treatments are refused or withdrawn by incompetent patients through mechanisms (advance directives or surrogate decision-makers) designed to allow patients to maintain their right to autonomy despite being incompetent. In these cases, families and clinicians reach a consensus decision to stop life support.

Sometimes, and there are limited data to indicate how often this occurs, families and physicians do not agree on the decision. Physicians do not have an absolute duty to fulfill surrogates' requests to stop life support, even when the surrogate is the durable power of attorney or has a copy of the patient's living will. However, the decision to overrule the clearly stated, informed, and rational request of a surrogate should be made very cautiously, and it should be a very rare event in clinical practice.

When discussing the decision to continue life-sustaining treatment for the current patient, clinicians have several responsibilities. They must inform the surrogate of the diagnosis, prognosis, and burdens of the proposed treatment. They must explain the principles of surrogate decision-making. Finally, they must elicit, from the surrogate, the patient's wishes in this situation as well as some explanation for how they arrived at their assessment of the patient's wishes.

All discussions with families about decisions to proceed with life-sustaining treatment in the ICU should be grounded in an understanding of the prognosis and treatment of the medical condition. Unfortunately, although ARDS has been described for almost 40 years, relatively few large, multicenter epidemiologic studies are available on which to base either short-term or long-term prognoses. Short-term prognosis appears to be more strongly related to the presence of comorbidity (e.g., patients with cancer, cirrhosis, and older patients have a worse prognosis) and the development of multiorgan failure than the severity of the lung injury. Although clinicians and families frequently become discouraged with prolonged mechanical ventilation, there is no evidence that patients who require prolonged ventilatory support, as long as they are spared multiorgan failure, have a poor prognosis. In the setting of bone marrow transplantation or cirrhosis with multiple organ failure, care of patients with ARDS may be futile.

With optimal management, mortality from ARDS in the modern era is probably around 30%. Survivors of ARDS have a decrement in their quality of life and pulmonary function, but few are profoundly debilitated from a pulmonary standpoint. ARDS does not appear to affect long-term mortality on its own.

Armed with this information, physicians should inform surrogates of the patient's prognosis. They should prepare families for what may be a prolonged course of mechanical ventilation. Family members should be encouraged not to focus on day-to-day changes in ventilator settings, such as administered concentrations of oxygen or settings of positive end-expiratory pressure, because most patients will have variability in these measures that do not reflect overall prognosis. Early in the course of ARDS, families can be prepared by informing them about clinical factors that portend a bad outcome (i.e., renal failure, liver failure, hemodynamic instability, and nosocomial infection). Families who have heard about these possibilities are better prepared for decision-making.

Family members of the current patient may rightfully choose to withdraw mechanical ventilation even after hearing all of the information about the prognosis and long-term outcomes of ARDS. The mere fact that the surrogate makes a decision that seems wrong is not sufficient grounds for questioning their competence or accuracy. Physicians should be cautious of being overconfident in their convictions about the best interests of the patient. There are ample data to show that physicians' judgments about the use of life support vary considerably, even when presented with identical cases. When clinicians disagree with surrogates, they should not loose the surrogates' trust and risk breaking the lines of communication. Once it is lost due to a hostile interaction, trust is extremely difficult to regain, and without it, there is little hope of a settlement.

Despite these efforts, some conflicts between family members and the health care team may prove very difficult to resolve. Contrary to some perceptions, civil lawsuits from end-of-life decisions in critical care are rare, and concern over legal liability should not be the physician's primary concern. Consultation with an ethics committee, ombudsmen, respected colleagues, social worker, or leader from the patient's religious or cultural group may all help to move the discussions toward resolution.

For the current patient, the physicians held a conference with the family to better understand their concerns. The physicians presented the outcome data on ARDS and reassured the family that the patient, at this point in his illness, had none of the poor prognostic signs. The physicians listened at length to the family explain why the patient had expressed such a specific wish about never being placed on a ventilator. The patient's father had died of emphysema on a ventilator after a prolonged illness, and the patient feared having the same death. The physicians explained that the current patient, a nonsmoker, did not have emphysema, but that it was possible that he would require prolonged mechanical ventilation for this illness.

Sometimes, family members may have fears that they are reluctant to express to physicians. In this case, an ICU nurse who had spent time with the patient's wife explained to the physicians that the wife was particularly afraid that her husband would survive but would require mechanical ventilation at home for the rest of his life. When the family was reassured that patients who survive ARDS rarely, if ever, require life-long mechanical ventilation, they agreed to continue mechanical ventilation. On day 23 of mechanical ventilation, the patient had a fever to 40.1°C, and ventilator-associated pneumonia was diagnosed. Despite the prompt initiation of broad-spectrum antibiotics, the patient progressed to develop septic shock and multiorgan failure. The physicians approached the family and explained the change in prognosis. A decision was made by the family in discussion with the medical team to withdraw life-sustaining treatment.

Clinical Pearls

1. Short-term prognosis of ARDS is influenced by age, comorbidity, and the development of multiorgan failure and less by duration of mechanical ventilation or severity of lung injury.

2. The physician should always his or her knowledge of the medical condition and personal biases about prognosis and burdens of care when contemplating the decision to override the family's wishes.

3. Replacing the surrogate decision-makers with a court-appointed guardian should only be considered when all attempts at negotiation and mediation have failed.

REFERENCES

1. Shellman RG, Fulkerson WJ, DeLong E, Piantadosi CA: Prognosis of patients with cirrhosis and chronic liver disease admitted to the medical intensive care unit. Crit Care Med 1988;16:671–678.
2. Asch DA, Hansen F-J, Lanken PN: Decisions to limit or continue life-sustaining treatment by critical care physicians in the United States: conflicts between physicians' practices and patients' wishes. Am J Respir Crit Care Med 1995;151(2 pt 1):288–292.
3. Heffner JE, Brown LK, Barbieri CA, et al: Prospective validation of an acute respiratory distress syndrome predictive score. Am J Respir Crit Care Med 1995;152:1518–1526.
4. Doyle RL, Szaflarski N, Modin GW, et al: Identification of patients with acute lung injury: predictors of mortality. Am J Respir Crit Care Med 1995;152:1818–1824.
5. Zilberberg MD, Epstein SK: Acute lung injury in the medical ICU: comorbid conditions, age, etiology, and hospital outcome. Am J Respir Crit Care Med 1998;157:1159–1164.
6. Rubenfeld GD, Crawford SW: Withdrawing life support from mechanically ventilated recipients of bone marrow transplants: a case for evidence-based guidelines. Ann Intern Med 1996;125:625–633.
7. Davidson, TA, Caldwell ES, Curtis JR, et al: Reduced quality of life in survivors of acute respiratory distress syndrome compared to critically ill controls. JAMA 1999;281:354–360.
8. Davidson, TA, Rubenfeld GD, Caldwell ES, et al: The effect of acute respiratory distress syndrome on long-term survival. Am J Respir Crit Care Med 1999;160:1838–1842.

Jason D. Christie, MD
Paul N. Lanken, MD

PATIENT 63

A 73-year-old man who fears suffocating yet requests withdrawal of life-supportive care

A 73-year-old man with chronic obstructive pulmonary disease (COPD) is admitted to the ICU with pneumonia, obtundation, and respiratory failure. He had required mechanical ventilation for four previous episodes of respiratory failure during the past 3 years. He would typically recover after 2 to 3 days of ventilatory support and return home after 7 days. Since his last discharge 10 months ago, however, his health has progressively declined. He now spends most days in one room using supplemental oxygen with his dog by his side. Because of severe dyspnea, he leaves his chair only to use a bedside commode.

His physician recently encouraged him to complete a durable power of attorney for health care and a living will. In completing his written advance directives, he selected his wife as his proxy and decided to accept mechanical ventilation for a future illness only if he appeared likely to recover his baseline health status. He would not want to stay on a ventilator for more than 1 week or undergo a tracheotomy. He told his physician that he prefers to be "made comfortable and allowed to die rather than becoming a prisoner kept alive indefinitely by a machine."

With the patient's advance directives in mind, his physicians decided to intubate and ventilate him for the present illness, because resolution of the pneumonia appeared possible. He received aggressive therapy with fluids, corticosteroids, bronchodilators, and broad-spectrum antibiotics. The pulmonologist, who knew the patient from past admissions, prescribed intravenous lorazepam and fentanyl to control agitation, dyspnea, and ventilator asynchrony.

On the fifth ICU day, the patient remained ventilator-dependent with oliguria and persistent fevers. His admission tracheal aspirate and blood cultures were positive for *Pseudomonas aeruginosa*. His physicians believed that the patient would not successfully wean from the ventilator soon and would most likely require prolonged, if not life-long, ventilatory support.

The pulmonologist and primary care physician arranged a meeting with the patient's wife, daughter, ICU nurse, and the hospital chaplain in the patient's room. Lorazepam and fentanyl had been discontinued, and the patient was calm, alert, and interactive. He could communicate by lip-reading, hand signals, and use of a letter board. The physicians discussed the nature of the patient's illness, its likely course, and his poor prognosis for breathing off the ventilator any time soon.

The patient made it clear he remained opposed to prolonged mechanical ventilation and requested that the ventilator be removed so that he could die. He indicated that his affairs were in order, he had made peace with his Maker, and he was ready to die. He stated his fear of feeling like he was suffocating if he were removed from the ventilator. The patient appeared to have intact decision-making capacity. His wife and doctors agreed with his request for withdrawal of life-supportive care. Initially, his daughter expressed some reservations that she did not want to "give up on Dad." She agreed, however, that it was his decision to make and stated her acceptance of his wishes.

Question: How would you manage this patient's request to be allowed to die?

Diagnosis: End-stage COPD with respiratory failure and ventilator dependency.

Discussion: Physicians who work in the ICU often face challenges in providing effective palliative care for patients who are withdrawn from life-sustaining therapy. In many instances, critically ill patients receive aggressive care to manage acute complications of advanced and irreversible underlying medical conditions. Unfortunately, life-sustaining interventions may only prolong the dying process and inflict unnecessary suffering when the probability of a meaningful survival becomes nil.

In such circumstances, a frank but sensitive dialogue between patients, families, and caregivers becomes critically important. This dialogue seeks to understand and communicate the patient's knowledge of the acute and underlying medical conditions, prognosis, and expectations of ICU care. Gaining a mutual understanding becomes an essential basis for formulating an appropriate plan of care for an individual patient.

Clinicians in the ICU always work to ensure that the goals of ICU care comply with their understanding of patients' life values and goals. Erring on the side of life is appropriate when a patient first presents with acute illness to an ICU, unless a do-not-resuscitate order is already in place. Within 1 or 2 days after ICU admission, however, the appropriateness of care should be discussed with patients who retain decision-making capacity or with members of the family and proxy decision-makers if patients can no longer enter into this dialogue. Ideally, the patient's primary care physician has already encouraged the patient in an outpatient setting to formulate and express treatment preferences regarding life-sustaining care.

Decisions to withdraw life-support in the ICU present special patient-care challenges. Most often, critically ill patients considered for the withdrawal of life support lack full decision-making capacity as a result of their critical illness. When patients can no longer participate in discussions, family members may have conflicts among themselves, with feelings of guilt and loss dominating their decision-making process.

A stepwise approach aids the decision-making process to determine the appropriateness of the withdrawal of life-supportive care. The success of these steps rests on the ICU team's ability to establish effective communication and mutual trust with the patient, family, and any surrogate decision-makers. The first step assesses the patient's decision-making capacity and identifies an appropriate surrogate decision-maker for patients who can no longer contribute to their treatment decisions. Next, members of the health care team clarify among themselves their recommendations and the medical facts upon which they base their recommendations. These facts, opinions, and recommendations are then presented to the patient and family. Conflicts among family members and ICU team members should be recognized and resolved if possible. In instances of continued conflict, the preferences of a fully informed, competent patient "trumps," in most instances, the preferences of the health care team and family, no matter how well intentioned they may be. Finally, the ICU team should plan and implement the withdrawal of life support with close attention to ensuring the patient's comfort and meeting other needs of the patient and family.

With the decision to withdrawal life-sustaining interventions, the primary goals of ICU care shift from life prolongation to comfort care. With this shift, however, nursing and physician involvement does not diminish in intensity. In fact, the initiation of palliative and end-of-life care often requires an increase in the time, commitment, concern, and effort that the ICU team expends. Alleviating suffering of an ICU patient who is being withdrawn from a ventilator is an active and often intensive process that requires close attention to details of symptom management, which includes the control of pain, dyspnea, and anxiety.

Certain symptoms, such as pain, anxiety, dyspnea, agitation, and delirium, occur so commonly at the end of life that ICU clinicians need to monitor patients closely for their presence. Although most ICU clinicians control these symptoms adequately with sedatives and analgesics during the maintenance of mechanical ventilation, often they underestimate medication requirements immediately before and after the withdrawal of life-supportive care. In this setting, the usual doses used for critically ill patients prove too small to alleviate the distress of dying. Such patients require a titration of medications—often to large doses by continuous intravenous administration—to achieve the desired effects. Moreover, intensivists should anticipate the pain, anxiety, and suffering of patients about to undergo the withdrawal of life-supportive care by initiating medications **preemptively** in sufficient doses to prevent dyspnea, anxiety, and other distress before they occur.

When withdrawal of mechanical ventilation is planned for a dying patient, an opioid, such as fentanyl or morphine sulfate, should be given by an intravenous bolus 30 minutes before ventilator withdrawal, followed immediately by a continuous infusion. A benzodiazepine, such as lorazepam, may be combined with the opioid to relieve anxiety further. The adequacy of symptoms relief should be reassessed before extubation and withdrawal of the ventilator. Some clinicians reduce the ventilatory support in a stepwise manner over 10–20 minutes to allow titration of opioids and sedatives to ensure adequate symptom control before extubation.

If a patient has previously received opioids, drug tolerance may have occurred, which will require higher opioid doses. For example, patients who have been receiving morphine at a dose of more than 10 mg/hr may require morphine boluses of 10–20 mg or more to achieve adequate palliation. In fact, no upper limit exists for dosing opioids to palliate dyspnea or pain for dying patients, so long as the physician's intent remains the relief of pain and suffering. Careful reassessments to determine the adequacy of therapy are required to justify upward titration of doses.

Pharmacologic and nonpharmacologic approaches exist for managing anxiety related to withdrawal of life-sustaining interventions. Spiritual concerns, unresolved family issues, interpersonal relationships, and fear of suffering or dying become heightened in anticipation of the withdrawal of life-support. Addressing these matters with patients can help relieve anxiety. By asking "what are you most afraid of?," physicians may allow the patient the opportunity to express their most important concerns. Giving patients sufficient time to be with family members, to put financial matters in order, or to say something to an important person provides patients with a sense of closure and control. Allowing extended visiting hours and visits by children or beloved pets can provide additional comfort to the dying patient. Little acts, such as putting the side rails of the bed down and turning off electronic monitors or alarms in the patient's room, help families to feel closer to the patient in a more natural setting. Visits by a hospital chaplain or a personal spiritual advisor should be offered and made available if desired.

Most patients benefit from the initiation of benzodiazepines for control of anxiety. When death is imminent, patients may experience an agitated delirium. Although benzodiazepines assist in combating agitation, haloperidol is the drug of choice for delirium.

Many of the events associated with dying create distress among family members. Forewarnings and explanations of the dying process can assist families in preparing for this experience. Many institutions provide families with brochures explaining the events that surround dying. Explanations that patients may experience episodes of delirium, "rattling" breathing from retained airway secretions, and the appearance of labored breathing combined with reassurances that medications will relieve the patient's distress help the family prepare for death. Because the exact moment of death cannot be predicted, caregivers should prepare the patient and family for this uncertainty by explaining that the dying process may take hours to days, and that death may not immediately follow the withdrawal of life support.

The current patient indicated a desire to be with his family and dog once more before he received sedation in preparation for ventilator withdrawal. With his family and dog in attendance, the patient was made comfortable with a fan blowing a cool breeze across his face. The vital sign monitors were turned off in the patient's room but left on at the nursing station. The physician ordered 8 mg of morphine by intravenous bolus, followed by a continuous infusion of 4 mg/hr as preemptive therapy for dyspnea. Lorazepam was given as a 2-mg bolus followed by a continuous infusion of 2 mg/hr. The pressure support on the ventilator was decreased over 10 minutes to 7 cm H_2O.

After the patient became comfortable in response to the medications, the family elected to leave the room while the endotracheal tube and ventilator were removed. The patient could initially respond to his family, but became somnolent yet arousable as he required increasing doses of morphine to control dyspnea over the next few hours. Later in the evening, the patient became unconscious and expired in no apparent distress with his wife, daughter, and dog by his side.

Clinical Pearls

1. Physicians should ask the question "What are you most afraid of?" to open a dialogue about end-of-life care.

2. Palliation immediately before and after withdrawal of life support can be an intensive process, requiring close attention to detail to control distressing symptoms of dyspnea, pain, anxiety, agitation, and delirium.

3. Before withdrawing life-supportive interventions, *preemptive* doses of opioids and sedatives should be given to prevent dyspnea and anxiety.

4. Dying patients should receive sufficient doses of opioids and sedatives to relieve suffering. No dose of drugs is too high as long as the intent of therapy is to relieve symptoms and not to accelerate death.

5. Even with the withdrawal of life-sustaining care, the exact time of death remains unpredictable. Patients and families should be informed that death may not occur immediately after removal of ventilatory support.

6. Clinicians should temporarily suspend ICU policies when necessary to allow patients to die as close as possible in the custom and setting of their choice. Nursing staff should accommodate rituals that help patients and families experience death. Visitation rules should be flexible to allow family, close friends, and important pets to attend to the patient.

REFERENCES

1. Quill T, Byock I: Responding to intractable terminal suffering: the role of terminal sedation and voluntary refusal of food and fluids. Ann Intern Med 2000;132:408–414.
2. Loewy E, Loewy R: The Ethics of Terminal Care: Orchestrating the End of Life. New York, Kluwer Academic/Plenum Publishers, 2000.
3. Foley K: Pain and symptom control in the dying ICU patient. In Curtis J, Rubenfeld G (eds): Managing Death in the Intensive Care Unit: The Transition from Cure to Comfort. New York, Oxford University Press Inc., 2001, pp 103–125.
4. Faber-Langendoen K, Lanken PN: Dying patients in the intensive care unit: forgoing treatment, maintaining care. Ann Intern Med 2000;133:886–893.
5. Hansen-Flaschen J: Sedation and paralysis during mechanical ventilation: treating distress and agitation. In Lanken PN, Hanson CW III, Manaker S (eds): The Intensive Care Unit Manual. Philadelphia, W.B. Saunders Co., 2001, pp 45–55.
6. DeLisser H, Lanken PN: End-of-life care. In Lanken PN, Hanson CW III, Manaker S (eds): The Intensive Care Unit Manual. Philadelphia, W.B. Saunders Co., 2001, pp 255–265.
7. Lanken PN, Wittbrodt ET: Palliative drug therapy for terminal withdrawal of mechanical ventilation. In Lanken PN, Hanson CW III, Manaker S (eds): The Intensive Care Unit Manual. Philadelphia, W.B. Saunders Co., 2001, pp 1089–1093.

Michael Frederich, MD

PATIENT 64

A 43-year-old man with squamous cell carcinoma of the face causing pain that is intermittently responsive to opioids

A 43-year-old man with a 2-year history of squamous cell carcinoma of the left ear has experienced disease progression, with the tumor now involving most of the left side of his face despite multiple operations. He complains of pain that is constant at a level of 4 out of 10 (4/10) and with intermittent crescendos to 10/10. The constant pain is described as aching and persistent, while the crescendos are described as shooting, stabbing, and burning.

Physical Examination: Blood pressure 90/60, pulse 86, respirations 24, temperature 37°C. General: thin, wasted, lethargic, and with obvious facial deformity. HEENT: left facial deformity with edema and erythema from the preauricular area to the submandibular area. The upper half of the left ear is absent and a dark eschar occludes the auricular orifice. The left side of the face is exquisitely tender to light palpation. Allodynia is present; touching the hair on the lower scalp just above, in front of, and behind the left ear is very uncomfortable. The buccal mucosa on the left has been invaded by tumor, and a strong odor is present. There are no signs of oral candidiasis or mucositis.

Clinical Course: An empiric trial of an oral broad spectrum antibiotic only slightly diminishes swelling and discomfort. Initial medications for pain include an NSAID (ibuprofen), an antidepressant (amitriptyline, for neuropathic pain), and oral morphine. The morphine is prescribed in a long-acting, controlled-release form taken routinely, with supplemental rescue doses of a short-acting, immediate-release oral form for breakthrough pain.

Although pain is controlled initially, increasing pain over the next several weeks requires escalating doses of oral morphine. The patient's regimen is changed to a parenteral form of morphine at a dose of 600 mg of long-acting, controlled-release oral morphine given every 12 hours (with an average of five additional 200-mg doses of short-acting, immediate-release oral morphine per day). Because this fails to control the pain, the parenteral morphine is converted to subcutaneous morphine. From a total morphine equivalent daily dose (MEDD) of 2200 mg of oral morphine, a 3:1 oral-to-parenteral conversion ratio results in a calculated subcutaneous morphine dose of 720 mg/day or 30 mg/hour. In addition, a bolus rescue dose of 10 mg every 20 minutes is ordered.

The patient experiences nausea and constipation that are palliated with appropriate medications. Escalation of the dose to 2400 mg of morphine per day causes confusion. Myoclonus is also noted. Despite this dosage and the side effects, his pain remains uncontrolled. He reports his baseline pain intensity to be 7/10 with crescendos to 10/10 over the left side of his face.

Question: What should be done with this patient's opioid regimen? Should opioid rotation be considered?

Diagnosis: Squamous cell carcinoma of the face, with nociceptive and neuropathic pain resistant to high doses of parenteral opioids.

Discussion: When a patient fails to receive satisfactory pain relief from high doses of morphine and experiences unacceptable opioid-induced side effects, opioid rotation may enhance the effectiveness and tolerance of pain control. Opioid rotation is the term used to describe a switch from one opioid drug to another. It may be useful in opening the therapeutic window and for establishing a better balance between analgesia and side effects.

Different mechanisms have been proposed to account for the effectiveness of opioid rotation for pain control. Prominent among these is altered interaction with opioid receptors. This mechanism probably explains the observed asymmetry in cross-tolerance among different opioids given at equianalgesic doses. In addition, accumulation of opioid metabolites may explain both the observed differences in analgesia and adverse effects in a clinical setting.

Cross-tolerance describes the phenomenon of tolerance to one drug resulting in tolerance to another drug. Cross-tolerance between opioids is incomplete. The benefit of rotating from one opioid to another depends on cross-tolerance to the analgesic effects being less than cross-tolerance to the adverse effects. In caring for the present patient, physicians had hoped that rotating to an opioid other than morphine would provide improved analgesia with fewer side effects.

Morphine is metabolized to morphine-3-glucuronide (M3G) and morphine-6-glucuronide (M6G). The M6G metabolite has analgesic properties and makes an important contribution to the analgesic efficacy of morphine. The M3G metabolite is devoid of analgesic activity but produces neuroexcitatory effects such as myoclonus and may cause confusion. These metabolites may accumulate in patients with normal or impaired renal function.

When pain is not well controlled with oral morphine, changing to parenteral or subcutaneous morphine is a logical next step. Relative concentrations of M3G and M6G in relation to morphine are greater after oral administration than after parenteral administration of morphine. Subcutaneous continuous administration of morphine is safe and effective. However, the present patient's pain did not respond to high doses of parenteral morphine, and intolerable side effects of myoclonus and confusion occurred. The need to rotate or change to a different opioid became apparent. But which opioid would be best?

Methadone is one alternative. It has the advantages of low cost and absence of known active metabolites. In addition, it is chemically quite different from other opioids. This may partly explain its observed efficacy in cases such as the one presented. deStoutz and coworkers found the benefit of opioid rotation to methadone was most significant in cases of myoclonus. Its relatively long half-life and a relatively unknown and perhaps variable equianalgesic dose compared with other opioids require a good deal of expertise in cancer pain management. Bruera and colleagues have observed that methadone is almost ten times more potent than suggested in equianalgesic tables when the MEDD is high.

However, there is another reason that might explain methadone's efficacy. Methadone is a racemic mixture of *levo-* and *dextro-* compounds. The L-isomer is an opioid, while both the L- and D-isomers have NMDA (*N*-methyl-D-aspartate) antagonist activity. Methadone may be more effective than other opioids in circumstances in which NMDA receptor activation develops, such as in patients whose pain has a neuropathic mechanism associated with tolerance. Morley has suggested that classifying some opioids as broad spectrum is justified. In addition to the varying abilities of opioids to promote tolerance at μ receptors, differences in the selectivity of other opioids such as methadone for other receptors could have an important bearing on their use as substituting drugs in opioid rotation.

It was decided to rotate the current patient's opioid from morphine to methadone. An equianalgesic ratio of 1:10 for methadone to morphine was used, as proposed by Bruera. Based on a total daily MEDD of 2400 mg, the patient's estimated dose was methadone 240 mg/day. The conversion was accomplished over 3 days, with the patient receiving one third of the final target dose of methadone each day while the morphine infusion was slowed by one third each day. The patient ultimately received methadone at 80 mg every 8 hours routinely. He was also allowed an additional dose of methadone 20 mg every 2 hours as needed for breakthrough pain. His myoclonus and confusion cleared in 3 days.

The patient's methadone dose required gradual titration upward to 100 mg every 8 hours routinely, and he remained comfortable at this dose. His amitriptyline was discontinued, and his facial pain was well controlled with the methadone alone.

Clinical Pearls

1. Opioid rotation, which is the changing from one opioid drug to another, is a useful technique for managing the variable qualities of opioids.

2. Opioid toxicities and side effects may be managed by rotating to a different opioid.

3. Analgesia may be improved by rotating to a different opioid.

4. Methadone is an opioid with NMDA antagonist activity that is useful in treating nociceptive and neuropathic pain. Because it has no known active metabolites, it may be less toxic than other opioids. It is more potent than previously thought, appearing to be ten times as potent as high doses of morphine.

REFERENCES

1. deStoutz ND, Bruera E, Suarez-Almazor M: Opioid rotation for toxicity reduction in terminal cancer patients. J Pain Symptom Manage 1995;10:378–384.
2. Bruera E, Pereira J, Watanabe S, et al: Opioid rotation in patients with cancer pain. Cancer 1996;78:852–857.
3. Vigano A, Fan D, Bruera E: Individualized use of methadone and opioid rotation in the comprehensive management of cancer pain associated with poor prognostic indicators. Pain 1996; 67: 115–119.
4. Fallon M: Opioid rotation: does it have a role? Palliat Med 1997;11:177–178.
5. Morley JS: Opioid rotation: does it have a role? Palliative Medicine 1998; 12: 464–466.
6. Mercadante S: Opioid rotation for cancer pain: rationale and clinical aspects. Cancer 1999; 86:1856–1866.

Peter Terry, MD

PATIENT 65

A 68-year-old man with severe COPD who wishes to forgo further invasive treatment but whose children desire aggressive care

A 68-year-old man with severe chronic obstructive pulmonary disease (COPD) is admitted to the hospital with an exacerbation of his underlying disease. He has been hospitalized for similar events three times in the past year, and each time trials of noninvasive ventilation failed, requiring intubation. After his third stay in the ICU, he was asked if he would want to be intubated in the future should another exacerbation occur. He was initially extremely reluctant to discuss the subject, but eventually stated that he did not want to be intubated again. He reiterated this wish 6 weeks following hospital discharge.

Physical Examination: Blood pressure 149/89, pulse 127, respirations 36, temperature 38.9°C. General: mildly obtunded, tachypneic and using sternocleidomastoid muscles to aid in respiration, which appeared labored. HEENT: unremarkable. Thorax: thin, barrel-shaped chest with inward movement of the lower costal margin, and periodic paradoxical abdominal wall motion with inspiration.

Laboratory Findings: Hct 42.4%, WBC 13,760/μL, creatinine 1.1 mg/dl. Arterial blood gases (room air): pH 7.28, PCO_2 68 mm Hg, PO_2 46 mm Hg.

When the patient's three children arrive at the hospital and are apprised of their father's illness and his wishes, all are adamant that the physician override their father's wishes. They request that all aggressive measures be taken, including intubation and mechanical ventilation.

Question: Whose request should be followed, that of the patient or his children?

Diagnosis: Severe COPD with an autonomous decision to forgo intubation and mechanical ventilation.

Discussion: The present patient, who will likely require intubation soon if his life is to be prolonged, has clearly stated his wishes in a verbal advance directive. At first glance, one would surmise that the appropriate course of action would be to acknowledge the children's concerns and request, but to ultimately ignore, their wishes. The concept of respect for patient's autonomous choices has permeated the teaching of medical ethics for the past several decades. And what decision could be a more momentous and persuasive expression of autonomy than that of a patient, fully informed by past experience, who specifically and repeatedly requests to avoid intubation and mechanical ventilation?

While the notion of autonomous decision-making has become ingrained in physicians' and medical ethicists' thinking, some have assumed that the right to make a decision is synonymous with actively exercising that right by making end-of-life decisions for themselves. In fact, there is evidence that many patients want to express their autonomy indirectly, by designating others to make decisions on their behalf. For example, in a study of men with newly diagnosed prostate cancer, many wished to be informed about their options for treatment but preferred that others make the final treatment decisions.

One might assume that were the present patient to be confronted with the fact that his children disagree with his decision, that he would still wish that his own stated preferences for treatment be honored. Evidence suggests that such assumptions may not always be correct. In two studies that have asked patients with terminal illness whether they would want to have their advance directive honored if a family member disagreed, more than half said that they would want to have their advance directive ignored.

As illustrated by the present case, physicians should realize from their experience that many patients do not wish to exercise this right in a direct manner. The appropriate first question to ask a patient when making end-of-life decisions is, "Who do you want to make these difficult decisions?," rather than "What decision do you want to make?" If the physician first asks the patient what decision he or she wants to make, the patient may presume that only they can make decisions, even though their preference would be for a loved one to do so.

In the care of the present patient, it is essential to assess his capacity to make decisions on this admission. If he is judged capable of making decisions, then he ought to be reminded of his prior request and asked whether he would like to designate his children to make decisions on his behalf or whether he wants to make decisions for himself, by himself. If he responds that he did not know that he could designate his children to make such decisions and expresses interest in doing so, he should be informed that his children currently do not agree with his decision to refuse intubation and mechanical ventilation. Regardless of the form of decision-making the patient chooses, physicians can then facilitate thoughtful and caring communication with the patient and his family. In situations in which the treating physician is confident that the patient understands the option of designating his children as surrogate decision-makers but chose to directly exercise this right himself, the physician has an obligation to respect his wishes. Here, too, the physician can skillfully extend emotional support to the children, encouraging them to spend time with their father and even giving them permission to gently express their reasons for wanting him to have aggressive care. The physicians should take care to emphasize that it is the patient's decision, and their responsibility is to respect his preferences. What should the physician do if the patient presents in an incapacitated state, unable to review his preferences or speak for himself, and the children disagree with their father's prestated wishes? It is important to hear the reasoning behind the children's objections. They may bring insights to bear on the patient's decision that the physician had not previously considered. For example, they may describe symptoms compatible with severe depression that the physician missed during hospitalization or outpatient visits, or they may describe conversations with their father that suggest his understanding of future intubations and ancillary treatment are not consistent with the norms of ICU treatment. If compelling reasons can be mounted by the children, then the physician must exercise judgment and may be right in suspending the patient's previous decision. Barring such evidence, however, the physician should honor the patient's request while advocating for respect for their father's autonomous right in discussions and counseling with his children.

Are the children's demands for more aggressive care such that the physician should be suspicious of their motives? Hardly. A number of studies have compared the decisions of patients, loved ones, and physicians who are presented with a number of end-of-life scenarios and asked what they believe patients would want in terms of end-of-life decisions. These studies show that the family, when they do err in judging what the patient would want, tend to be more aggressive than the patient would be, while physicians tend to be less aggressive than the patient. Such observations may explain why disagreements arise between physicians and loved ones concerning end-of-life decisions in unconscious patients who have not stated their wishes.

The current patient was asked if, when he made his decision, he knew that he could have opted for his children to make a decision on his behalf. When he said no, he was asked if he would want them to do so, knowing that they disagreed with his decision to forgo ventilation. When he heard that they wanted more aggressive treatment, he immediately agreed to be intubated if necessary. He subsequently underwent intubation and mechanical ventilation and was successfully extubated 72 hours later.

Clinical Pearls

1. Many patients do not want to be actively involved in end-of-life decisions, preferring that their families make decisions on their behalf.

2. When discussing end of life decisions with a patient, first ask, "Who do you want make decisions about your care?"

3. When patients are informed that loved ones disagree with their end-of-life decision, they will often ask that their previously stated wishes be ignored.

REFERENCES

1. Schgal A, Galbraith A, Chesney M, et al: How strictly do dialysis patients want their advance directives followed? JAMA 1992;267:59–63.
2. Davison BJ, Degner LF, Morgan TR: Information and decision-making preferences of men with prostate cancer. Oncol Nurs Forum 1995;22:1401–1408.
3. Terry PB, Vettese M, Song J, et al: End-of-life decision making: when patients and surrogates disagree. J Clin Ethics 1999;10:286–293.

Frank J. Brescia, MD

PATIENT 66

A 54-year-old woman with severe pain from metastatic cancer whose needs exceed a hospital's palliative care resources

A 54-year-old woman comes to the hospital emergency department with increasing back pain, confusion, and difficulty walking over the past 24 hours. The patient has a 3-year history of breast cancer with known disease in her bones, lung, and pleural cavity. Despite multiple chemotherapeutic and hormonal agents, research protocols, as well as radiation treatments to painful sites, the patient's disease has progressed. She recently was placed on hospice home care and has been living at home with her only child, an unmarried son. The patient is followed by several different physicians, but has not been seen in several weeks.

She is treated in the emergency department with pain medications and is discharged home. There is no direct communication with her attending physicians. No diagnostic studies are ordered. The following day, her pain and confusion worsen and she can no longer ambulate. Her medical oncologist arranges admission to the hospital.

Physical Examination: General: obese woman with obvious pain; confused, somnolent, mildly agitated, mild dehydration. Lymph nodes: none. HEENT: PERLA, tongue dry. Chest: clear. Cardiac: tachycardia. Abdomen: distended with palpable bladder. Neurologic: cranial nerves intact; disoriented; unable to move lower extremities, weakness in both upper extremities, and unable to test sensory level; bilateral Babinski's reflex.

Laboratory Findings: Hct 22%, calcium 12.8 mg/dl, BUN 58 mg/dl, creatinine 1.2 mg/dl, albumin 2.4 g/dl.

Hospital Course: The patient is admitted to the oncology unit, where she receives high-dose steroids, intravenous fluids, pamidronate, and analgesics. A Foley catheter is placed. An emergency MRI of the cervical/thoracic spine confirms extensive destruction with instability of the cervical spine and spinal cord compression at C4–5. Neurosurgical and radiation consultations are obtained, and the patient is placed in a halo apparatus.

Despite radiation and steroids, no improvement is noted in her neurologic deficit. Pain remains a problem, and members of the nursing staff are uncomfortable about escalating her opioid doses for fear of respiratory difficulty. The patient is unable to make decisions for herself, and her son is hostile to the staff refusing to allow a DNR order.

Question: How can this patient's care be better coordinated?

Diagnosis: Advanced metastatic breast cancer with nonresponsive spinal cord compression of the cervical spine.

Discussion: It is widely accepted that care for patients approaching death needs to be improved. Many clinicians caring for dying patients have feelings of helplessness, frustration, and sadness. Many experience a profound sense of failure. This final phase of progressive chronic illness is often poorly managed by the health care system, with fragmented and inadequate services, conflicting and confused goals and expectations, and at times frank negligence. Indeed, studies suggest that as many as 40% of chronically ill patients may die with unrelieved symptoms.

Over 2 million patients die each year in the United States, which is approximately 1% of the population. Today, the typical American lives longer and, unlike a century ago, will succumb from a chronic illness—with these illnesses imposing multiple, complex needs on the healthcare system in the months or years before death. Increasing numbers of Americans die away from their homes. Sites of death vary by the age of individuals and their locations across the country, with the Pacific coast and mountain states having the fewest deaths ($< 40\%$) occurring in hospitals. With the establishment of the Medicare benefit for home hospice services in the early 1980s, it seems reasonable to expect that more deaths in the future will occur at home. In 1998, for example, more than twice the number of patients elected hospice care over conventional care than did in the previous 6-year period. Despite these changes, however, more people die in hospitals (50–60% of total deaths) than anywhere else.

The experiences of the current patient sadly highlight the major deficits in care. She was superficially evaluated in the emergency department, which failed to diagnose spinal cord compression, a common problem of advanced breast cancer. Also, the hospital lacked a coordinated program to manage her needs for palliative care. This health care system failed to recognize and appropriately manage her problems, and inadvertently it contributed to the difficulties in her last days by preventing continued home care with her son. Several practical solutions to her hospital experience could have helped: appropriate skilled, competent staff; good communication and early access to care; and case management within a multidisciplinary approach to all the complicated physical, emotional, and social needs that eventually arose.

Hospitals and local health care systems have multiple missions that include the early diagnosis of disease at a stage that allows curative care and the prevention of untimely deaths. If that goal is not feasible, other goals include restorative care to prolong life and reduce disfigurement, disability, and discomfort. Conventional acute health care institutions have difficulty addressing the needs of patients approaching death (e.g., reducing unnecessary tests and procedures, providing emotional and spiritual concerns, relieving pain, and comforting family members as death draws near). These health care systems often do not assess or adequately document patients' wishes for care in circumstances of disease progression. It is incorrect to assume that dying at home is always superior to dying in a hospital. The difficulty of witnessing increasing distress of a loved one may cause family members to seek, or demand, hospitalization. The burden of total 24-hour care for lengthy periods is enormous. In addition, caring for seriously ill patients at home is complicated by the difficulty of conducting diagnostic studies or palliative procedures.

Terminal cancer patients, regardless of the setting (home, hospital, nursing home), appear to share a common three-step decline the last weeks of life (15 weeks, 8 weeks, and 2 weeks before death), with increasing functional dependency as death approaches. The specific features that ultimately necessitate terminal hospitalization in patients with advanced cancer (i.e., patient demographics, family dynamics, type of physician caring for the patient, geographic location, disease, trajectory of progression) all remain ill defined.

It is easy to understand the need for developing a comprehensive hospital-based program for end-of-life care. Recognition of current deficiencies often arises through patient, family, or staff complaints, ethics consultations, sentinel events (such as the current patient's case), or the observations of interested and concerned hospital staff who advocate change.

There are also several caveats to consider in trying to improve the delivery of care for patients at the end of life. It is important to remember that patients and loved ones are worried about their immediate practical needs, not a program's agenda. Although system-based interventions may be straightforward, it may prove difficult to improve patient outcomes, due, for instance, to the institutional bias against use of opioids. Improving communication, caring, continuity, comfort, and closure—things that matter most to people—go a long way to help patients die with less suffering in hospitals.

From these simple concepts more specific questions arise: How good is communication at the institution? How are patient preferences documented and honored? What provisions exist for incurably ill children, minorities, or non-English-speaking patients? How does the system handle the most difficult patients, including those who are hostile or who suffer from agitated dementia or long-standing psychiatric problems? How is care provided to patients who are acutely injured and not expected to survive? What expertise does the hospital have to manage pain and other symptoms, as well as emotional issues? Have physicians and other clinical staff been trained in skills of breaking bad news? What are the institution's physical accommodations for dying patients and their families? Are policies and rules conducive to visiting dying patients—are rules relaxed to allow extended stay, children, or special foods? Are the ICU and other specialty services (oncology, pediatrics, neurology) able to identify special needs required for their patients as well as identify and help ease the stress of families and staff? Are spiritual needs talked about, and are they ever formally assessed and addressed? Does the health system have appropriate tools for assessment of pain and other physical complaints, clinical guidelines for common problems, and proper chart documentation? Are there ongoing educational programs and quality improvement efforts that address the needs of patients with advanced, incurable illness? Finally, is there a method to examine the quality of end-of-life care and family support provided by the health system?

Program development to remedy deficiencies at the end of life requires energy and commitment by the institution to identify problem areas and to change the operational systems and culture of health care delivery. Commonly, a task force of concerned, informed, and influential individuals from within the institution's hierarchy is necessary to develop a vision, mission, and intervention plan. Procedures and policies are necessary that embrace and maintain an environment that supports openness and change. Reflecting the nature of palliative care, the nature of this type of organizational intervention must be interdisciplinary. Optimally, programs should be organized horizontally across hospital or academic departmental lines, avoiding duplication, fostering collaboration, and helping to save expenses and conserve resources. Reimbursement challenges need immediate attention to address financial issues. Effective strategies require creative and practical solutions and will differ from institution to institution. Each clinical program exists in the unique culture of the larger health system and community, but it is often im-

portant for the survival of a program to have a strong departmental base within the hospital or health system. This may require that the program is centered within a politically strong department, such as medicine, oncology, or neurology, or it may require the development of a separate department or division of palliative care. Some have suggested that the hospital subsidize pain, supportive, and palliative care programs through the clinical divisions that do the best financially.

Walsh, at the Cleveland Clinic, has openly published a business plan that worked for his oncology-based program. This approach proceeds from an analysis of the "market environment," defining the strengths and weaknesses for the institution. Program assessment, operational requirements, financial possibilities, as well as public relations all are required for planning. Will the new program manage all end-of-life diagnoses, or will it evolve incrementally as the program grows? Will there be a consultative team to see all hospitalized patients scattered throughout the system? How many clinicians are needed, and how will after-hours clinical care be provided? Are there enough patients and needs to have dedicated palliative care beds? Should this be covered under acute care reimbursement or the hospice benefit? Should these patients, by the nature of care, all have DNR orders?

The business plan can be utilized as a marketing tool, a means to help recruit new staff and a constant internal resource. The program will need to demonstrate high standards of excellence, including presence, availability, adaptability, competency, caring, resourcefulness, and financial independence. It must not be seen as a "soft" program but as a facilitating influence that makes receiving care and the dying experience easier for patients in its care. Patient care, education of families, teaching of house staff, as well as research must all become part of the mission. Finally, the health system's leadership must support the program in tangible ways, directing public relations and fund development resources to assist with the program's sustained development.

With the current patient, because of her increasing medical and nursing needs, her mental agitation, and her son as the only caregiver at home, she is discharged after 96 days to a nursing home a great distance from her home. She expires 1 week later. The acute care hospital in which she received care subsequently has embarked on efforts to establish an integrated palliative care and pain service that will provide comprehensive end-of-life care.

Clinical Pearls

1. Despite recent increases in the number of people dying at home, hospitals remain the place where most Americans die.

2. The goals and expectations of acute hospital care often conflict with the needs of the dying, causing patients to have pain and other symptoms inadequately managed.

3. Multiple questions need to be addressed when deciding to develop a comprehensive end-of-life program of care, including competency, comfort, compassion, communication, continuity, and closure.

4. A formal business plan worked out by a task force supported by hospital administration is a necessary first step in designing a quality improvement plan and a palliative care program.

REFERENCES

1. Walsh D, Gombeski WR, Goldstein P: Managing a palliative oncology program: the role of a business plan. J Palliat Support Med 1994:9(2):109–118.
2. Brescia FJ: Specialized care of the terminally ill. In DaVita VT, et al (eds): Cancer: Principles and Practice of Oncology. Philadelphia, J.B. Lippincott, 1997.
3. Manfredi PL, Morrison RS, Morkis J: Palliative care consultations: how do they impact the care of hospitalized patients? J Palliat Support Med 2000:20(3):166–172.
4. Lynn J: Serving patients who may die soon and their families. JAMA 2001:285:925–922.

Mary Beth Happ, PhD, RN

PATIENT 67

An 80-year-old man in respiratory failure who repeatedly removes catheters and tubes

An 80-year-old man presents to the emergency department with a 2-week history of shortness of breath, right-sided chest pain, decreased appetite, weight loss, and coughing. He had previously enjoyed an active life and close partnership with his 69-year-old wife. His past medical history is unremarkable.

Physical Examination: Blood pressure 178/57, heart rate 105, temperature 37.8°, respirations 38. General: thin. Chest: clear. Cardiac: normal.

Laboratory Findings: Chest radiograph: right lung mass abutting the chest wall. Chest CT: solid, peripheral mass in the right middle lobe. Pulmonary function tests: normal. Fine needle aspiration: nondiagnostic.

Hospital Course: The patient desires aggressive care and undergoes a right thoracotomy. Intraoperative biopsies demonstrate a spindle cell neoplasm with invasion of the chest wall. A lobectomy and regional chest wall resection are performed, but his postoperative course is complicated in the surgical ICU by pneumonia and hypotension, which require continued mechanical ventilation. On two occasions during the first postoperative week, the patient pulls out his endotracheal tube, which is replaced because he has difficulty breathing on his own. After 11 days of mechanical ventilation, a tracheotomy is performed, and the patient is transferred to the medical ICU for weaning from mechanical ventilation.

Because of persistent pneumonia, a bronchoscopy is performed to evaluate his airways. Several tumor deposits are seen proximal to the right middle lobe bronchial stump. Three weeks after surgery, the patient appears unlikely to wean successfully from mechanical ventilation. He frequently tugs at his catheters and, over a 3-day period, pulls out his jejunostomy tube, tracheostomy tube, and central venous catheter. All require reinsertion. His mental status fluctuates between periods of complete lucidity, lasting 8 to 24 hours, and episodes of confusion and agitation, which require soft constraints. On several occasions, he mouths the words, "I want to die," to the nurse as he reaches for the ventilator tubing. In the presence of his wife, however, he acquiesces to her encouragement to continue life-sustaining treatments.

Question: Do the patient's efforts to remove catheters and tubing represent his directive to discontinue life-sustaining treatments?

Diagnosis: Spindle cell lung carcinoma in an elderly patient who cannot be weaned from the ventilator.

Discussion: Treatment interference, also known as device disruption, device self-removal, or self-extubation, represents a serious management problem for patients at the end of life. Underlying delirium, restlessness, agitation, and pain combined with discomfort caused by catheters and tubes are common causes of *unintentional* treatment interference. Although most closely associated with patients hospitalized in acute care settings, treatment interference also poses problems in home and long-term care facilities for patients who receive intravenous medications, tube feedings, and supplemental oxygen. Patients who wear ostomy or catheter appliances also are at risk. Adverse outcomes of unplanned device removal include local tissue trauma and swelling, bleeding from removal of intravascular catheters, aspiration on removal of airways and nasogastric tubes, respiratory failure, and death.

Treatment interference also may represent *intentional* efforts by patients to communicate their healthcare wishes to families and caregivers. Distinguishing between intentional and inadvertent removal of treatment devices requires frequent, careful assessment by the patients' bedside nurses. Through these assessments, healthcare providers can identify the best means for communicating with patients or for understanding the behavioral expressions of noncommunicative patients, including those encumbered with airway appliances or affected by illnesses that interfere with articulated speech. Therapeutic effectiveness can be fostered by consistency in assigning patients professional caregivers, especially nurses. Clinical familiarity further promotes the recognition of patient behaviors that may sometimes represent subtle efforts to communicate treatment preferences.

The loss of a patient's ability to speak is a major clinical event. In addition to engendering emotional pain, fear, and anxiety among patients and family members, it complicates the assessment and treatment of pain and other distressing symptoms at end-of-life. Augmentative and assisted communication techniques (e.g., picture boards, writing pads, magic slates, electronic communication devices) can often enhance communication. As with the current patient, however, patients in ICU settings are often too weak to write legibly and are forced to rely on feeble gestures, head nods, and mouthing words to communicate.

The nurses who cared for the current patient during his long ICU stay considered a variety of reasons, both unintentional and intentional, for his removal of devices. On some occasions, his disruptive behavior appeared to be unintentional and a result of delirium. On other occasions, the nurses believed that his interference with treatment was a desperate expression of a fear of dying and a desire for closer attention. In some cases, the nurses interpreted his actions as a wish to end his life-sustaining care. They also considered that his removal of the endotracheal tube, followed later by the tracheostomy tube, represented an effort to talk.

In the ICU, agitated patients are often managed with physical restraints, such as soft wrist bands attached to the bed frame, to prevent treatment interference. Physical restraints, however, present risks for physical, psychological, and emotional injury and raise serious ethical concerns, especially when used for end-of-life care. Moreover, a routine application of physical restraints may obscure the efforts of some patients to communicate the treatment preferences that their treatment interference represents.

Family members at the bedside can serve as a watchful extension of the nurses to prevent treatment interference, thereby avoiding physical restraints. Family members can hold hands, offer verbal reminders, and provide comfort and reassurance for patients at risk for unintentional treatment interference. They also can communicate with patients whose treatment interference represents an expression of their wishes. When family members or friends of dying patients are unavailable, trained volunteers or paid companions can perform this function.

Other restraint-free techniques to prevent treatment interference are listed in the table. Commercial appliances, such as detachable sleeves and protective shields, camouflage intravenous insertion sites. A variety of stabilizers and holders secure gastrostomy, endotracheal, and tracheostomy tubes and prevent self-removal. Dressings, paper tape, long sleeves, and binders can also hide some devices. Diversionary techniques to prevent treatment interference keep a patient's hands occupied. Their use should be individualized to the patient's interests and abilities.

Comfort measures targeted to device insertion sites can relieve the pulling sensation from the weight (torque) of tubing. Measures directed toward other sources of discomfort can decrease generalized patient distress and agitation that might otherwise result in treatment interference. For instance, the present patient repeatedly tugged on his bladder catheter early in one nursing shift. After several verbal reminders to the patient, the

Table: Non-restraint Strategies to Prevent
Treatment Interference*

Explanation and reminders
   Frequent verbal explanation
   Guided visualization of device
   Written reminder (post a sign)
Distraction and diversion
   Activity apron
   Occupational therapy consult
   Writing tools
   Reading material
   Gadgets/stress balls
   Photo albums
   Washcloths, towels to fold
   Empty tubing/packaging
   Music/television
Camouflage
   Long-sleeved gowns
   Generous tape, elastic wrap, or dressings at
     site
   Commercial device -(e.g., protective,
     cushioned sleeve or IV site guard)
   Abdominal binder
Comfort and positioning
   Repositioning/specialty mattress
   Tube stabilizer
   Augmentative communication
   Analgesia/sedation
   Aromatherapy
   Massage/touch therapies
Technologic reduction
   Discontinue nonessential devices
   Intravenous adaptor
   Replace with less restrictive/less intrusive
     device
Environment
   Maximize visualization
   Videocamera
   Noise reduction
   Family presence
   Sitter/companion

*Adapted with permission from Happ MB: Using a best prac-
tice approach to prevent treatment interference in critical care.
Prog Cardiovasc Nurs 2000;15:60.

nurse examined the catheter tubing and noticed
that it was kinked, which had resulted in bladder
distension. Repositioning the tubing remedied the
behavior.

In interpreting the meaning of treatment interference, it should be recognized that seriously ill patients may at times express fears and treatment preferences to their professional caregivers that they
cannot share with their family members. Although
the present patient designated his wife as his
spokesperson, he confided in the nurses his desire to
discontinue mechanical ventilation and other life-
sustaining care. Patients may choose nurses, physicians, and other health care personnel as "compassionate strangers" to receive profound end-of-life
messages. This route of communication might represent a patient's decisional ambiguity, a "test" of a
previously unacceptable thought or feeling, or an effort to relieve family members of the decisional burden. Such revelations to health care professionals
present opportunities to expand the dialogue to include the patient and family members.

Interpretations of disruptive behavior as a refusal of further life-sustaining care, however,
must be made with caution. Such interpretations
should arise from intimate clinical knowledge of
the case, including the patient's present clinical
condition, prognosis, and neurologic status as
well as the context of the patient's past verbal
wishes, written directives, and psychological state.
The current patient's nonverbal behavior and efforts to communicate his wish to die spurred a
bedside conference involving the patient, his wife,
attending physician, and nurse. Using a variety of
assistive communication techniques, the patient
made his preference for treatment withdrawal understood by his wife in a consistent and credible
way. Although the patient did not have a living
will, his wife recalled his previous wishes not to
be "kept alive on machines" if he were terminally
ill. His physician shared with the patient and his
wife the patient's poor prognosis.

With his wife and adult children in attendance at
the bedside, the patient's wishes were honored. He
was able to express final sentiments to his family
("thank you" and "I love you") by mouthing words.
Humidified oxygen was administered via a tracheal
mask in place of mechanical ventilation, and a continuous intravenous morphine sulfate infusion was
titrated to relieve signs of dyspnea and discomfort.
He became unresponsive and died 6 hours later.

Clinical Pearls

1. The causes of treatment interference are varied and may change over the course of acute or long-term treatment. Frequent reassessment by healthcare providers is needed to understand the cause and meaning of a patient's behaviors.

2. Interventions to prevent treatment interference in seriously ill patients should be directed toward the possible causes or meaning of the behavior. Interventions must be individualized to a patient's unique situation, clinical condition, prognosis, and functional and psychological status, as well as long-held values and previous stated preferences.

3. In some cases, disruptive behavior that interferes with treatment may represent a behavioral directive to discontinue life-sustaining treatments. Such interpretations must be made with caution and only by clinicians with close, direct knowledge of the patient. Assigning meaning to a nonverbal patient's behavior is made easier when the interpretation is consistent with a patient's past verbal and written directives about treatment limitation.

REFERENCES

1. Strumpf NE, Evans L: Physical restraint of the hospitalized elderly: perceptions of patients and nurses. Nurs Res 1988;37:132–137.
2. Jablonski RS: The experience of being mechanically ventilated. Qual Health Res 1994;4:186–207.
3. Sullivan-Marx E: Psychological response to physical restraint use in older adults. J Psychosoc Nurs 1995;33(6):20–25.
4. Williams CC, Finch CE: Physical restraints: not fit for woman, man, or beast. J Am Geriatr Soc 1997;45:773–775.
5. Happ MB: Treatment interference in acutely and critically ill adults. Am J Crit Care 1998;7:224–235.
6. Wunderlich RJ, Perry A, Lavin MA, Katz B: Patients' perceptions of uncertainty and stress during weaning from mechanical ventilation. Dimens Crit Care Nurs 1999;18:2–8.
7. Happ MB: Preventing treatment interference: the nurse's role in maintaining technologic devices. Heart Lung 2000;29:60–69.
8. Happ MB: Using a best practice approach to prevent treatment interference in critical care. Prog Cardiovasc Nurs 2000;15:60.
9. Happ MB: Interpretation of nonvocal behavior and the meaning of voicelessness in critical care. Soc Sci Med 2000;50:1247–1255.
10. Elstrom K, Padilla G, Doerling L, Brenner M: Relationship of self-extubation to outcomes in medical intensive care unit (MICU) patients. Am J Crit Care 2001;10:203–204.

Sarah Johnston, MD

PATIENT 68

**A 73-year-old man with a history of stroke, COPD, and arterial insufficiency
of the leg whose son requests discussion of end-of-life care**

A 73-year-old man complaining of pain in his right foot is brought to the office by his son. His past medical history shows an ischemic brainstem stroke 3 years previously, chronic obstructive pulmonary disease (COPD), mild dementia, hypertension, and noncompliance with medications. He has a 100-pack-year smoking history and continues to smoke whenever he can obtain cigarettes. Six months previously, he moved to an assisted care facility, after which, his son notes, he has been more compliant with his medications, is eating better, and is in improved spirits.

Physical Examination: Blood pressure 178/95, pulse 96, temperature 37.5°C, body mass index (BMI) 18. General: thin, cachectic, alert, and oriented. Extremities: right foot is cool, without palpable pulses, with redness of all five toes. Neurologic: Mini-Mental Status Examination (MMSE) 19/30. The patient's gait is ataxic. His speech is slurred.

The patient's son expresses concern that his father's health is deteriorating and asks if there should be a discussion about his future and end-of-life care.

Question: When and how should the physician initiate and participate in the discussion about this patient's end-of-life care?

Diagnosis: A patient with severe COPD and degenerative conditions who needs assistance in discussing end-of-life care.

Discussion: A series of investigations have provided helpful insights into the patterns and preferences of patient-physician communication regarding advance care planning. Most patients and physicians believe that either party may initiate the discussion about end-of-life care, but both groups think it is the physician's responsibility to do so. Patients believe that this discussion should be initiated earlier in the patient-physician relationship and earlier in the course of disease than do physicians. Most patients believe the discussion should occur in the outpatient setting rather than in the hospital. Most patients think that others, particularly close family members, should be included in the discussion. There is no reliable way to predict whether and how an individual patient's preferences might vary from these majority views, and therefore, advance treatment planning discussions must be individualized.

Early patient-physician discussions about end-of-life care are beneficial. They enhance the patients' sense of being cared for and being in control, and they reduce depression. These benefits persist over time and may help subsequent advance planning discussions with proxies. They also enhance the relationship between the patient and physician.

With the current patient, the physician should initiate a discussion about the patient's future and end-of-life care. The patient should be asked if he wishes for his son to be included in the discussion. He should be asked if he has a written advance directive or a power of attorney, and if so, a copy should be obtained. Naming of a surrogate decision-maker and having treatment preferences in writing are high priorities for many patients and can be helpful in discussions and care planning. Additional key features of this first discussion include emphasizing the supportive role of the physician and exploring the patient's thoughts about preferences for end-of-life care. During this first discussion, it is important to focus on the patient's thoughts about the end of life, general goals, and priorities. The physician's supportive role can be emphasized.

Several factors make it difficult for people to make detailed end-of-life decisions far in advance. First, a patient's preferences may understandably change over time. Secondly, preferences expressed for hypothetical scenarios may not predict decisions in subsequent real situations. It is, therefore, essential that the first discussion about end-of-life care not be the last. Most patients believe these discussions should occur over several outpatient visits. Because patients' medical and psychosocial circumstances change over time, the discussion about end-of-life care should be viewed as an ongoing, dynamic process of communication and shared decision-making.

The current patient reported that his son was his power of attorney and that his lawyer had a written advance directive on file. Following discussion of his prognosis, he chose noninvasive evaluation of his right leg circulation. Unfortunately, he developed gangrene of the right foot several days later and required a below-the-knee amputation. Postoperatively, he became very confused. His BMI dropped to 17. The physician held another discussion with the patient and his son to elicit their preferences for nutritional support and end-of-life care.

When discussing the risks and benefits of specific interventions such as nutritional support, the physician should recognize that most patients prefer a more active role for the physician in medical decision-making than do physicians. Significantly more patients than physicians think that the patient and physician should share in decision-making, rather than expecting the patient to make a decision alone. More patients than physicians believe that the physician should give recommendations in addition to facts.

Following the discussion, including a recommendation from the physician, the patient and his son agreed to a plan of oral nutritional supplements and continued monitoring of the patient's nutritional status. The patient required nursing home care, physical therapy to adapt to the amputation and prosthesis, and ongoing nutritional assessment, but over the course of the next several months, he recovered his baseline BMI and cognitive status.

Clinical Pearls

1. Although some patients may initiate the discussions, responsibility for initiating advance care planning discussions generally rests with physicians.

2. Patients prefer that their physicians share in their medical decisions and offer recommendations, rather than merely providing information and leaving it to patients to decide.

3. Patients vary in their preferences for end-of-life discussions and decisions; advance care planning must be individualized.

4. Advance care planning is an ongoing process of patient-physician communication and shared decision-making.

REFERENCES

1. Johnston SC, Pfeifer MP, McNutt R: The discussion about advance directives: patient and physician opinions regarding when and how it should be conducted. Arch Intern Med 1995;155:1025–1030.
2. Miles SH, Koepp R, Weber EP: Advance end-of-life treatment planning: a research review. Arch Intern Med 1996;156:1062–1068.
3. Johnston SC, Pfeifer MP: Patient and physician roles in end-of-life decision making. J Gen Intern Med 1998;13:43–45.
4. Balaban R: A physician's guide to talking about end-of-life care. J Gen Intern Med 2000;15:195–200.
5. Steinhauser KE, Christakis NA, McNeilly M, et al: Factors considered important at the end of life by patients, family, physicians, and other care providers. JAMA 2000;284:2476–2482.

Bradley A. Sharpe, MD
Steven Z. Pantilat, MD

PATIENT 69

A 56-year-old woman with metastatic breast cancer and new hypercalcemia admitted to a hospitalist

A 56-year-old woman with a history of breast cancer metastatic to the liver and mild hypertension treated with atenolol presents with weight loss, fatigue, nausea, and anorexia. Three years ago, she had a right lumpectomy and axillary node dissection and received radiation and chemotherapy. She currently takes tamoxifen. She was well until a week before admission when she noted progressive fatigue, lethargy, and anorexia. On the day of admission, she developed nausea and worsening fatigue. She has no neurologic complaints and no fevers or chills.

Physical Examination: Blood pressure 121/76, pulse 105, temperature 36.8°C. General: thin, sleepy but cooperative. Chest: clear to auscultation. Cardiac: tachycardic without murmurs, S_3 or S_4. Abdomen: non-tender. Neurologic: oriented +3, symmetric and nonfocal.

Laboratory Findings: WBC 5200/μL, electrolytes normal, creatinine 1.5 mg/dl (0.6–1.2 mg/dl), calcium 14.2 mg/dl (8.7–10.1 mg/dl), phosphorus 3.4 mg/dl (2.4–4.6 mg/dl), albumin 3.2 g/dl (3.4–4.7 g/dl). Liver function tests: normal. Chest radiograph: normal.

Hospital Course: The patient was admitted to the care of a hospitalist and received 4 liters of normal saline in the first 24 hours and intravenous pamidronate, followed by a furosemide diuresis. The hospitalist contacted her primary care physician of 24 years, who confirmed her past medical history and medications. The primary care physician also stated that she thought the patient wanted to be a "full code." On admission, the patient told the hospitalist that she had never discussed end-of-life care or code status before.

Question: What is the role of the hospitalist in end-of-life care?

Diagnosis: Hypercalcemia of malignancy and no prior end-of-life discussions.

Discussion: Hospitalists are physicians who provide inpatient care in place of a patient's primary care physician. Hospitalist systems are expanding rapidly, in large part because they promote greater efficiency and expertise in the different realms of patient care—they allow hospitalists to focus on the inpatient setting and free primary care physicians to focus on the outpatient setting.

Although these systems can improve care, they also introduce discontinuity when patients are sickest and require hospitalization. With this transfer of care, medical and psychosocial information not easily found in a computerized medical record or paper chart -(such as code status) can be lost. Also, as is the case with the current patient, when a patient becomes acutely ill, she must rely on a new physician whom she does not know. Because the majority of Americans die in hospitals, scenarios such as this one will become increasingly common, and hospitalists will come to play a major role in providing end-of-life care.

In this case, the woman is admitted with hypercalcemia of malignancy. Overall, her prognosis is very poor; the average survival for patients with cancer who are hospitalized with hypercalcemia is 30 days. In addition, her chance of surviving an in-hospital cardiopulmonary arrest is less than 1 in 200. Unfortunately, she never discussed her wishes concerning resuscitation before this hospitalization. Thus, the hospitalist caring for her must address her diagnosis, prognosis, and preferences for care.

The lack of a prior relationship between hospitalists and their patients creates challenges in addressing advance directives. First, it requires patients to discuss life-and-death matters with doctors they have never met before. They cannot rely on the trust and comfort provided by a longstanding doctor-patient relationship. Secondly, patients may be so ill that they are unable to communicate clearly. Finally, hospitalists do not know the patient's baseline functioning or prior goals and values.

Despite these disadvantages, there are also a number of advantages to the relationship between hospitalists and patients that may foster effective discussions. First, as with the current patient, admission to the hospital typically signals a decline in a person's clinical condition, providing a natural opening for discussions of code status. Second, hospitalists can approach discussions about advance directives as a standard part of the admission evaluation, helping to dispel fears that such a topic reflects unspoken prognostic pessimism. Third, hospitalists, who are accustomed to communicating with critically ill patients on a daily basis, may offer patients a realistic estimate of survival, avoiding the tendency to overestimate the prognosis that has been observed in primary care practice. Such information influences patient decision-making. Fourth, given their daily interactions, hospitalists can have frequent discussions, allowing the patient to consider options and clarify issues over a few days rather than weeks to months. In addition, as a result of addressing these issues routinely in their care of many seriously and terminally ill patients, hospitalists may develop an expertise in discussing advance directives and do-not-resuscitate orders in hospitalized patients. Increasingly, hospitalists are developing skills in communication, shared-care planning and decision-making, as well as in symptom management, that are critical to the care of patients with advanced, life-threatening illness. Their unique role and site-based practice position them to provide valuable contributions toward improving the overall end-of-life care for hospitalized patients.

For patients with a poor prognosis for long-term survival, hospitalists should have an open, honest, and empathic conversation about their wishes surrounding life-sustaining interventions. It is essential that such discussions address code status initially and revisit the issue as the patient's clinical status changes. Furthermore, hospitalists should have these discussions routinely at the time of admission, since the vast majority of patients for whom decisions are made to limit life-sustaining treatment are competent when admitted.

Although hospitalists can and should play an active role in discussing advance directives, they should also encourage primary care physicians to be as involved as they would like in these decisions. Over a third of primary physicians state that they want to have input into these discussions. Hospitalists should contact primary physicians at the time of hospitalization to learn of any previous discussions and current code status. In addition, when the primary physician is at a distance from the hospital or cannot otherwise visit in person, hospitalists should encourage them to speak with the patient by phone.

The current patient was admitted with hypercalcemia of malignancy and has a poor prognosis. On the night of admission, the hospitalist contacted the primary physician, who was comfortable with the plan and with the hospitalist's addressing the patient's wishes regarding resuscitation. With hydration and pamidronate, the patient felt subjectively better, although her calcium levels remained difficult to control.

In a thoughtful, caring, nonthreatening manner, the hospitalist discussed her prognosis and likely survival from an in-hospital cardiac arrest. Although initially upset and devastated by the news, the patient understood her condition and agreed with the hospitalist's recommendation that, in the event of a cardiac arrest, she be allowed to die peacefully and that the hospitalist should write a "do not attempt resuscitation" order. The hospitalist had daily discussions with her about her condition and her options for further interventions. On the third hospital day, the primary care physician and hospitalist together talked with the patient about the possibility of hospice care. She was discharged to home hospice the next day.

Clinical Pearls

1. Hospitalists play a crucial role in providing appropriate care at the end of life.

2. The lack of a prior relationship between hospitalists and patients presents challenges, but also opportunities, for discussing advance directives.

3. Hospitalists should routinely address advance directives and preferences for care with patients at the time of admission and as the clinical status changes.

4. Hospitalists should involve primary care physicians in all end-of-life decisions and discussions.

REFERENCES

1. Lo B, McLeod GA, Saika G: Patient attitudes to discussion life-sustaining treatment. Arch Intern Med 1986;146:1613–1615.
2. Danis M, Southerland LI, Garrett JM, et al: A prospective study of advance directives for life-sustaining care. N Engl J Med 1991;324:882–888.
3. Tulsky JA, Chesney MA, Lo B: How do medical residents discuss resuscitation with patients? J Gen Intern Med 1995;10:436–442.
4. The SUPPORT Principal Investigators: A controlled trial to improve care for seriously ill hospitalized patients: the study to understand prognoses and preferences for outcomes and risks of treatments (SUPPORT). JAMA 1996;274:1591–1598.
5. Pantilat SZ, Alpers A, Wachter RM: A new doctor in the house: ethical issues in hospitalist systems. JAMA 1999;282:171–174.
6. Pantilat SZ, Lindenauer PK, Katz PP, Wachter RM: Reach out and touch someone: primary care physician experiences and communication with hospitalists. Presented at the Annual Meeting of the Society of General Internal Medicine, May 1, 1999.
7. Cristakis NA, Lamont EB: Extent and determinants of error in doctors' prognoses in terminally ill patients: prospective cohort study. BMJ 2000;320:46–47.

Lawrence J. Schneiderman, MD

PATIENT 70

A 60-year-old man admitted to the ICU with metastatic mesothelioma whose son demands continued aggressive life-supportive care

A 60-year old man with metastatic malignant mesothelioma is admitted to the ICU for severe short-ness of breath and chest pain. During the previous 2 months, he has become progressively bedfast, cachectic, and anorectic. In the ICU, the patient requires high-dose morphine to control his pain. He is intubated, mechanical ventilation is initiated, and intravenous vasopressors are administered for hypotension.

During the following several days, it becomes apparent that the patient is ventilator-dependent. The ICU team develops a consensus that comfort care has become the appropriate goal of treatment. The son, however, demands all possible life-sustaining treatments, including attempted cardiopulmonary resuscitation if the patient experiences a cardiac arrest. Meanwhile, the son spends hours on the phone seeking information on access to other possible treatments, such as laetrile and endostatin.

The hospital has a policy that defines medically futile treatment and outlines steps to be taken in the event of a dispute between parties involved in decision-making. The policy defines futile treatment as "any treatment that has no realistic chance of providing a benefit that the patient has the capacity to appreciate (as distinguished from producing physiologic effects limited to parts of the body), or merely preserves permanent unconsciousness or cannot end permanent dependence on medical care that is available only in an intensive care unit." The policy also states that "although a particular treatment may be futile, palliative or comfort care is never futile."

Question: Should the physicians follow the son's wishes to continue aggressive life-sustaining treatment that they regard as futile, or should they emphasize comfort care?

Diagnosis: Terminal metastatic malignancy with no realistic chance of survival outside the ICU.

Discussion: Medicine today has the power to achieve a multitude of effects. For the current patient, the available treatments include the infusion of drugs to prevent hypotension, ventilator support to manage respiratory failure, and CPR to reverse cardiac arrest. The physician's charge, however, is to provide not merely an *effect* upon some part of the body, but a *benefit* to the patient as a whole. A patient is neither a collection of organs nor merely an individual with idiosyncratic desires. Rather, a *patient* (from the Latin word "to suffer") is a person who seeks the *healing* (meaning "to make whole") powers of the physician.

Although physicians try to achieve a patient's (or surrogate's) desired goals, there are times when these goals do not comport with medical goals. For example, artificially maintaining the blood pressure in this patient is an example of an effect that merely prolongs the dying process without restoring consciousness and granting him, at the very least, the capacity to appreciate the effect as a benefit.

Some argue that physicians should not make such "value judgments." They claim that only physiologic futility is "value neutral," and hence physicians should keep the vasopressor infusion going as long as it has any effect on the patient's blood pressure and that physicians should carry out all the other interventions demanded by the son. However, to specify physiologic objectives as the goals of medicine is not "value neutral" but rather a value choice which has strayed far from the patient-centered tradition of the medical profession.

Occasionally, a grieving loved one will say "Do everything!" when asked what should be done for a dying patient. "How can you be absolutely certain there won't be a miracle?" In fact, one can never be absolutely certain. At most, one can only be certain "beyond a reasonable doubt," as the law recognizes in a criminal trial in which a person's life is also at stake. One can only conclude after observing many failures that the future success of a treatment is not reasonably likely. But after how many failures?

Here, one must keep in mind the denominator—all the seriously ill patients who will be put through painful, burdensome, life-sustaining efforts in hopes of achieving a miracle. When do the odds violate professional standards based on principles of non-malfeasance (avoiding harms with no benefits) and proportionality (assuring that the benefits are not severely overweighed by the burdens and risks)? When does CPR become a futile act of crushing the heart and breaking ribs? Physicians can empathize, but physicians cannot do more than nature allows. Indeed, the very meaning of "miracle" depends on the premise that "the things which are impossible with men are possible with God" (Luke 18:27).

Invoking medical futility, however, does not grant physicians the power to act "unilaterally" and "arbitrarily" in making end-of-life decisions. It requires a scrupulous attention to the best available evidence and to principles and professional standards, along with a respectful communication and application of dispute resolution procedures that allow all values and wishes to be expressed. These conditions limit and equalize the powers of all parties: patients, loved ones, and physicians.

Are physicians obligated above all to prolong life? Those who claim this obligation are probably unaware that this claim is not supported by the classical tradition of medicine. The Hippocratic physician sought to assist nature in restoring health, alleviating suffering, and avoiding futile treatments. Indeed, Hippocratic physicians shunned claims of life-prolonging powers in order to escape the taint of charlatanism.

At this point in the current patient's illness, the physicians are acting within the Hippocratic tradition by seeking to avoid futile treatments and instead provide treatments that alleviate suffering. They should accept the son's actions as manifestations of grief and love (and possibly guilt), and they should try to enlist him in better efforts to express these feelings by participating in the comfort care. Recognizing that the manner of death is in their power, the physicians should emphasize that "doing everything" now means doing everything possible to ensure a peaceful, dignified, pain-free death. By contrast, if they were simply to yield to the son's unrealistic demands, whether from misguided notions of their obligations or from fear of lawsuits or "bad headlines," the physicians would be corrupting their moral obligations to the patient.

Medicine, as any profession, must propose its standards of practice, which society may accept, modify, or reject. This hospital, along with many others, has defined medical futility and provided procedures for dispute resolution. One expression of society's response takes place in the courts. Although physicians should not expect the courts to give them prior permission to forgo futile treatment (because the courts will want the opportunity to examine all the facts *after* the action is completed), nevertheless courts have sided with physicians who have withdrawn futile treatments after careful deliberation and due process. Indeed, hospitals are likely to find the legal system willing (and even eager) to defer to well-defined and procedurally scrupulous processes for the internal resolutions of futility disputes.

In the current case, the healthcare team spent several days with the son and the rest of the family in order to make a reasonable accommodation to their needs to grieve and come to terms with the patient's dying. The family was given a date at which time anyone who wished could be present with the patient in a private setting when all life support and monitors would be withdrawn. This date gave the son sufficient time to seek transfer of the patient or court intervention, which he chose not to do. Because the patient was ventilator- and vasopressors-dependent, the physicians could reasonably predict the patient would not linger after withdrawal of ventilatory support. He died peacefully in the presence of the family.

Clinical Pearls

1. A patient (from the Latin word "to suffer") is a person who seeks the healing powers of the physician. The physician's duty is to provide not merely an effect upon some part of the body, but a benefit to the patient as a whole.

2. Physicians can empathize with grieving family members, but physicians cannot do more than nature allows. They cannot ethically offer futile treatments in hopes of a miracle.

3. Invoking medical futility requires scrupulous attention to the best available evidence and to principles and professional standards, as well as a respectful communication with family members in the application of dispute resolution procedures.

4. Physicians should accept loved ones' unrealistic demands as manifestations of grief and love (and possibly guilt) and try to enlist the family in better efforts to express these feelings by participating in comfort care treatments. Physicians should emphasize that "doing everything" also means doing everything possible to ensure a peaceful, dignified, pain-free death.

REFERENCES

1. Schneiderman LJ, Jecker NS: Wrong Medicine: Doctors, Patients and Futile Treatment. Baltimore, Johns Hopkins University Press, 1995.
2. Schneiderman LJ, Faber-Langendoen K, Jecker NS: Beyond futility to an ethic of care. Am J Med 1994;96:110–114.
3. Schneiderman LJ: The futility debate: effective versus beneficial intervention. J Am Geriatr Soc 1994;42:883–886.
4. Schneiderman LJ, Capron AM: How can hospital futility policies contribute to establishing standards of practice? Cambridge Q Healthcare Ethics 2000;9:524–531.
5. Johnson SH, Gibbons VP, Goldner JA, et al: Legal and institutional policy responses to medical futility. AHA J Health Law 1997;30:21–47.

Mark R. Tonelli, MD, MA

PATIENT 71

A 35-year-old man with end-stage cystic fibrosis who wants to know if completing an advance directive is important

Near the end of a routine clinic visit, a 35-year-old man with end-stage cystic fibrosis ($FEV_1 <$ 20% predicted, PCO_2 55 mm Hg) mentions that his lawyer offered him an opportunity to complete a "health care directive" as part of the service of writing a property will. He deferred at the time but now wonders whether he should complete these or some other documents to ensure that "I don't die a miserable death." He has decided not to pursue lung transplant evaluation and understands that he is likely to die within the next year or two. He expresses a willingness to complete any type of directive that would limit pain and suffering associated with dying, but also states that his quality of life is currently acceptable and that he wants to go on living as long as that is the case. He is estranged from his parents, who live in another state, and is not married.

Question:　What sort of advance directive, if any, should this patient be advised to complete?

Diagnosis: Advanced cystic fibrosis in a patient who needs to initiate and communicate his end-of-life planning.

Discussion: Advance directives have been promoted as tools that allow individual patients to anticipate certain types of medical decisions, planning for a future when they will be unable to directly participate in the decision-making process. Instructive directives (e.g., living wills) outline specific preferences regarding future care under certain circumstances. Proxy directives (e.g., durable power of attorney for health care) designate a surrogate to make medical decisions for the patient in the event of future incapacity. Ethically, such documents are seen as a way to project and protect individual autonomy in situations where the ability to choose autonomously is lost. Legally, advance directives, in one form or another, are recognized in all 50 states. In addition, the Patient Self-Determination Act requires that all hospitals receiving federal funding inform patients about the availability of advance directives and inquire as to whether any have been completed.

Unfortunately, the promise of advance directives has not been borne out in practice. Most large studies, including the SUPPORT study ("Study to Understand Prognoses and Preferences for Outcomes and Risks of Treatment"), have failed to find any difference in outcome measures, including length of ICU stay, cost, and percentage of people undergoing resuscitative efforts before death, when comparing those with and without instructive advance directives. Many potential reasons for the lack of effectiveness have been suggested, but the primary problem centers on the fact that instructive directives are inherently ambiguous and lack the same moral weight as contemporaneous decisions. As such, directives rarely can stand on their own as an accurate and meaningful representation of what an individual would want in a particular clinical situation, one that is always more complex and nuanced than anticipated in a directive. In addition, many advance directives are now completed without the consultation of medical professionals, as in the current case, leaving real concern among clinicians as to whether basic standards of informed consent are met.

Improving upon advance directives has proven difficult. Two possible approaches can be taken in an attempt to avoid the ambiguity of standard instructive directives. The first is to define very clearly the conditions that must be met before these instructions take force, avoiding the use of ambiguous terms such as "terminal condition," "incurable illness," and "prolonged dying." The feasibility of such an approach depends, to a large degree, on the predictability of the natural history of a disease. For instance, a patient with amytrophic lateral sclerosis (ALS) will undoubtedly face a time when mechanical ventilation is needed. Although multiple scenarios would need to be addressed, an advance directive specifically dealing with questions of "if," "when," and "how long" mechanical ventilation should be employed would be both feasible and likely to impact the course of care. Other disease-specific advance directives have been offered, though none has yet been clearly shown to effect change in end-of-life care.

The second approach involves stipulations regarding specific care that hold in all clinical contexts. For instance, a Jehovah Witness' refusal of blood products, even if it would result in loss of life, does not demand interpretation by a clinician. Likewise, a portable "do not attempt resuscitation" (in some states known as an "EMS/No CPR" order) instructs others not to initiate CPR regardless of the circumstances. The major limitation of such directives is that very few individuals wish to preclude specific interventions regardless of circumstance. Even those with chronic or life-shortening diseases may wish for invasive or intensive care so long as there is a significant chance of returning them to what they feel is an acceptable quality of life.

Advance directives, then, appear to be neither necessary nor sufficient to ensure that care at the end of life is consistent with the patient's goals and values. When patients perceive them as sufficient, directives themselves can sometimes be a barrier to important discussions between patients and caregivers about end-of-life care.

Acknowledging the limitations of advance directives, however, does not mean that addressing patient concerns and respecting patient values is unimportant. Rather, recognizing that advance directives fail to change outcomes should only serve to encourage physicians to take the time to explore the fears, hopes, and values of individual patients facing life-threatening illness. As it has become clear that advance directives alone do not help improve the care at the end of life, thoughtful physicians and researchers have begun to focus on a more inclusive concept of advance care planning. Advance care planning often includes the completion of advance directives, but really it focuses on the process of communicating the patient's goals and values to health care providers and surrogate decision-makers. In thorough advance care planning, directives serve as a way to promote discussion and elucidate values rather than being seen as an end in themselves.

In the current case, the patient's question regarding advance directives serves as a starting point for serial discussions dealing with the issues likely to be faced in the coming months. The patient's conception of a "miserable" versus a "good" death is explored, as is his conception of what constitutes an acceptable quality of life. Specific therapies, particularly mechanical ventilation, are discussed in order to understand under what context such interventions would be appropriate. Given the estrangement between the patient and his parents, the patient identifies a trusted friend as his surrogate decision-maker and completes a durable power of attorney for healthcare.

In addition, the patient is encouraged to discuss his goals and values with his surrogate as well as to explore options for resolving the conflict with his parents. The patient expresses a desire to undergo any intervention, including mechanical ventilation, if there is a reasonable chance of returning to his previous level of functioning. He understands that decisions regarding when that time is reached might be made by his surrogate and his physician. Other than the durable power of attorney for health care, no other advance directives were seen as necessary or appropriate.

Clinical Pearls

1. Advance directives are neither necessary nor sufficient to improve the care through the end of life.

2. Instructive directives may be most useful and appropriate in diseases with a predictable natural history or when particular interventions are not desired regardless of the circumstances.

3. Proxy directives are often more useful. They are particularly appropriate when a patient feels that the person who best understands his goals and values is not the person to whom decision-making responsibility would fall under state law.

4. Advance care planning focuses on process, rather than simply the completion of documents. Eliciting the goals and values of individuals and encouraging communication with family and caregivers are more important than completion of legalistic documents in end-of-life care.

REFERENCES

1. Emanuel L, Danis M, Pearlman R, Singer P: Advance care planning as a process: structuring the discussions in practice. J Am Geriatr Soc 1995;43:440–446.
2. Tonelli MR: Pulling the plug on living wills: a critical analysis of advance directives. Chest 1996;110:816–22.
3. Teno J, Lynn J, Wenger N, et al: Advance directives for seriously ill hospitalized patients: effectiveness with the patient self-determination act and the SUPPORT intervention: Study to Understand Prognoses and Preferences for Outcomes and Risks of Treatment. J Am Geriatr Soc 1997;45:500–507.
4. Tierney WM, Dexter PR, Gramelspacher GP, et al: The effect of discussions about advance directives on patients' satisfaction with primary care. J Gen Intern Med. 2001;16:32–40.
5. Prendergast TJ: Advance care planning: pitfalls, progress, promise. Crit Care Med. 2001;29(2 suppl):N34–39.

INDEX